YOGA FOR HAPPY M

Simple techniques for getting your spark back and enjoying parenthood again

by Puran Prem Kaur

To Anand,
Love & Light,
Puran Prem Kaur
xxx

"Happiness is your birthright"

~ Yogi Bhajan, PhD, Master of Kundalini Yoga

First published in Great Britain by Practical Inspiration Publishing, 2016

ISBN (print): 978-1-910056-36-3

ISBN (ebook): 978-1-910056-37-0

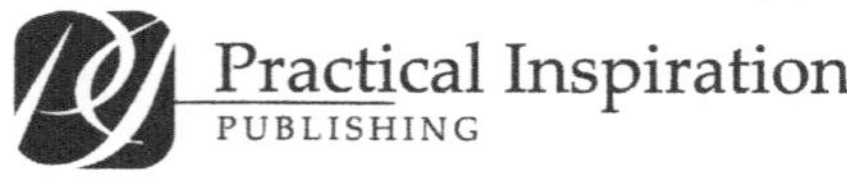

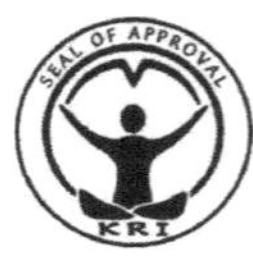

This publication has received the KRI Seal of Approval. This Seal is given only to products that have been reviewed for accuracy and integrity of the sections containing the 3HO lifestyle and Kundalini Yoga as taught by Yogi Bhajan®.

This book is dedicated to my children, Ben and Jack,
with eternal love and gratitude

The exercises in this book are designed to be safe for most people provided they carefully follow the instructions. The benefits attributed to these exercises come from the centuries-old Yogic tradition. Results will vary due to physical differences and the correctness and frequency of practice. All liability is disclaimed in connection with the use of the information in individual cases. If you have any doubts as to the suitability of the exercises for you personally, please seek medical advice from your GP.

Contents

"Becoming a mother is a journey and along the way you confront things within yourself you never thought you would, that in fact you didn't even know were there – and no one can truly prepare you for it. You are the child's first teacher, and for the first three years of her life, your aura and your child's auric field are one. From the first day of the child's life your life, your rhythm, even your waking and sleeping hours are no longer decided by you. The challenges you face are real. At times you are tested on every level – emotionally, physically and mentally. Yet at the same time you experience an overwhelming sense of devotion and unconditional love. Imagine this innocent child looking so lovingly at you – you! This is the beginning of a long journey, the greatest journey you will ever take in your life."[1]

~ The Kundalini Research Institute

[1] *I Am a Woman: Essential Kriyas for Women in the Aquarian Age* (Kundalini Research Institute; 2009), p.136

Foreword

By Guru Dharam Khalsa, BAcC RCHM, Director International School of Kundalini Yoga (iSKY)

A challenging experience of parenthood inspired Puran Prem Kaur to seek a complementary means of navigating difficult postnatal circumstances. She found Kundalini Yoga and is now sharing the fruits of her journey with others.

Although the title specifically targets mothers, this delightful book could be for anyone who would like to apply time-tested yogic techniques to alleviate stress, insomnia, anxiety, guilt and anger while promoting body confidence, vitality, a strong immune system and hormonal balance.

The text is clear, the layout well presented and the photographs ably demonstrate the poses. The tone of the book is astutely judged and there is plenty of interesting information but the emphasis is, quite correctly, on gaining self-empowerment through your own experience of practice.

While yoga is now a very popular activity, there are few publications which manage to demystify an esoteric discipline, while retaining a sense of its depth and intrinsic potential, and communicating in such an accessible tone and in everyday language.

Puran Prem has achieved this balance admirably and has made an important contribution to the propagation of practical Kundalini Yoga into the lives of mothers and, I suspect, others everywhere!

Introduction

When my second son was a few months old, I found myself and my family in crisis. My eldest son had reacted very badly to having a brother who took up some of my time with his requirements for milk and clean nappies, and launched an extreme, often violent, protest. This included refusing to wash or eat properly for months or to sleep for more than four hours a night. The baby was hospitalised twice during his first five months due to serious illness; by the second admission, I had been diagnosed with Postnatal Depression. I was offered nothing other than antidepressants which created all kinds of other problems, when what I really needed was more sleep and some help with managing my elder son's emotional needs.

I was exhausted but it wasn't just physical exhaustion. I was deeply unhappy and more stressed than I had ever been in my life. I resented my children and their constant demands. I felt bitter that becoming a mother had meant swapping a lucrative and meaningful career for conflict and loneliness, while my then husband's career had flourished. The more difficult my children became, the less time other people wanted to spend with them – increasing my isolation and deepening my depression. My objective every day was simply to survive and, in order to do that, my emotions began to switch off.

In the depths of this crisis, I stumbled across a reference[2] to a psychological illness called Parental Burnout that I had never heard of before. It was described as a condition in which a parent (assumed to be the mother) wakes up each morning dreading the daily responsibilities that come with having children, wishing she could run away, and has to force herself to put the children's needs first. The parent feels guilty about resenting the children's presence.

I was fascinated – the description encapsulated my own feelings exactly – but bizarrely I could find almost no further information about it. Parenting charities I contacted had never heard of it and there were no books written about it. This seemed to confirm what I suspected: lots of unhappy women struggled to look after

2 *Parental Burnout* by Kenneth N Condrell PhD, originally published on the Fisher Price website.

their young children but nobody really wanted to talk about it.

At least I finally knew what was wrong: physical and mental exhaustion had led me to an emotional breakdown, a type of burnout. As with all burnout conditions, I was desperately trying to escape the situation I had found myself in and had started to shut down. The problem was, unlike burnout in the work environment, I couldn't follow the example of Graham Greene's Querry and take myself off to a remote part of Africa to hide.[3] I couldn't even take a day off. There were two young children who needed me 24/7. And as much as I struggled to look after them, I loved them deeply and didn't want to give up on them or on myself as their mother. Somehow we had to survive, so I had to find some energy from somewhere.

Although a lot has been written about exhaustion, energy and depressive conditions, I found it difficult to find healing techniques that fitted in with the realities of raising young children. A book about boosting energy might suggest, for example, a brisk walk every evening before dinner – an effective technique in itself but totally impractical for someone housebound with young children. This lack of appropriate information only served to increase my sense that I was living on a different planet from everyone else.

At my lowest point, by what seemed like chance, I found **Kundalini Yoga**. This unusual form of **Yoga**, brought to the West by **Yogi Bhajan**, offered simple and practical techniques that did fit in with the restrictions of parenting. Unlike other forms of Yoga that were developed by people who deliberately isolated themselves from society in order to focus exclusively on their spiritual development, Kundalini Yoga was specifically designed for householders: people with familial and work commitments that also needed to be met. People who were short of time.

Kundalini Yoga as taught by Yogi Bhajan® gave me many tools with which I could increase my personal energy levels and begin to heal myself.

I discovered I was far from unusual in becoming so physically and emotionally exhausted, with no real support being offered and few people even seeming to notice. I know now that behind closed doors many exhausted women with young children struggle along, day in and day

[3] *A Burnt-out Case* by Graham Greene, in which he coined the phrase "burnout" (first published in the UK by William Heinemann, 1960)

out, sometimes for years. We are encouraged to hide our emotions about how we really feel about parenting, to push them down inside ourselves and carry around a carefully constructed mask. But one of the most important lessons I learned from this difficult period in my life is that suppressing emotions is very dangerous and eventually leads to physical and mental ill-health. Our emotions are an important part of who we are and we experience them for a reason. If we can acknowledge and understand them, they can warn us when change is needed and help us find the way out.

Kundalini Yoga doesn't take away the pains of the human existence, but it gives us a toolkit for managing those pains to the best of our ability, regaining our energy and enjoying life again.

It is important to note I am not oblivious to the needs of dads. Their role has changed enormously over the last fifty years and, like mums, they are still working out exactly what that role is. We are at a critical point in the way we raise our children and we will only make real progress if we work together. But the needs of dads are different in some key ways, so this book focuses on mums.

The purpose of this book is to share just some of the techniques and theories from the vast Kundalini Yoga canon that can help mums who are burning out to get their spark back. It can only be regarded as an introduction to a huge body of teachings that have been passed down through the ages. The suggested exercises are not intended to replace but to supplement any other medication or treatment you may be having or considering. I hope also to raise awareness about Parental Burnout and to encourage a more open discussion about the realities of parenting so we can improve them for both parents and children.

How to Use This Book

This book is arranged thematically around the main emotional and physical difficulties that women with young children tend to face. I discuss each of these themes and provide a short questionnaire so you can check which applies to you. There is then an introduction to what the Kundalini Yoga teachings tell us about these specific issues, plus some lifestyle and dietary tips from the teachings. I have included some suggested points for reflection; Yoga is essentially about self-awareness, and Kundalini Yoga itself is sometimes referred to as the Yoga of Awareness. It teaches us about our bodies, what our physical limitations are and how we can go beyond them. But it also teaches us about our minds and our emotions. It enables us to develop our **Neutral Mind** so we can take an objective view. In the midst of what can seem like chaos in the world of raising small children, it is still possible to step back and look at how we can help ourselves.

In each chapter I also suggest a breathing practice, a **kriya** (or set of exercises) and a **meditation**. You can concentrate on just one chapter if there is a particular area causing you concern, or you can work your way through the book. Practising a kriya and a meditation every day would be ideal, but a set three times a week would still be a great start. If you cannot fit in the whole recommended practice in a chapter, then just do the breathing exercise or the meditation. Even three minutes a day of Kundalini Yoga can start to initiate change.

Words defined in the Glossary at the end of the book are highlighted in **bold** the first time they appear.

I send this book to you with love and I wish you light, happiness and peace. And many a good night's sleep!

Puran Prem Kaur xx

Chapter 1
Allowing the Sunshine In:
How to fit Yoga into Busy Lives

Is Yoga for You?

When I was about the age my oldest son is now, I found my dad practising Yoga in the sitting room. I had no idea what it was at the time and I don't remember ever hearing anyone, including my parents, talk about it back then. Only a few years ago one of my first teachers, commuting to work by train, felt compelled to hide her Yoga books behind more conventional reading matter.

Just how much things have changed in the last few years was highlighted recently when we celebrated the United Nations' first International Day of Yoga (21st June 2015). This was an historic event not just because it was the first day dedicated to Yoga on a global scale, but because it was also the first time all 177 countries that comprise the UN agreed unanimously on something! Such is the power of Yoga to elevate people.

Yoga in the western world is no longer regarded as just for hippies. It is no longer even regarded as unusual (although Kundalini Yoga could probably still be described as a little unconventional). But there do remain many misconceptions. In a recent survey I conducted of people without personal experience of Yoga, the most common perception was it is all about "stretching". Those who had a little experience were aware it relates to "postures", "breathing" and "well-being". Most were aware there are a variety of benefits to this ancient practice, with the most commonly quoted being "relaxation", "stress reduction", "flexibility", "core strength" and "calmness". These are great benefits for sure, but they could all be considered side-effects of the real purpose of Yoga.

My survey revealed what I suspected to be the case: there are many people who know Yoga would be good for them but who haven't yet tried it. Two of the most commonly stated reasons for this were "lack of flexibility" and "fear of looking silly". One of the advantages of this introduction to Yoga you are holding in your hands is that nobody else need see what you look like when you start! And as you will shortly discover, flexibility is not a prerequisite of a Kundalini Yoga practice.

What is Kundalini Yoga?

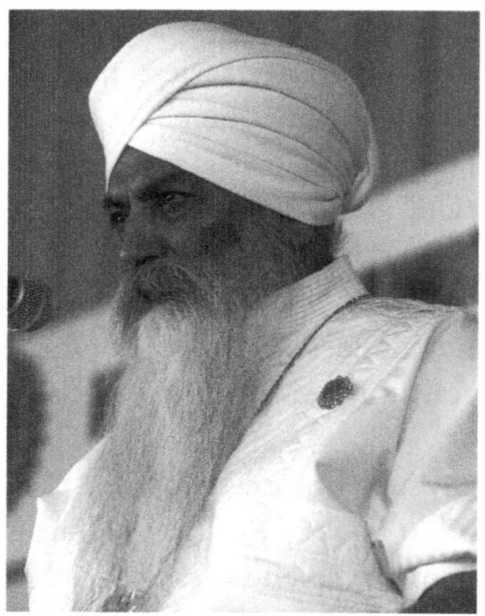

Yogi Bhajan at summer solstice - copyright Gurumustuk Khalsa

There are now so many different styles of Yoga being taught it can be difficult to know where to start. Fortunately Kundalini Yoga, which Yogi Bhajan (pictured) introduced to the West in one of his first public appearances on 5th January 1969, is accessible; regardless of age, gender and physical or mental condition there is something for everyone. Kundalini Yoga gives us a comprehensive array of breathing techniques, dynamic and static physical exercises or postures (**asana**), meditation techniques and mantra. A Kundalini Yoga practice can be relaxing, physically demanding and deeply spiritual – all at the same time. It is an ancient practice which has survived for many thousands of years. Despite these deep roots Kundalini Yoga remains highly relevant in the demanding modern world, giving us the tools to survive and thrive, keeping us supple and fit, and empowering us to fight the many psychological illnesses that currently prevail.

If we choose to embrace the teachings fully, Kundalini Yoga gives us an entire lifestyle, encompassing what and how we eat, how we manage our relationships with others, and even how and when we sleep. This powerful tradition enables us to discover our inner light or true potential, the meaning of our lives, and to connect our individual consciousness with the Universal Consciousness: the real purpose of practising Yoga.

"The difference [between Hatha Yoga and Kundalini Yoga] is only a matter of time and rate of progress. The purpose of the two approaches is the same; only Kundalini Yoga is direct, quick, and a perfect practice for the modern household."

~ Yogi Bhajan[4]

[4] *The Aquarian Teacher* by Yogi Bhajan, PhD (Level One Instructor Manual; Kundalini Research Institute; 2003), p.33

Kundalini Energy

A detailed explanation of the nature of **Kundalini energy** is outside of the scope of this book. Suffice it to say there is a pool of powerful energy lying at the base of every human spine, whether the owner practices Yoga or not. It is therefore available to everyone as long as they have the tools to access it and allow it to rise up through the spine correctly. Kundalini Yoga as taught by Yogi Bhajan® is safe as long as you follow the instructions as given (including **tuning in** with the **Adi Mantra** as detailed below) and don't do any of the recommended exercises for longer than the times specified. See "Before You Begin" below for more information.

If you would like to learn more about the theory of Kundalini energy, there are some excellent books and websites referred to in the Further Reading and Music Sources section.

Finding time for Yoga

Young children take up a lot of time and it can feel as though there aren't enough hours in the day as it is. How are you also going to find time for Yoga? In the afore-mentioned survey, when asked why people who were aware of the range of benefits of Yoga had not yet tried it, the most common reason given was "lack of time". The good news is that even 5 minutes a day can make a difference and for some people it is better to do a small amount every day than a longer practice only every now and again. Yogi Bhajan taught we should *"Always do some **sadhana** no matter how short."*

Although 2 ½ hours in the early hours of the morning is considered to be optimal, it is unlikely someone who is new to Kundalini Yoga is going to jump straight in the deep end and be able to sustain such a practice over time, especially if they have young children. Yogi Bhajan said, *"If we are to learn to run, we must first learn to walk."* He advised that a daily practice can grow but for some people it is better to start off slowly, a little at a time: *"Build slowly and constantly at a pace you can maintain, but definitely do something!"*[5]

As well as setting aside time exclusively for Yoga there are many ways you can incorporate yogic practices into your daily life – multi-tasking, in other words! Here are my top tips:

- While sitting at a desk or driving: check your posture. Are you sitting as upright as possible? Is your chin tucked slightly in so the neck is long,

---

[5] *Sadhana Guidelines: Create Your Daily Spiritual Practice* (Kundalini Research Institute; 2007), p.68

rather than scrunched? Is your chest lifted? Are your shoulders relaxed? Is your abdomen relaxed? We can use a lot of energy just by holding tension in the body;

- While watching television: sit on the floor in **Easy Pose** (see page 6) or **Rock Pose**. Use a cushion under the hips rather than collapsing the spine into the sofa;
- Before going to sleep: do a few minutes of Left Nostril Breathing (see pages 27-28);
- While washing up or ironing: chant a **mantra**;
- When putting clothes into the washing machine: do some Crow Pose squats (see pages 29-30);
- In the bath: practise **Breath of Fire** (see page 8)
- In the shower: sing the Long Time Sun song (see pages 18, 156 and the link on my website which can be found at www.karmaparent.com/mantra). The acoustics in the bathroom will amplify the sound beautifully!
- Check your breathing whenever you remember during the day, even if it's just for a minute or two. Are you breathing slowly and deeply through the nose, keeping the mind and emotions calm, or is your breathing shallow, creating unnecessary stress? Is the **Navel Point** moving out on the inhale and in and up on the exhale? Are you exhaling completely before taking the next inhale? After checking you are breathing naturally with the diaphragm (wearing clothing that is loose around the belly makes this much easier!) take one or two long deep breaths (see page 7 for an explanation of **Long Deep Breathing**). Eventually a healthier breathing pattern becomes automatic.

Practising Yoga with Children

Depending upon the age of your children there are many yogic practices you can share with them. My energetic sons, aged 8 and 5 at the time of writing, love doing Frogs (see page 42) and Cat-cow exercises (see page 13), Leg Lifts (see page 131), Cobra (see Sun Salutations in Chapter 2) and Triangle (see page 122). Long Deep Breathing and singing the Long Time Sun Song together helps to keep my youngest son in his bed when it's time to settle down! In fact, if I ever forget to sing it to either of my children they are quick to remind me: "Mummy, what about the song?"!

With time, Yoga becomes so much a part of your life you no longer need to fit it in because it's just part of who you are. I often say to my students that during the class we are simply practising for when we get out into the real world: Yoga doesn't stop when we get off the mat and that is exactly the point of doing it. It becomes part of who we are, our attitudes towards life and towards other people, the way we respond to the challenges life throws at us, the decisions we make and the paths we choose to take. It enables us to find and empower the person we really are: the **true Self** so often hidden away under layers of habitual patterns, social conditioning and fears.

Before you begin

There are a few basic points to bear in mind before you begin any Kundalini Yoga practice:

- If possible, avoid eating for two hours beforehand as any breathing or physical work is more comfortable on an empty stomach;

- Wear clothing which does not restrict the navel area and in which you can move easily. White or light-coloured clothing is recommended because it is said to expand the **Aura**[6] (I have felt my Aura shrink immediately after putting on black clothing). Covering the spine is recommended during meditation;

- Yogi Bhajan recommends tying long hair up, and covering the head with a non-static, natural cloth like cotton to allow the Kundalini energy to flow unimpeded;

- The only equipment you will need is a non-slip mat and possibly a cushion and a blanket. Yogi Bhajan also recommends sitting on an animal skin or a wool blanket as these are non-static and insulate your psycho-electro-magnetic field from the electromagnetic field of the Earth. Many Kundalini Yoga practitioners sit on a sheepskin for this reason (animal-friendly alternatives are available);

- If you are pregnant or on the first couple of days of your **Moon Cycle** do not do Breath of Fire, **Root Lock**, any **inversions** (such as Shoulder Stand) or other exercises that put pressure on the navel area (specifically Bow Pose, Camel Pose, Locust Pose, Sat Kriya and strenuous leg lifts[7]). The recommendation during pregnancy is you should do whatever feels right during the first three months. For the remainder of the pregnancy there are a few specific kriyas

6 *I Am a Woman*, p.xi

that are recommended, with some adjustments, which are outside the scope of this book. Walking for 3-5 miles per day is also recommended;

- If you have given birth within the last six weeks, practising Kundalini Yoga is not recommended.

There are a few key techniques that come up time and again so I will explain them here.

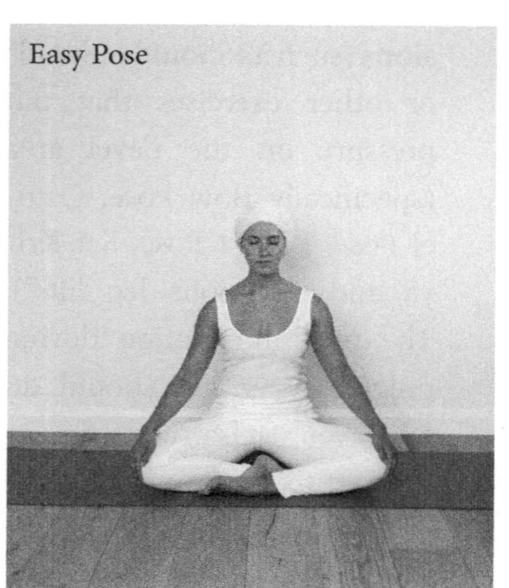
Easy Pose

Sitting in Easy Pose

Many of the exercises, especially meditations and breathing practices, involve sitting in Easy Pose. Sit with the legs crossed, one heel tucked up into the groin, and the other foot on the floor in front so the ankles are not actually crossing each other.

If that doesn't feel comfortable for you (despite the name, Easy Pose isn't easy for everyone!), try sitting in Half-Lotus Pose or even on a straight-backed chair as long as it gives you firm support.

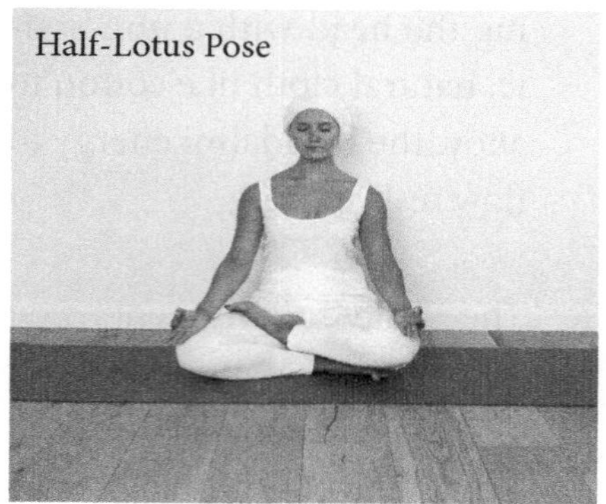
Half-Lotus Pose

However the legs are positioned, ensure you pull the spine up straight and lift the chest. Tuck the chin in slightly so the neck is long. Relax the shoulders and the abdomen. Imagine a golden thread is running from the base of your spine all the way up through the neck and out the top of the head, holding your spine completely straight.

Gyan Mudra

A **mudra** is a hand position and Gyan Mudra, which stimulates knowledge and wisdom, is used

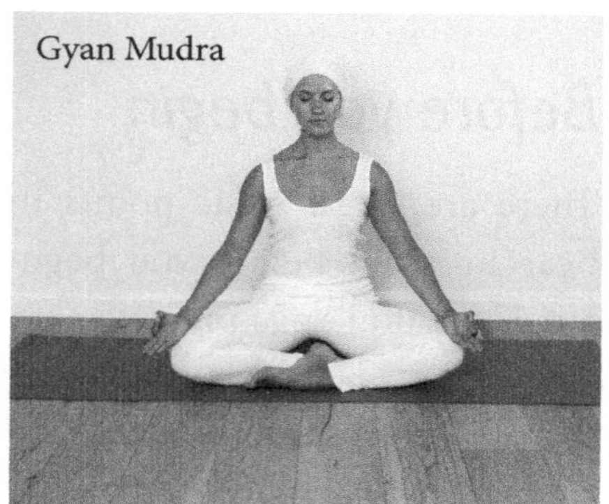
Gyan Mudra

[7] *Kundalini Yoga: The Flow of Eternal Power* by Shakti Parwha Kaur Khalsa (Time Capsule Books; 1996), p.197

frequently in Kundalini Yoga. The thumb and index finger touch each other with the other fingers extended so the palm is largely open.

Long Deep Breathing

Long Deep Breathing uses the full capacity of the lungs by utilizing all three sections or chambers: the abdominal or lower chest, the chest or middle chest, and the clavicular or upper chest.

We can practise this breathing technique in three parts: lie on the back with the left hand on the abdomen and the right hand on the chest.

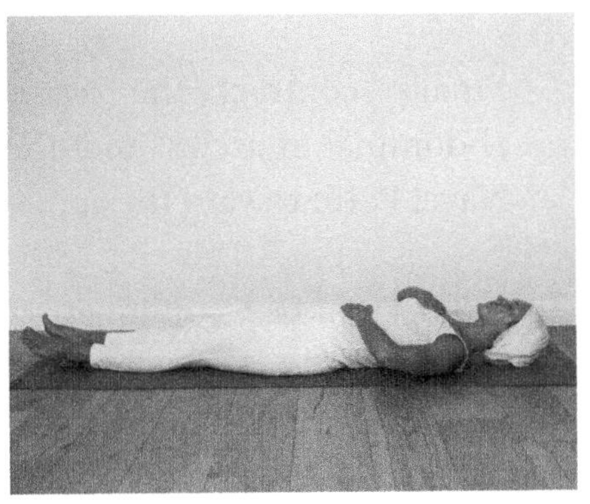

Inhale by first relaxing and filling the abdomen. The hand on the abdomen will rise towards the ceiling. On the exhale, the hand lowers steadily. The other hand monitors the chest to ensure it remains still and relaxed. Next move the hands to the ribs.

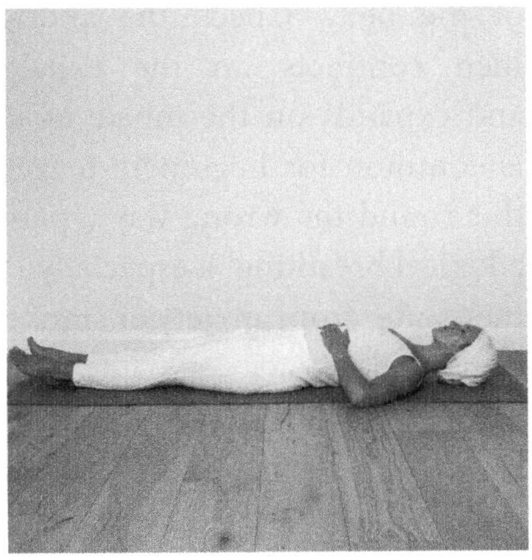

Expand the chest and feel the hands expand outwards. The ribs themselves expand in all directions and the lower ribs, the floating ribs, expand more than the upper, fixed, ribs. Compare the depth and volume of this breath with the isolated abdominal breath. Exhale completely without using the abdomen. Then contract the navel and keep the abdomen tight. Without inhaling, lift the chest. Now inhale slowly by expanding the shoulders and the collarbone. Exhale as you keep the chest lifted.

In Long Deep Breathing we combine these three actions into one smooth inhale and exhale: we start with an abdominal breath then add a chest breath and finish by lifting the upper ribs and collarbones and breathing into the upper chest. All three are done in one smooth motion. As you exhale, let the upper chest deflate first then the middle chest then finally pull the abdomen in and up as the Navel Point pulls back toward the spine. On the exhale, keep the spine erect and steady: do not bend it or collapse the chest area.

Start by practising for 3 minutes a day.

Breath of Fire

One of the foundational breath techniques in Kundalini Yoga, Breath of Fire accompanies many postures. Breath of Fire should not be done if you are pregnant or on the first couple of days of your Moon Cycle; substitute with Long Deep Breathing instead.

To practise Breath of Fire sit with a straight spine and place the hands on the abdomen. Focus on the Navel Point. Exhale powerfully through the nostrils and simultaneously pull in the navel. As you inhale, the navel is released. The inhale and the exhale are of equal length with no pause between them. There is a flutter to the movement, as the diaphragm moves up and down, rather than the abdomen moving in and out.

Breath of Fire can take some time to learn and it can be helpful to start slowly. Try panting like a dog through the mouth, then close the mouth and continue the movement with the breath moving through the nose rather than the mouth. After some practice, you can breathe fairly rapidly (2 or 3 breaths per second).

Don't exaggerate the pumping of the belly. Check the abdomen contracts on the exhale and expands on the inhale as it is common for beginners to get this round the wrong way ("paradoxical breathing"), especially if they suffer from anxiety or smoke heavily.

Start by practising for 3 minutes.

See my website for a demonstration: www.karmaparent.com/about-me.

Root Lock (Mulbandh)

Root Lock is very similar to the pelvic floor exercises which are discussed in great detail in antenatal classes! It is frequently applied at the end of an exercise, or series of exercises, to crystallise the effects. It pushes the Kundalini energy up through the spine. To practise applying the Root Lock imagine a lift or hydraulic lock at the base of the spine:

- First contract the anus. Feel the muscles lift upward and inward;
- Next contract the area around the sex organs. This is experienced as a slight lift and rotation inward of the pubic bone, similar to trying to stem the flow of urine through the urethral tract;
- Finally contract the lower abdominal muscles and the Navel Point toward the spine.

Root Lock is the combination of these three actions, applied together in a smooth, rapid, flowing motion.

Tuning in

Tuning in before any Kundalini Yoga practice prepares us mentally. It links us with the **Golden Chain** of Teachers who have come before us, including Yogi Bhajan and his own spiritual Teacher, **Guru Ram Das**. It reminds us of the rich body of Kundalini Yoga teachings available to us and of the Teacher within us all.

Sitting in Easy Pose, press the palms together in front of the body, thumbs against the sternum, forearms parallel to the ground. The eyes are closed, the focus on the **Brow Point**, between the eyebrows. We tune in with the mantra *Ong Namo Guru Dev Namo* which we chant three times in the pattern below, each repetition on one breath:

See my website for a demonstration: www.karmaparent.com/mantra.

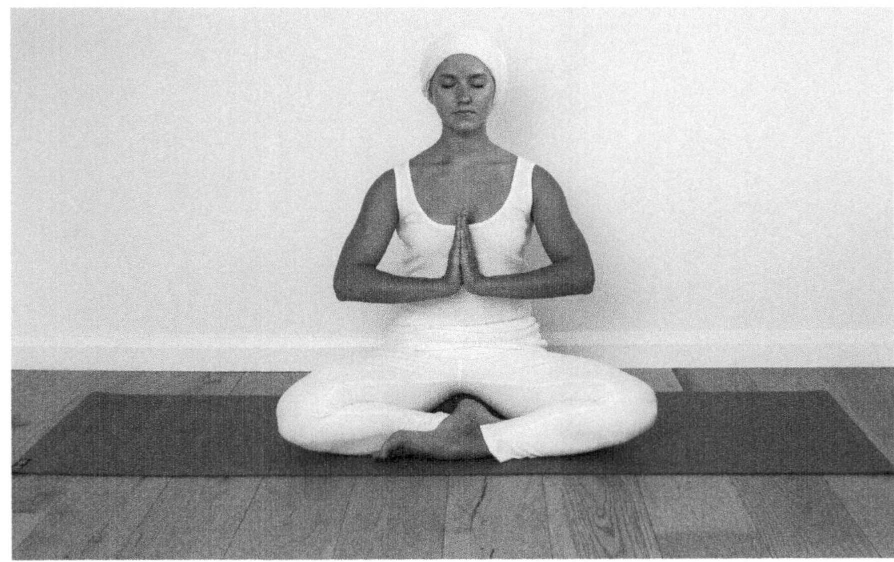

You are now ready to get started.

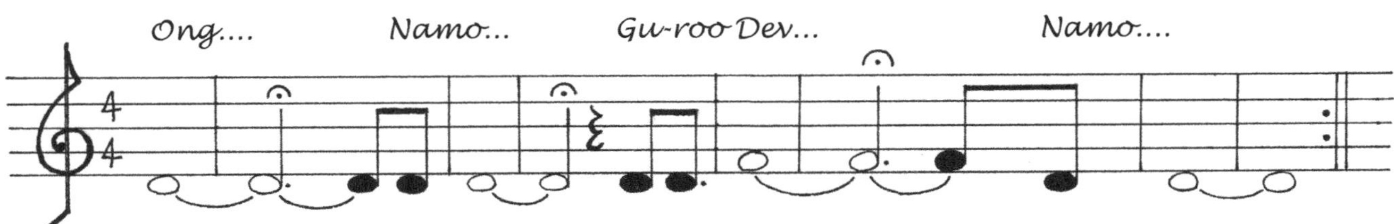

Chapter 2
Getting Warmed Up:
Preparing for a Kundalini Yoga Practice

Warming up

Although Yogi Bhajan did not generally teach warm-up exercises, he did acknowledge that there were times when a warm-up would be useful. Before any physical practice it is sensible to bring some gentle movement to the spine, the muscles and the joints, especially if you have been inactive for a while. In this chapter you will find three different warm-up sets you can use depending upon how much time you have and which appeals to you the most.

It is also a good idea to set an intention every time you begin a practice. What would you like to achieve today? What is important to you right now? Dedicate your practice to someone. Or visualise yourself feeling the benefits of the kriya you are about to do. For example, if you are going to do a set to improve the immune system, visualise yourself completely fit and healthy.

During each exercise

Focus at the **Third Eye**, the point between the eyebrows, unless instructed otherwise. Kundalini Yoga often uses dynamic movement in a posture; coordinate any instructions relating to the breath with the movement. Focus on the exercise rather than thinking about your To Do list and go deep within. Hear *Sat* on the inhale and *naam* on the exhale[8]. Exercises are usually given for a specific amount of time; if you find yourself struggling to complete one imagine you are doing it for someone you love.

Concluding an exercise

Unless instructed otherwise, inhale and hold the breath while

[8] *Sat Nam* (pronounced *Sat Naam*) is a mantra used frequently in Kundalini Yoga; it means "Truth is my identity"

maintaining the posture you have been working on and apply the Root Lock. Repeat this up to three times then exhale completely and apply the Root Lock. Again, repeat this up to three times then relax.

Between exercises

Relax for a few moments afterwards. Go within and observe the effects of the exercise you have just done.

Music

Music is sometimes used in a Kundalini Yoga practice and some of the kriyas include references to pieces of music with a specific beat or mantra. I have listed sources for purchasing these in Further Reading and Music Sources.

Warm-up set 1

This set of warm-up exercises takes just 5 minutes. If you are only planning to do a meditation then this short set will make it more comfortable for you to sit still for a few minutes.

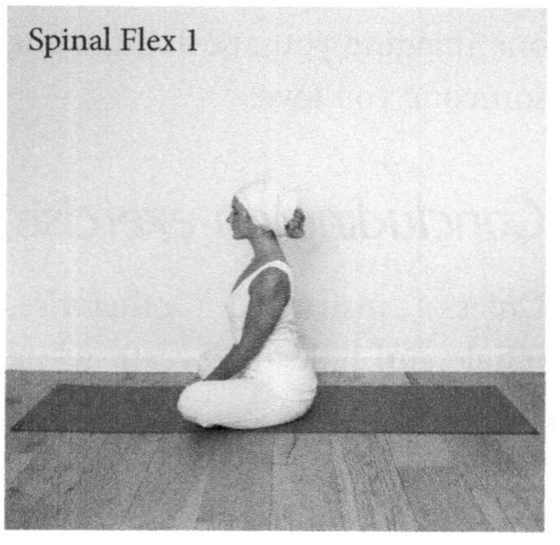

Spinal Flex 1

Spinal Flex

Sitting in Easy Pose, hold on to the front ankle and flex the spine forward and backward. Inhale as you come forward, keeping the head up and opening the chest, and exhale as you move backward. As you inhale forward imagine someone is behind you pulling your shoulder blades together. As you exhale backward, round the shoulders forward but without collapsing the back. The head and shoulders stay relatively still; the movement is in the spine. Continue for 1 minute.

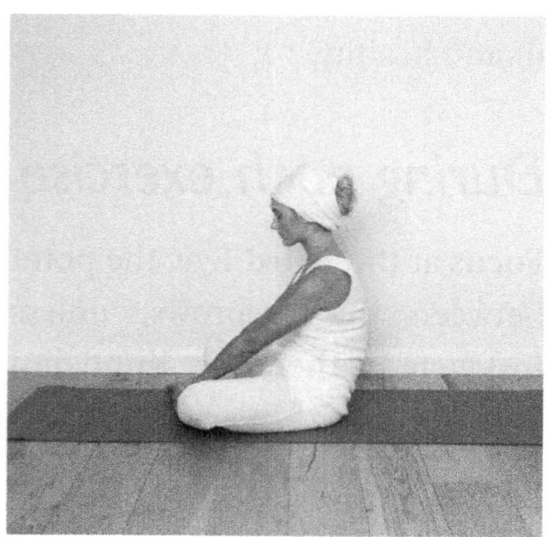

Continue the flexing of the spine for a further minute with the hands on the knees in Gyan Mudra and the arms straight.

These two exercises will flex different sections of the spine.

CAT-COW

On all fours, with the hands underneath the shoulders and the knees underneath the hips, exhale and round the spine. Inhale and drop the spine, opening up the chest as you raise the head, keeping the eyes closed to protect the optic nerve. Continue for 2 minutes. This exercise flexes the spine more deeply and stimulates the **Throat Chakra**.

LIFE NERVE STRETCH

Sit with the legs stretched out in front. Hold the big toes in finger lock: the index and middle fingers hooked round the big toes, the thumbs pressing on the toenails. Exhale and, lengthening the spine, bend forward from the navel. Inhale, using the legs to push up. Keep the chin tucked in and don't lead with the head: lead with the Navel Point, the head following. If you can't reach the

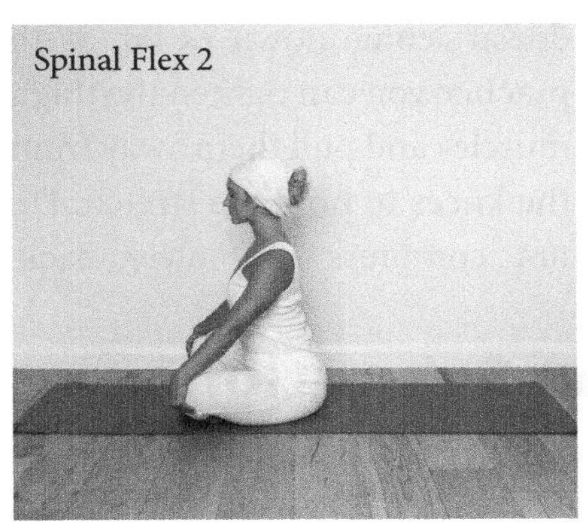

Spinal Flex 2

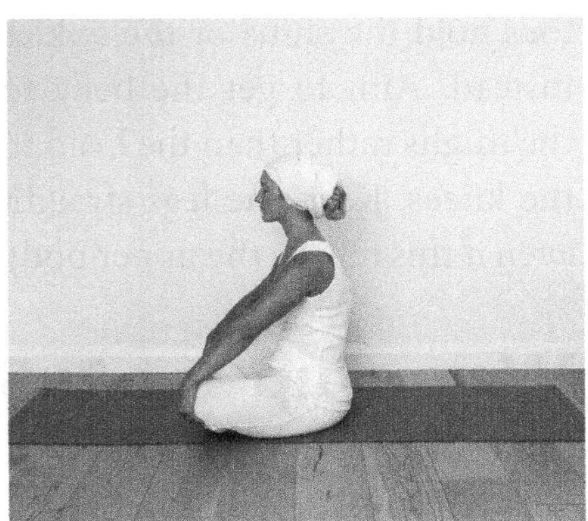

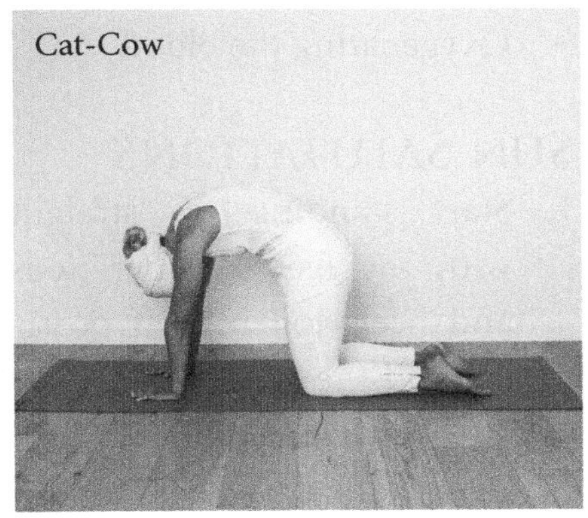

Cat-Cow

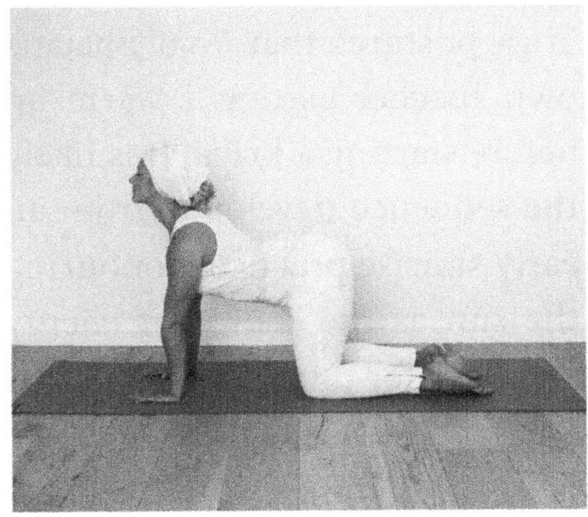

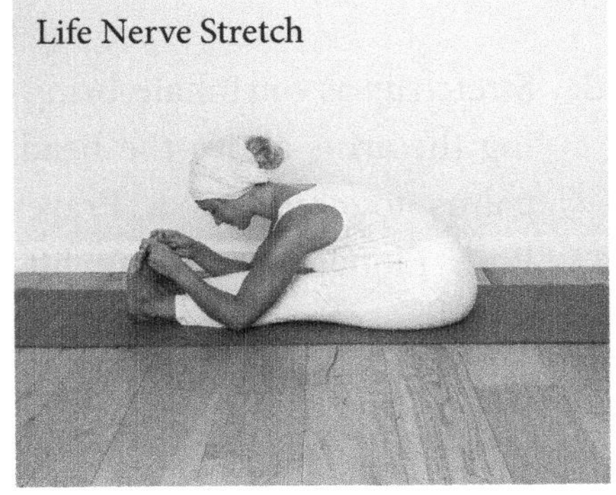

Life Nerve Stretch

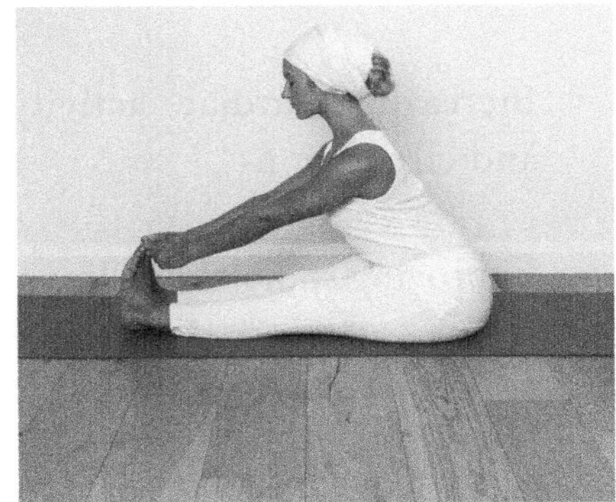

toes hold the shins or the ankles instead. Aim to get the belly to the thighs rather than the head to the knees. Keep the legs straight even if this means the upper body doesn't come down as far. With practice you can tighten the thigh muscles and pull them away from the knees to hold the stretch. Do not compress the lower back. Continue for 1 minute. This exercise stretches the hamstrings and is great for the sciatic nerve.

Warm-up set 2: Sun Salutations

Surya Namaskara, or Sun Salutations, are a very well-known set of Yoga postures that Yogi Bhajan's own Teacher used as a warm-up before starting a kriya. It is likely the sequence developed from an early sunrise practice, honouring the sun as the source of energy and light for the world.

A set in themselves, the benefits of Sun Salutations include:

- Increasing cardiac activity and circulation
- Improving spinal flexibility
- Massaging the inner organs
- Aiding the digestive system
- Exercising the lungs
- Oxygenating the blood

Sun Salutations

1. Start standing up straight with the feet together, toes and heels touching if possible and the weight distributed evenly between both feet. Arms hang down by the sides with the fingers touching.

2. Stretch up as you inhale, bringing the arms above the head, palms touching in a Prayer Pose. Elongate the spine, lifting the chest and making sure the shoulders are relaxed and the neck is not crunched. Look up to the hands.

3. Exhale and hinge forward from the hips, keeping the spine straight for as long as possible, elongating it as if reaching forward with the top of the head. When the spine cannot be held straight any longer, relax the head as close to the knees as possible, keeping the knees straight and bringing the hands down to the floor. If possible, the palms are on the floor, either side of the feet, with the fingertips in line with the toes. Gaze at the tip of the nose.

4. Inhale and look up, straightening the spine but keeping the hands or fingertips on the floor.

5. Exhale and bend the knees, stepping the right foot back to come into a lunge position like an athlete on a starter's block.

6. Step the left foot back to join the right so the legs are straight out behind. Elbows are bent, tucked into the ribcage, and the palms are flat on the floor under the shoulders, fingers spread. The body forms a straight line from the forehead to the ankles, evenly balanced on both sides. Don't push forward with the toes.

7. Inhale, straighten the elbows and arch the back, coming into a Cobra Pose. Stretch through the upper back and try to keep the feet together if possible to protect the lower back. Point the forehead to the sky and gaze at the tip of the nose. Fingers are still spread wide.

8. Exhale and lift the hips so the body is balanced in an inverted v-shape. Feet and palms are on the floor, elbows and knees straight, fingers spread. Gaze towards the navel and hold this posture for five deep breaths.

9. Inhale and step the right foot forward, aiming to bring it between the hands.

10. Step the left foot forward to join the right foot. Inhale and look up, straightening the spine but keeping the hands or fingertips on the floor.

11. Exhale and relax the head as close to the knees as possible in a forward bend.

12. Inhale and come all the way up into a standing position with the arms stretched above the head.

13. Exhale and return to the starting standing position.

In the next round, at position 5, step the left foot back first and at position 8, step the left foot forward first.

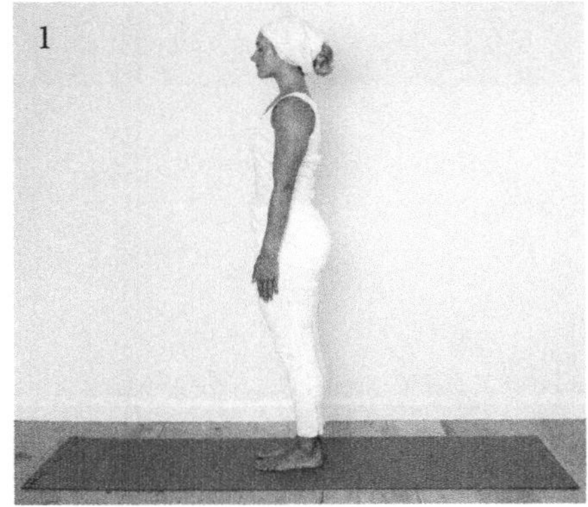

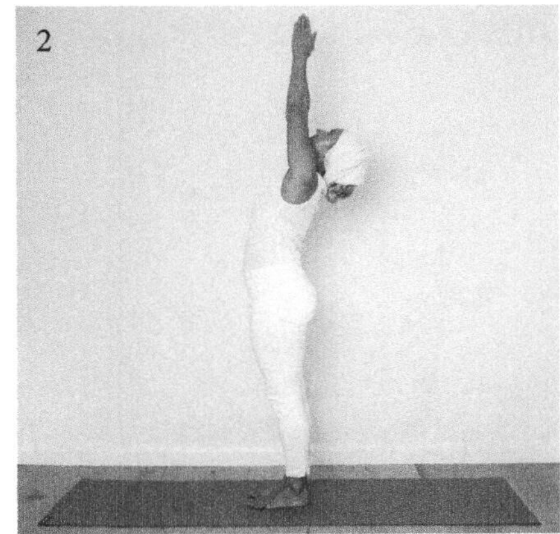

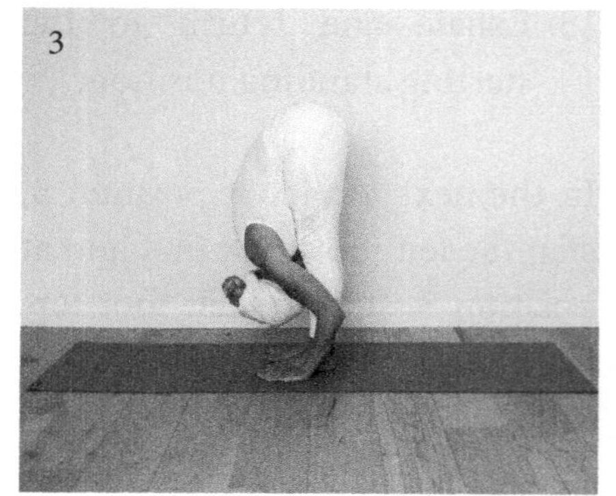
3

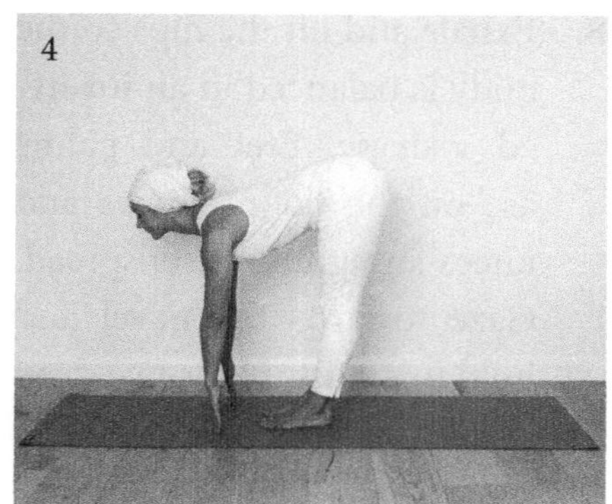
4

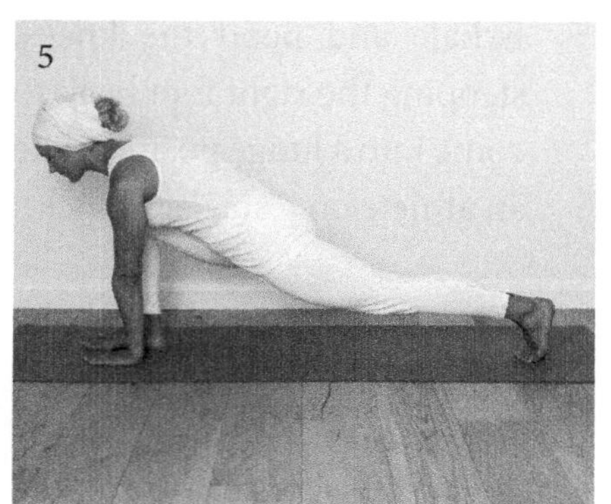
5

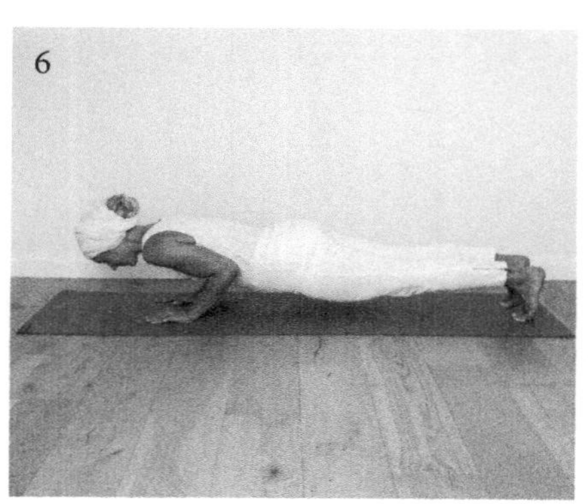
6

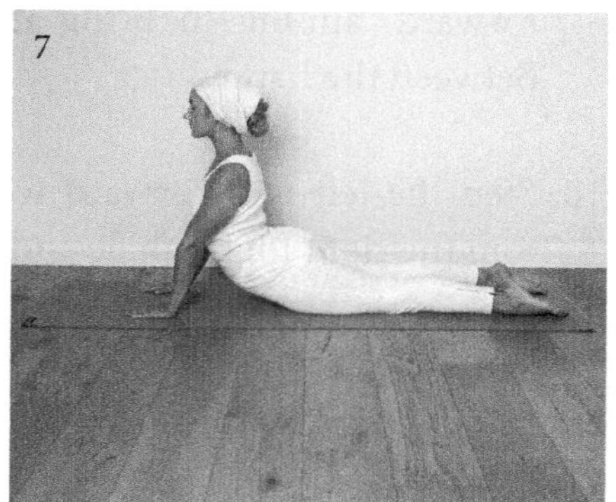
7

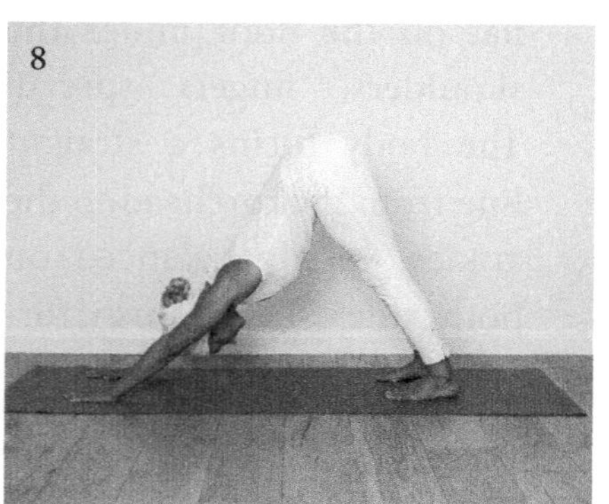
8

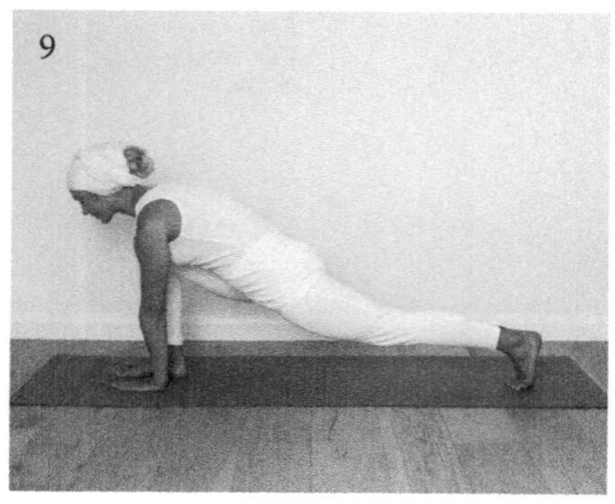
9

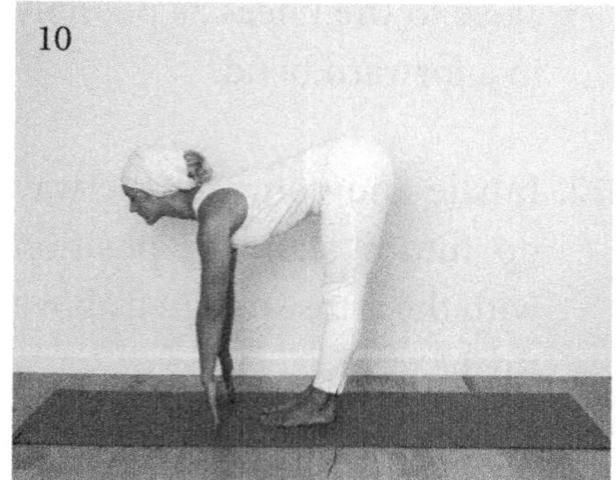
10

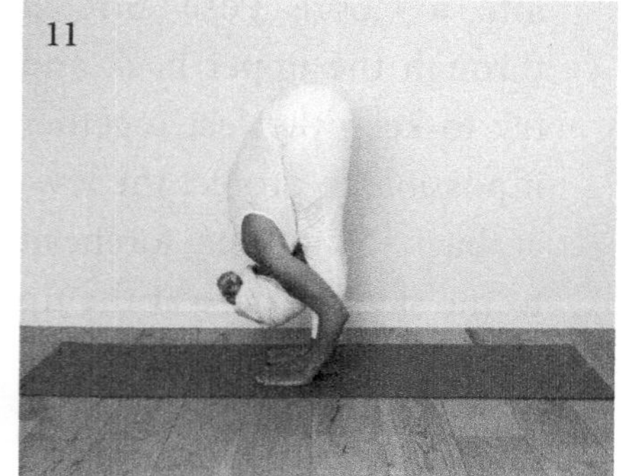
11

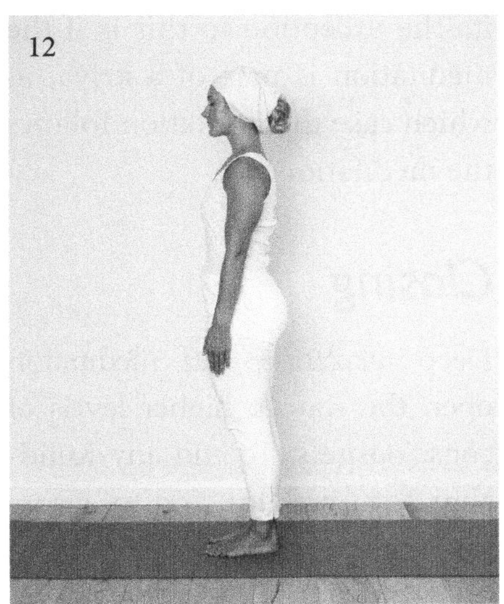

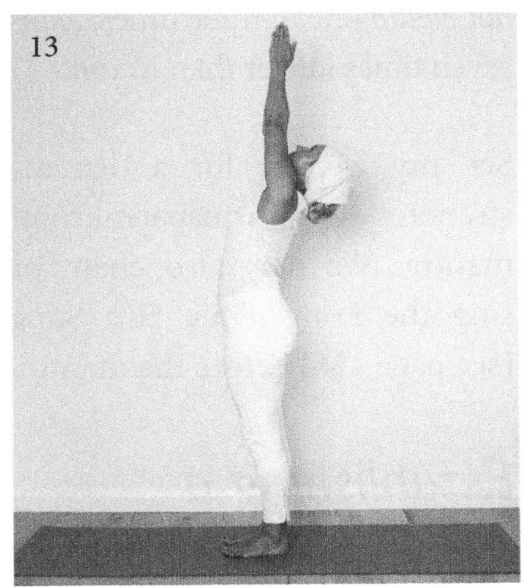

Warm-up set 3

The cardiovascular kriya called Complete Workout for the Elementary Being (also known as Har Aerobic Kriya) can also be used a warm-up set (see pages 140-142).

At the end of your practice

A period of relaxation is important to allow your body to absorb the effects of the practice you have done. When time is short, just a couple of minutes of relaxation are better than nothing. See Chapter 3 for more on relaxation.

Corpse Pose

The body can start to cool down quickly after even a short Yoga practice. Cover yourself with a blanket and lie flat on your back with palms facing upward. Make sure the spine is straight, the shoulders are placed evenly on the ground and you have nothing underneath your neck or head. Check the ankles are not crossed and the feet are hip-width apart, falling naturally out to the sides. Close the eyes and consciously tense and release each part of the body, starting with the toes and working your way up to the facial muscles. Ideally a period of relaxation should last between 5 and 7 minutes[9] unless the set you have just done states otherwise.

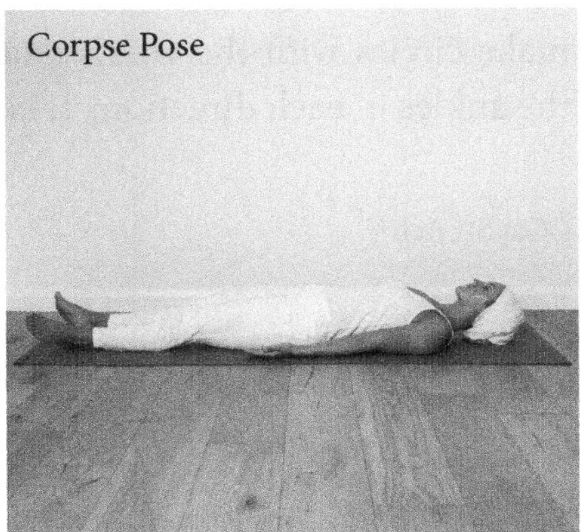
Corpse Pose

[9] *Sadhana Guidelines*, p.62

For some people, lying in Corpse Pose can make them feel vulnerable so it can be difficult to relax. Covering yourself with a blanket may help, or sitting in Easy Pose with the eyes closed is a good alternative.

Coming out of Relaxation

Always come out of a period of relaxation slowly and mindfully. Focus on deepening the breath. Gently begin to bring some small movements to the body: wriggle the fingers, wriggle the toes and make circles with the wrists and the ankles in each direction. Take the arms overhead and stretch. Still lying on the back, come into a Cat Stretch, bringing the right knee to the chest and taking it across the body in the direction of the floor so the right knee drops over to the left side. The arms are stretched out to the sides. Turn the head to look towards the right hand. Repeat on the other side.

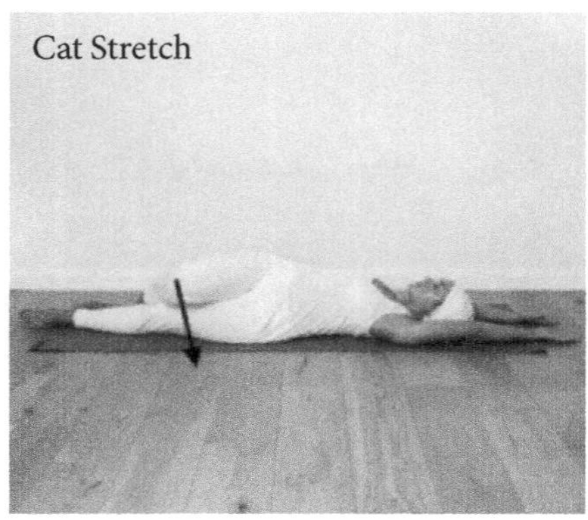
Cat Stretch

Bring both knees to the chest. Rub the soles of the feet together and the palms of the hands together. Place the soles on the floor and the palms over the eyes. Then hug the knees to the chest again and rock gently from side to side to massage the lower back. When you are ready, roll onto one side, or rock back and forth a few times on the spine, to come up to a sitting position.

Meditation

A meditation is usually done after the period of relaxation when you are in the best frame of mind for it. The exception to this is if the meditation is part of a kriya, in which case the relaxation follows the meditation.

Closing

Deep relaxation and meditation open the way to higher levels of consciousness. To end any Kundalini Yoga practice, and to ensure we are alert enough to go back into the world, we close our practice with a mantra. We chant the words *Sat Naam* one to three times; *Sat* is seven times longer than *Naam*.

See my website for a demonstration: www.karmaparent.com/mantra. We may also chant or sing the Long Time Sun Song (see page 156) before the mantra.

Establishing a Regular Practice

Little and often is for many people the easiest way of establishing a regular practice. Anchor your practice to your daily routine so you are more likely to remember to do it and more likely to fix it as a habit in your day. For example, upon waking, once you have dropped the children at school, before lunch or your evening meal, or before getting ready for bed. Choose a time when you are least likely to get distracted. Switch off all screens and phones! Just 40 days of regular Kundalini Yoga practice can create profound transformation but you do need to concentrate. Try keeping a journal relating to your practice. It doesn't have to be much: just noting down what you have done each day and any observations helps to keep you motivated as it's easy to see the progress you make. It's also a good place to record any questions you may have for your teacher next time you come to class.

Chapter 3
By the Light of the Moon:
Improving Sleep

"Things come out of you in three ways: in anger, in love and in your tiredness. [Mostly] you mess up when you are tired. Your energy is weak, you have no defenses and you fall apart."

~ Yogi Bhajan[10]

Most parents of young children are sleep-deprived to some extent. Adults are said to need between 8 and 10 hours of sleep every night but this can seem an impossible dream for parents. They get woken regularly during the night and are unable to have any catch-up sleep at the weekends. Any problems with insomnia (that pre-date the children or have developed since, due to anxiety for example) are even more troublesome when the hours (or minutes) available for sleeping are already limited.

Sleep deprivation makes looking after yourself and your children much harder. It makes the processing of emotions more difficult. It can seriously affect relationships between partners, between parents and their children, and between parents and their other relatives and friends. In the survey I conducted (see Chapter 1), almost half of the women who responded said lack of sleep had a direct impact on their intimate relationship because once they had struggled through the day and the children were asleep in the evening, they had run out of energy for any quality time with their partner.

Prolonged sleep deprivation is also linked to serious mental health problems including psychosis and bipolar disorder. A 2007 study at Harvard Medical School and the University of California at Berkeley using MRI scans revealed sleep deprivation causes the brain to become

[10] The Teachings of Yogi Bhajan, 12th July 1989

incapable of putting an emotional event into the proper perspective and making a controlled, suitable response.[11]

Fortunately, regular practising of Kundalini Yoga reduces the amount of sleep you need. Yogi Bhajan taught that adults really only need 5–6 hours' sleep a night – as long as they are getting the right kind.[12]

According to Yogi Bhajan there are four stages of sleep:

1. Tossing, turning and worrying;
2. A light dream, "reverie" stage;
3. Dream state, which is an energy-draining stage; and
4. The deep, dreamless sleep state, which is the only sleep that rejuvenates us and the only sleep we actually need.

The important one, the deep sleep state, only lasts a maximum of two and a half hours but most of us take some time to get to that point and some time to come out of it.

Is this You?[13]

- Do you have trouble getting to sleep even when you are tired?
- Do you wake in the night for no apparent reason? Or do you wake earlier than you need to still feeling tired?
- Do you find it difficult to get out of bed?
- Do you have dark circles or puffiness under your eyes?
- Are you irritable and moody? (also see Chapter 9)
- Do you drink caffeine all day? (also see Chapter 12)
- Do you suffer from frequent coughs and colds? (also see Chapter 11)
- Do you suffer from poor concentration and memory? While we sleep, toxins that build up in the brain during the day called beta amyloids are cleared at a rate 10 times greater than during

---

[11] Yoo, Seung-Schik, Gujar, Ninad, Hu, Peter, Jolesz, Ferenc, Walker, Matthew (2007), "The human emotional brain without sleep – a prefrontal amygdala disconnect" in *Current Biology* **17** (20): R877–R878 doi:10.1016/j.cub.2007.08.007. PMID 17956744

[12] *Kundalini Yoga: The Flow of Eternal Power*, p.108

[13] See the NHS website for more detail on the risks associated with lack of sleep: www.nhs.uk/Livewell/tiredness-and-fatigue/Pages/lack-of-sleep-health-risks.aspx

wakefulness. This is also the time when information is uploaded and consolidated into our long-term memories;

- Do you find it hard to lose weight (see also Chapter 13)?
- Is your blood sugar creeping up? Inadequate sleep is a cause of insulin resistance;
- Is your blood pressure increasing? Our blood pressure is usually 15 points lower when we are asleep ("nocturnal dipping"). Prolonged sleep deprivation is linked to heart disease and if you are consistently getting less than seven hours of sleep, you may develop high blood pressure.

Reflection Points

- Can you get to bed half an hour earlier than usual? If you have a partner, are the nocturnal duties being shared fairly? Can you have a half-hour nap during the day when the baby sleeps? There are many examples of people (highly driven ones, admittedly) who managed for years with much less night-time sleep than the average person by having a short daytime nap as well: John F. Kennedy, Winston Churchill, Margaret Thatcher, Leonardo da Vinci, Salvador Dali, Marie Curie and Thomas Edison to name just a few;
- Is your room dark enough?
- Are stimulants (alcohol, caffeine, sugar, nicotine or drugs) disturbing the quality of your sleep?
- Is your diet exacerbating sleep problems? If you eat within three hours of going to bed your body will still be digesting. If you eat too early in the evening, do you tend to wake during the night or too early the next morning? Eating too much can also disturb your sleep. Do you find certain foods are easier to digest at night than others?
- Are you dehydrated? Tiredness can be a symptom of dehydration. We lose around 1.5 litres of water a day (through the skin, lungs and gut as well as through our urine via the kidneys), and women who are breastfeeding lose even more. Adequate hydration results in pale to light yellow urine (dark yellow indicates under-hydration and totally clear indicates over-hydration);
- Are you getting enough exercise during the day? Incorporating some cardiovascular exercise into your day reduces fatigue. Exercise uses up the adrenalin and other hormones the body produces

under stress and also relaxes the muscles. Try the Har Aerobic Kriya (see Chapter 13);

- Do you race around doing jobs or use screens (television, tablet, smartphone) right up until the point when you try to sleep? Try having a "switch off" time at 9pm: some time to chat to your partner, do some gentle stretching, listen to relaxing music, read something inspirational, have a bath or write your diary. If you are feeling overloaded, make a list of all the things you need to do so you can sleep knowing nothing will be forgotten.

Yogic Viewpoint: Relaxation

Many people first come to Yoga because they are aware they need to learn how to relax. Despite the amount of non-working time many people have – compared with the hours people worked during the Industrial Revolution for example – modern lifestyles don't tend to incorporate much genuine relaxation. This is especially true when we have young children to look after 24/7. Many of the tools we use for relaxation, such as watching television, engaging with social media and drinking alcohol, don't tend to be very effective. The immediacy of technology (instant messaging, 24-hour news) and all our supposed time-saving gadgets seem to fuel our modern addiction to being constantly busy!

Proper relaxation is essential for our physical and mental well-being. It helps us release patterns of what Yogi Bhajan called "commotional living": the self-defeating emotions we experience such as anxiety, anger and hopelessness which are generated by our inner emotional dialogue. These are often what prevent us from getting to sleep and sleeping soundly. Letting go into a truly relaxed state helps us to release these negative emotions. Commotional living also drains the reserve energy of the nervous system. People who rarely switch off can often seem quite agitated and "nervous". They cannot sit still for a moment; they are constantly "on the go". Not surprisingly, they often have trouble sleeping. Learning to relax teaches us how to manage stress. It releases rigid patterns we hold deep in our muscles and our blood flow.

Yogic Methods of Relaxation

Stretching

Stretching, especially deeper stretching after cardiovascular exercise, allows energy to flow unrestricted through the body and untangles any areas of tension, leading to greater relaxation. Examples of poses we often use in Kundalini Yoga that enable this kind of deep stretching are Triangle Pose and Life Nerve Stretch.

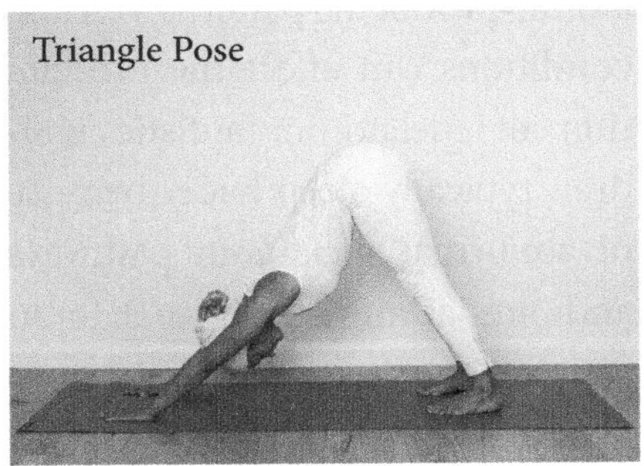
Triangle Pose

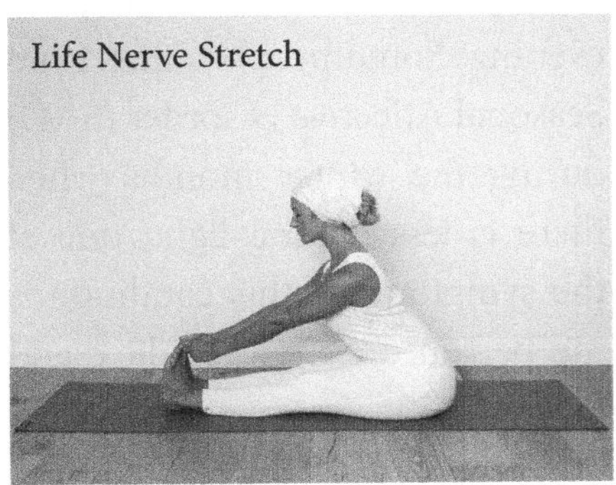
Life Nerve Stretch

Conscious relaxation

If you tend to feel groggy after a daytime nap, try lying in Corpse Pose for up to 15 minutes instead. Consciously relaxing the body while keeping the mind alert is revitalising. You can also listen out for children while you are doing it. While they are busy, watching a favourite programme for example, or the baby is asleep, go upstairs and take a few minutes to revitalise yourself.

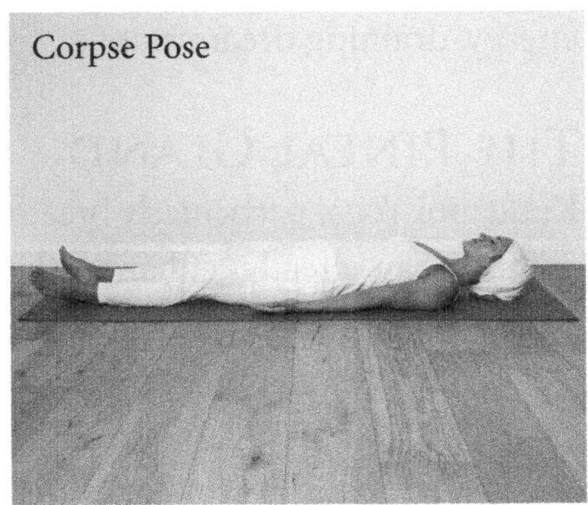
Corpse Pose

Breathing techniques

Two breathing techniques particularly useful for encouraging relaxation are Left Nostril Breathing and Long Deep Breathing. Use these whenever you get the opportunity; the more you practise them, the easier it becomes to switch into a more relaxed state when needed.

Breathing techniques are also useful for oxygenating the blood, which helps to prevent tiredness. Yogi Bhajan taught that although we are supposed to have 21 per cent oxygen in our blood, we normally live on just 15 or 16 per cent. He advised doing **pranayama** and Breath of Fire in particular every three or four hours, just for a minute or two, to oxygenate the blood and balance yourself.[14]

Relaxing Postures

The best posture for deep relaxation is Corpse Pose. Lying with the legs up against the wall is also very relaxing and great for preventing varicose veins too.

[10] The Teachings of Yogi Bhajan, 12th July 1989

Yogi Bhajan's Specific Recommendations Before Going to Sleep

Yogi Bhajan gave us the following routine to induce deep sleep:[15]

1. Lie on your stomach and turn your head so your right cheek is on the pillow. This will free up your left nostril to bring in cooling, soothing and calming energy;

2. Start long, deep breathing through your nose, keeping your mouth closed. Think the sound *Sat* as you inhale, and *Naam* as you exhale;

3. After a few long, deep breaths use your arm or hand to completely block off your right nostril. Continue breathing through your left nostril;

4. When you feel yourself starting to get drowsy, turn over onto your back or however you wish to sleep. It is better for your heart and digestion to sleep on your right side than the left. Continue long, deep breathing.

As soon as your breathing becomes regular and slow you will go quickly through the preliminary stages of sleep and almost immediately reach the deep dreamless sleep state, avoiding the energy-draining dream state.

The Pineal Gland

Kundalini Yoga, particularly breath control, can greatly enhance the activity of the **pineal gland.**[16] We will look at the pineal gland again in Chapter 12 but in relation to sleep, this tiny gland in the brain has one particularly important function: the production of melatonin. When it functions normally, this hormone is produced by the light-sensitive gland (which Yogi Bhajan referred to as a "sunspot")[17] with the onset of darkness and helps us to sleep.

These days, artificial light is available to us throughout the night which, as shift workers know only too well, confuses our natural melatonin-producing patterns. Certain conditions can affect the production of melatonin; autistic children typically sleep badly because of abnormal melatonin pathways and are administered melatonin supplements to help them to sleep during the night. Blind people often take melatonin during the evening. Some people suffer from Seasonal Affective Disorder (SAD) during the winter months when there is less natural light; one of the symptoms of this condition is the person does not produce and

---

15 *Kundalini Yoga: The Flow of Eternal Power*, p.112

16 *The Aquarian Teacher*, p.165

17 Lecture given in Los Angeles on 12th May 1987 (*www.libraryofteachhings.com*)

regulate melatonin properly. Blue light, which is emitted from televisions, tablets and personal computers, is particularly disruptive to melatonin production[18].

Top Tips for Improving Sleep

- Avoid caffeine which disturbs sleep patterns[19]
- 108 Frogs (see pages 42-43) just before retiring can knock you out cold. Start with 26 and work up gradually;
- Wash your feet in cold water and then dry them vigorously with a towel to prepare the nervous system for sleep[20];
- Splash some cold water on the forehead to make you really sleepy[21];
- Brush the root of the tongue as well as the teeth to clear out mucous pockets at the back of the throat[22];
- Long deep breathing through the left nostril for 3-5 minutes will relax you;
- If you have to get up in the night with young children, keep the lighting as low as possible and don't switch your tablet or smartphone on.

Yoga Set for Improving Sleep

Breathing Exercise

Left Nostril Breathing

Sitting in Easy Pose with the spine straight, use the right thumb to gently block off the right nostril. The other fingers point straight up. Inhale and exhale deeply through the left nostril. Continue for 3 minutes.

The left nostril (and the left side of the body generally) is connected to the right hemisphere of the brain. Isolating the breathing through the left nostril only is very

---

18 Advice from Harvard Medical School *http://www.health.harvard.edu/staying-healthy/blue-light-has-a-dark-side*

19 *The Aquarian Teacher*, p.165

20 *Kundalini Yoga: The Flow of Eternal Power*, p.110

21 *The Aquarian Teacher*, p.248

22 *Kundalini Yoga: The Flow of Eternal Power*, p.110

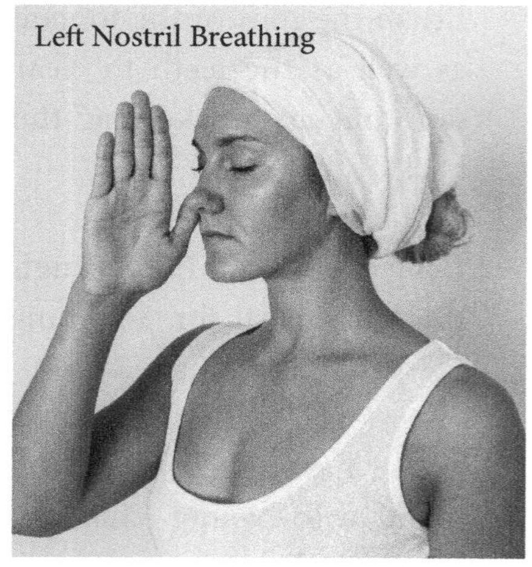
Left Nostril Breathing

calming, so ideal before going to sleep or when you just need to relax a bit. At any one time, we breathe through a dominant nostril which alternates every 90 to 150 minutes[23]. So when you first start isolating the breathing to one nostril, it can be challenging if that is not the dominant nostril at that particular time. It gets easier with practice.

Kriya

KRIYA FOR CONQUERING SLEEP[24]

1. Sit on the heels with the palms on the thighs. Keep the spine straight and lean back 30 degrees from the vertical. Hold the posture with Long Deep Breathing for 1 minute. Inhale, exhale and relax.

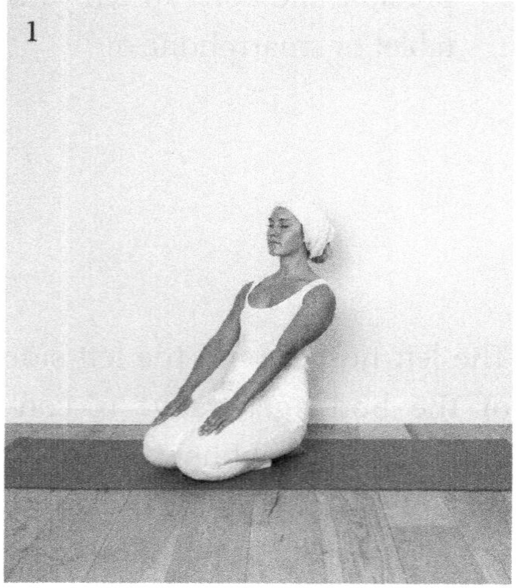

1

2. Still sitting on the heels, fold the arms across the chest and hold on to the elbows. Rotate

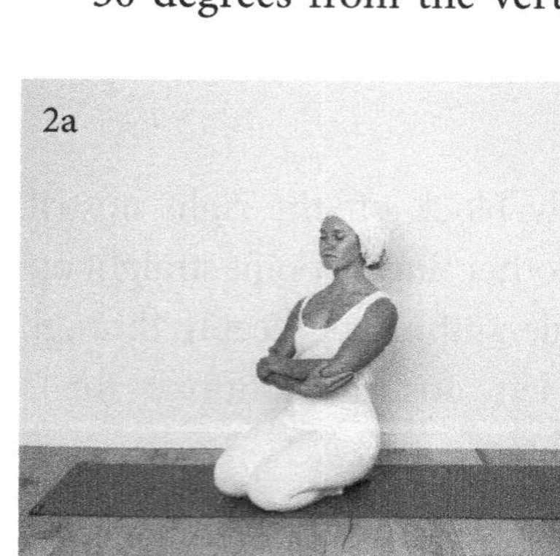
2a

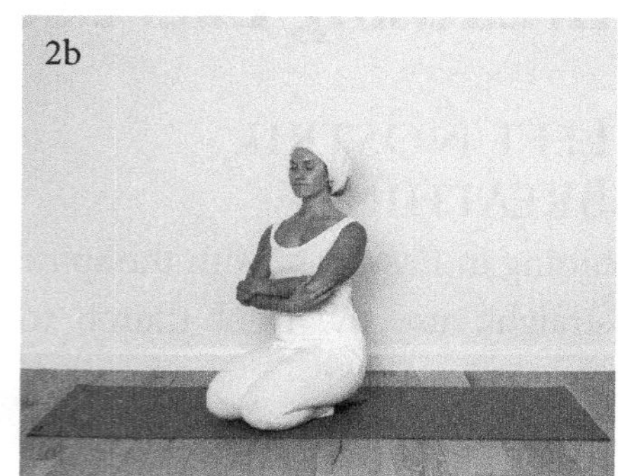
2b

[23] *The Aquarian Teacher*, p.96

[24] *Sadhana Guidelines*, pp.132-133

the torso in a circle from right to left (anticlockwise). Continue for 3 minutes.

3. Body Drops: Immediately extend the legs in front of you. Put the hands on the ground next to the hips. With the inhale, lift the hips and the heels off the ground. With the exhale, drop the body. Complete 20 of these body drops.

   Author's suggestion: Try your best, and make sure you keep the back straight.

4. Repeat exercise #2 for 3 minutes.

5. Do 15 body drops.

6. Bridge Pose: Sit with the knees bent and the hands, palms flat, slightly behind the hips. The feet are flat on the ground about two fists apart. Press the hips up and let the head relax back. Hold the pose for 1 minute with normal breathing. Continue with Breath of Fire for 1 minute. Inhale, exhale completely, and hold the breath out as you apply Root Lock. Inhale, exhale and relax.

7. Do 10 body drops.

8. Repeat Bridge Pose for 1 minute with Breath of Fire.

9. Relax completely on the back for 2 or 3 minutes.

10. Come into Bridge Pose and raise the right leg 60 degrees. Point the toes forward. Begin a powerful Breath of Fire for 1 minute. Inhale deeply, exhale completely, and apply Root Lock. Repeat the exercise with the left leg raised. Relax.

11. Crow Pose: squat with the feet flat on the ground. Extend the arms in front, parallel to the ground, with the palms facing

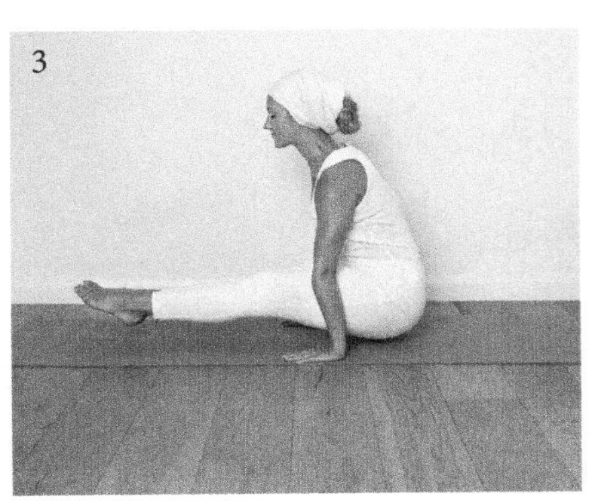
3

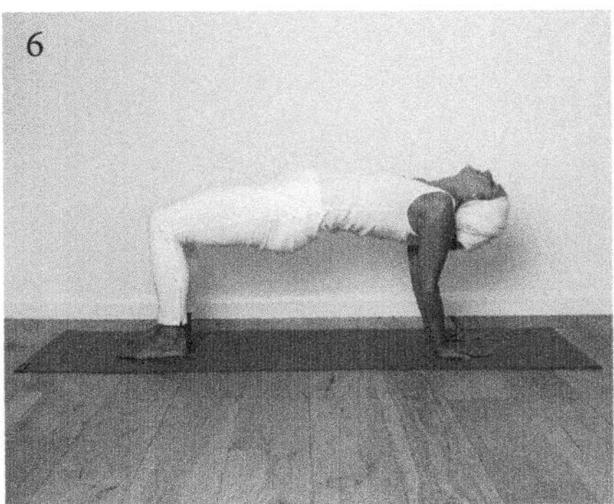
6

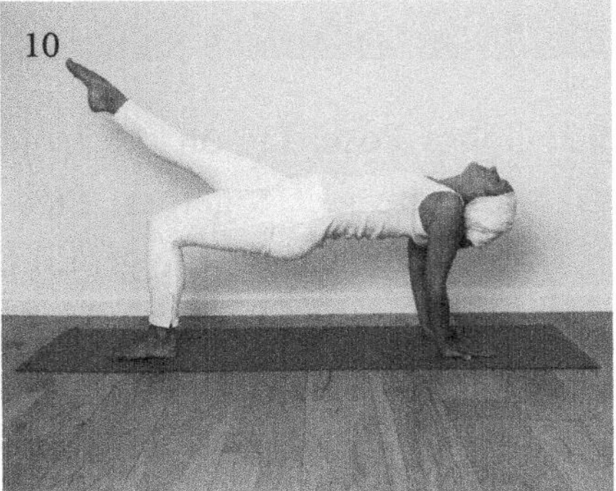
10

down. Inhale deeply and stand up, then exhale completely as you squat down. Keep the spine as straight as possible. 10 repetitions.

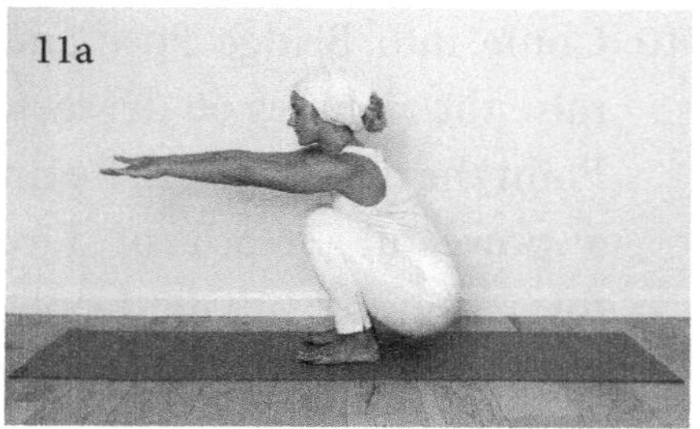
11a

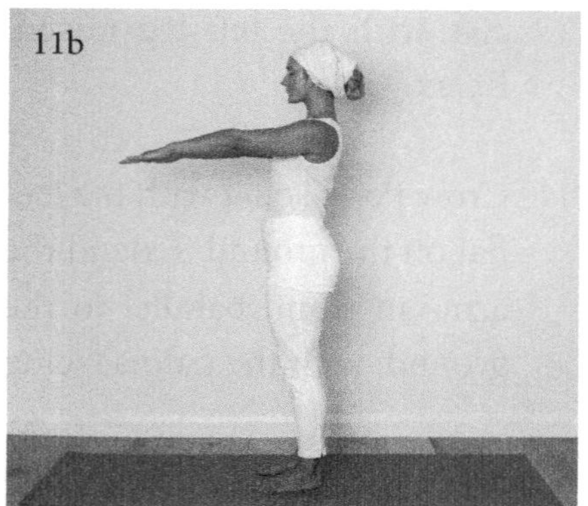
11b

12. Cobra Pose: Lie on the front with the feet together. Place the palms flat on the ground, underneath the shoulders. Push up, straightening the arms, so the upper body rises from the ground. The pelvis stays in contact with the ground. Keep the feet as close together as possible to protect the lower back and the eyes closed to protect the optic nerve. Hold for 1 minute with normal breathing. Then kick the buttocks with one heel for 1 minute. Each time the heel strikes the buttocks, exhale slightly. Then kick with the other heel for 1 more minute. Relax.

Author's suggestion: If the back is not flexible enough to keep the hips on the ground, place the forearms on the ground instead of the hands (Sphinx Pose).

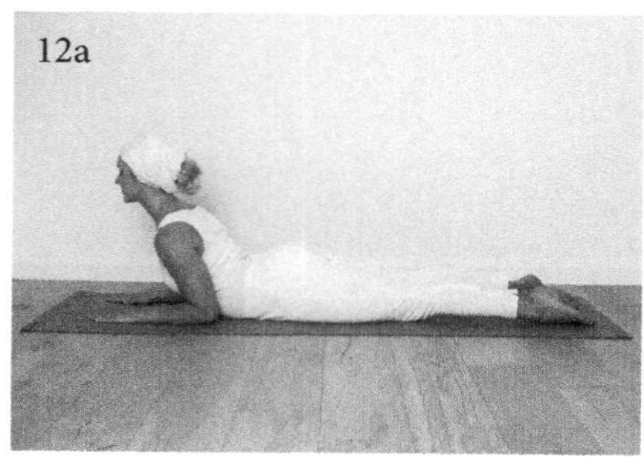
12a

13. Sit on the heels in Rock Pose. Extend the arms straight over the head with the palms flat together. Bring the hands halfway down toward the top of the head so that the elbows are slightly bent. Raise the eyes up and focus on the centre of the skull on the pineal gland and project through the crown of the head for 1 minute.

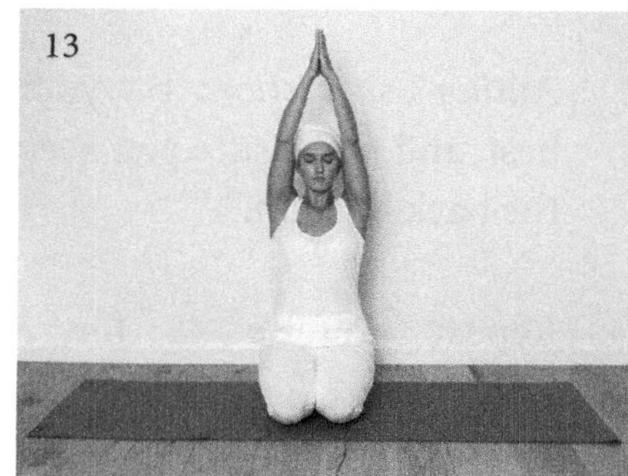
13

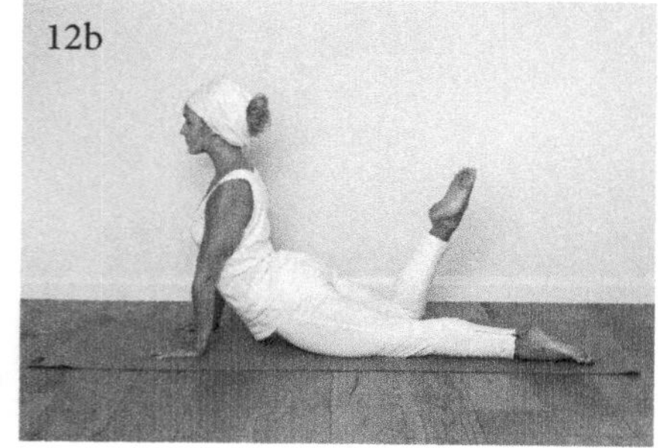
12b

Meditation

SHABD KRIYA FOR DEEP SLEEP AND RADIANCE[25]

If this meditation is practised on a regular basis, once a week or even every night, your sleep will be deep and relaxed. The control of the rhythm of the breath strengthens the nervous system and regenerates the nerves.

Sit in Easy Pose with a straight spine. The hands are in the lap in Buddha Mudra: palms up, right hand resting on top of left. The thumbs touch and face forward. The eyes focus at the tip of the nose and are about 9/10ths closed so that only a tiny amount of light enters.

Inhale in 4 equal parts through the nose, i.e. the inhale is divided into 4 "sniffs". Mentally vibrate *Sa Ta Na Ma* in time with the four sniffs. Hold the breath and mentally chant 4 repetitions of *Sa Ta Na Ma* (ie 16 counts).

Then exhale in 2 equal strokes, mentally projecting *Wahe Guru*. Continue for 5 minutes and gradually work up to 11 minutes.

Note: this meditation can make you very spacey and dreamy and will often put you to sleep before you complete the allotted time!

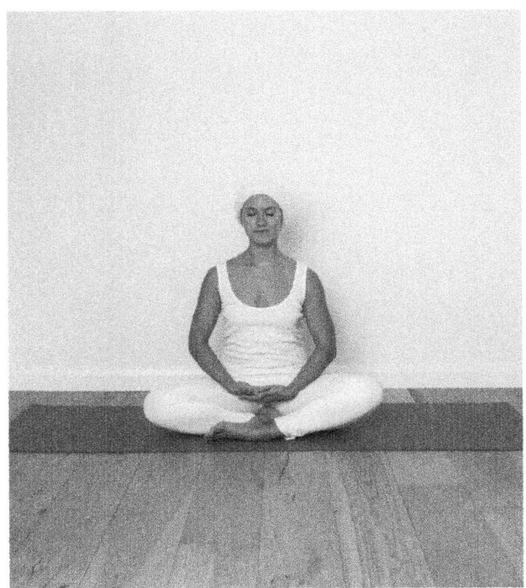

[25] From a public lecture given by Yogi Bhajan on 1st April 1974 (*www.libraryofteachings.com*)

Chapter 4
The Energy of the Sun:
Boosting Energy

"If you just breathe in the upper part of the lungs and breathe out… [you] suffer a lot of energy lapses… [if you don't breathe in the lower areas of the lungs to properly oxygenate the blood] you barely survive. Symptoms are that you get exhausted very soon and get fatigued very fast."

~ Yogi Bhajan[26]

When my energy is high, I love being a parent. I love pretending to be the Kissing Monster and chasing my two excitable and hyperactive sons around the house trying to kiss them while they run around shrieking in mock terror. I love running races in the park with them, jumping in puddles and going on spontaneous adventures through the woods together, or sharing a picnic in the garden. I love hiding underneath one of their beds with them, reading stories by torchlight. This is parenthood at its best and it's what I imagined when I first wondered what it might be like to have children. It's the image we are fed through the television, through advertising, in the photos our friends post on social networking sites: happy, smiling children and happy, smiling parents, released from the mundanity of adult life to enjoy the fun of childhood again.

When my energy is low – when I have not had enough sleep or when I am ill – it's a very different picture. Neither of these factors earns me a minute's break from the responsibilities of 24-hour childcare as a single parent. The childcare just gets much harder: I no longer have the strength to think of an imaginative way to break through my youngest son's irrational tantrum and am therefore more likely to inflame the situation by snapping at him.

[26] *Praana Praanee Praanayam*, p.64

When we don't have the energy to meet the demands of life – demands which are high when we are caring for young children – we experience stress. Stress in turn creates more exhaustion as well as various physical and mental health consequences. All parents of young children need energy to cope with the demands of parenting.

Adults all have different energy levels and we all experience fluctuations in those energy levels for different reasons. As we have seen in the previous chapter, the amount of energy we have does not depend exclusively on how much sleep we get – or don't get – but also factors such as the quality of that sleep, what we eat and drink, whether we are sufficiently hydrated and how stressed we are. Yogi Bhajan taught that the depth and rate at which we breathe also has a massive impact on our energy.

Where does our energy come from?

Understanding the source of your energy will help you to take any opportunities for recharging that present themselves. If you are introverted (like approximately 25% of the population) you obtain your energy from inner sources. If you are extroverted (like the remaining 75%) you collect your energy from your external environment. It is possible to be a bit of both; you can work out which you tend to be using "Is This You?" below.

You are also likely to find things easier if you can understand where your children stand on this spectrum because if they are sourcing their energy effectively, they are less likely to be tired and difficult at home.[27]

High Sensitivity

Another factor that affects our energy levels is how sensitive we are to external stimuli. A highly sensitive person can easily, and sometimes quite suddenly, become overwhelmed and exhausted. An estimated 15-20 per cent of the population are very sensitive to stimulation including subtle sounds, sights or physical sensations such as pain: anything that wakes up the nervous system. It can be external, such as noise, it can come from our own body (e.g. muscle tension, hunger, sexual feelings), or it can be memories, thoughts, fantasies or plans.[28]

---

[27] See *Raising Your Spirited Child: a guide for parents whose child is more intense, sensitive, perceptive, persistent and energetic* by Mary Sheedy Kurcinka (Harper; 1991) for a detailed discussion of this topic

[28] *The Highly Sensitive Person: How to Thrive When the World Overwhelms You* by Elaine N. Aron (Element; 1999), p.8

The level of stimulation need not be dramatic but can build up through repetition until one quite minor stimulation can feel like the last straw. It is easy to see from this how high sensitivity can present challenges in the parenting arena. A highly sensitive person who has been looking after noisy young children and refereeing their squabbles all day may reach breaking point by tea-time. A highly sensitive person who has been at work all day may really need some quiet time at home to recover, but instead faces the noise and stress of bath-time with children who are over-excited because they haven't seen her or him for a few hours.

Illness

There are also certain physical disorders that can lead to exhaustion, such as adrenal fatigue, chronic fatigue syndrome and hypothyroidism, and it's important to seek medical advice if you think that might be the case for you. Yoga can help boost thyroid function with exercises involving the neck: neck rolls (see Kriya for Disease Resistance in Chapter 11), Cobra Pose (see Sun Salutations in Chapter 2) and Cat-Cow (see Warm-up set 1 in Chapter 2).

Hormonal Fluctuations

For women, our monthly cycle and other hormonal issues also affect our energy levels. See Chapter 10 for a discussion on the subject of hormones and how to balance them.

Is this You?

- Do your energy levels tend to dip at a particular time of day, such as mid-afternoon?
- Do your energy levels tend to dip at a particular point in your monthly cycle?
- Do you find it hard to get out of bed in the morning even if you have had a reasonable amount of sleep?
- Do you feel you don't have the energy to perform simple tasks or to do things you would like to do?
- Are you suffering from stress?
- Are you aware of any problems in relation to your thyroid function?

Are you an introvert?

- Do you find being in a large group for an extended period exhausting?
- Do you prefer having dinner with the family or one special friend rather than a large group?
- Is your physical space important to you?

- Do you feel revitalised by solitary activities such as reading and writing?
- Do you find noise and interruptions difficult?
- Do you solve problems by thinking them through yourself before ever talking about them with anyone else?
- Do you need time to reflect before answering a question, often feeling frustrated with yourself for not sharing an answer you realise you knew?

If you answered "Yes" to several of these, you are predominantly an introvert.

Are you an extrovert?

- Do you enjoy and need to interact with other adults?
- Do you feel exhausted when you have spent too much time alone or only with young children?
- Do you solve problems by talking them through with other adults?
- Do you find introverted children bewildering and encourage them to leave their room and play with other children?
- Do you frequently worry that you talk too much and don't listen enough?
- Do you love parties?

If you answered "Yes" to several of these, you are predominantly an extrovert.

Reflection Points

- If you are predominantly an introvert, you are likely to feel much better after a busy day with the children if you spend some quiet time reading once they are in bed. You will probably find it helpful to make sure the weekend is not packed with play dates and other busy activities but includes some quiet time, or perhaps a walk in the woods with the children rather than a trip to a busy playground;
- If you are predominantly an extrovert you need time with other adults, so if you have to spend a whole day with young children, you are likely to feel much better if you call a friend for a chat in the evening or make sure your weekend includes lots of opportunities for getting out of the house and socialising with other parents and their children;
- Can you get outside more to boost your energy levels with some extra oxygen?

When my boys were younger, it was really hard to take them outside anywhere because they always ran off – in different directions! Rather than deciding which one I would rather keep, I had to find easier places to take them: enclosed back gardens (trampolines in particular); a playground enclosed with heavy gates; a playground with water jets (which neither of them would ever willingly leave); a skate park with their scooters (which again neither would ever choose to leave);

- Remembering the old adage "a change is as good as a rest", can you have a change of scenery even for a short while? Could you take the children to a different park from usual?

Yogic Viewpoint: The Importance of the Breath

Breath gives us life; we cannot live long at all without it. And although it is something we do automatically from the moment we are born, most of us don't breathe correctly. It is very common for people to breathe in a shallow, erratic way, through their upper chest. As we have already seen, some people even breathe the wrong way around, pulling the belly in when they inhale.

One of the causes of poor breathing is stress, which results in a shallow breathing pattern with a faster breath rate. This in turn causes chronic tension, weak nerves and susceptibility to more stress. This sets the scene for illness and breakdown in one or another of the body systems.

Insufficient oxygen levels in the body also make us vulnerable to the development of cancer. Dr Warburg won his first Nobel Prize in 1931 for proving that although cancer has countless secondary causes, the primary cause is low oxygen levels, which prevent the cells from producing energy. Cells that cannot produce energy aerobically cannot produce enough energy to function properly and therefore lose the ability to do whatever they need to do in the body.

So it is no exaggeration to say that of all the positive changes a person can make in their life, learning to breathe deeply and completely is probably the most effective for increasing health and vitality. It also enables us to feel more connected in our lives and to develop our higher consciousness.

Once we start to think of the breath in broader terms than simply respiration, we realise that the breath and its movements are connected to the movements of all the emotions and thoughts. How many times do we take a deep breath when faced with challenging behaviour from our children? The mind, and therefore our reaction to the behaviour, follows what is going on with the breath.

Pranayam, the yogic science of controlling and conserving **prana**, our life force, through breathing techniques which change the physical, mental and energetic states of our lives, is central to the practice of Kundalini Yoga.

GENERAL ADVICE ABOUT PRACTISING PRANAYAM[29]

- Practise on an empty stomach, but not when you are so hungry it distracts you;
- Keep your posture correct: spine straight, chest lifted and chin in. Keep space in your upper body so the primary breathing muscles can do their jobs;
- Carefully follow all the instructions as given; do not improvise. You may shorten the practice but do not increase it;
- Be as relaxed as you can. Check yourself for areas of unnecessary tension: abdominal muscles, facial muscles, throat and tongue (do not stiffen or press it against the palate or teeth unless instructed to do so). Keep the lips relaxed when appropriate. Allow energy to flow freely through all your major joints (ankles, knees, hips, vertebrae, shoulders, elbows and wrists);
- Keep aware of the sound and flow of the breath so it remains rhythmic and unforced;
- Don't exceed your comfortable limits. Don't strain or hurt yourself in an effort to do a kriya. Start at a reasonable level and pace and allow yourself to grow into the full time and intensity.

THE CHAKRAS AND ENERGY

"Men of great knowledge actually found out about the chakras – their

[29] *Praana Praanee Praanayam*, p.V

workings, their petals, their sounds, their infinity, their co-relationship, their powers. They found that the life of a human is totally based on these chakras. They developed into a whole science. This total science gave birth to Kundalini Yoga. That is how Kundalini Yoga was born."

~ Yogi Bhajan[30]

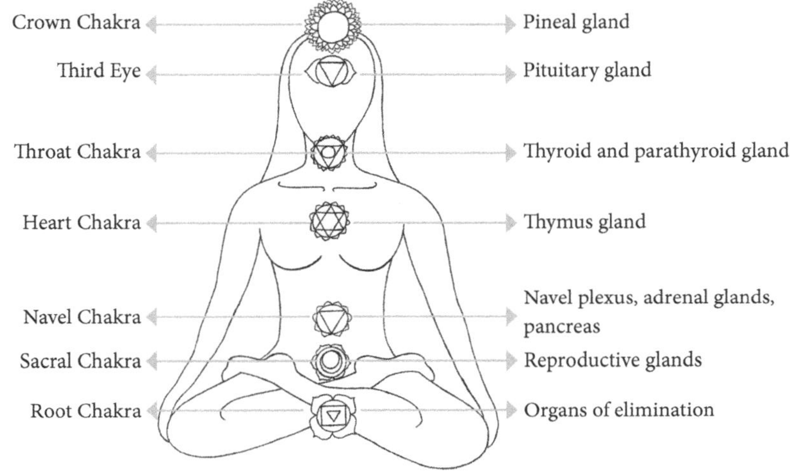

The **chakra** system is fundamental to the technology of Kundalini Yoga. There are hundreds of chakras, or energy centres, in the body and in Kundalini Yoga we focus on the seven major ones – the **Root Chakra**, the **Sacral Chakra**, the **Navel Chakra**, the **Heart Chakra**, the Throat Chakra, the Third Eye and the **Crown Chakra** – plus the Aura (which Yogi Bhajan referred to uniquely as the eighth chakra). The chakras are vortices of energy, invisible to most people; those who prefer something more tangible will be interested to know they correspond with areas in the endocrine system, or to **nerve plexes** in the Physical Body, as shown above. The eighth chakra corresponds with the electro-magnetic field known to surround the human body.

It can be helpful to consider the characteristics of individual chakras, although it is important to note they are all interconnected. It is possible for individual chakras to be closed from time to time, or to function less than optimally (either too weak or too strong). Kundalini Yoga assists prana in clearing blocks to the natural flow of energy through the system.

When we feel we need a boost of energy, this may be an indication that the Navel Chakra is not functioning optimally. Located

[30] *The Aquarian Teacher*, p.183

in the abdominal area, specifically the area of the **solar plexus** and the Navel Point, this chakra is associated with the navel plexus, liver, gall bladder, spleen, digestive organs, pancreas and **adrenal glands**. It was via an umbilical cord through this area that we were once attached to and nurtured by our own mothers and it is where we continue to hold a reserve of energy throughout our lives. This is what is said to travel down to the base of the spine to become the Kundalini energy. By strengthening our Navel Chakra through Kundalini Yoga, we are building up that reserve of energy.

The Throat Chakra, associated with the **thyroid gland**, may also be sluggish. Lethargy is often indicative of poor functioning of the thyroid. Chanting strengthens the Throat Chakra, as do all exercises that stimulate the thyroid.

Top Tips for Instant Energy

- Comb your hair with a wooden comb;[31]
- Take a cold shower! Yogi Bhajan was an expert in the science of **hydrotherapy**, and taught that a cold shower opens up the capillaries and flushes out the organs, which then get a rich supply of blood when the capillaries close again. He cautioned women to cover their thighs when taking a cold shower so as not to upset the calcium-magnesium balance, and to avoid it altogether if they are pregnant or menstruating or suffering from a fever, rheumatism or heart disease;[32]
- Splash some cold water between the eyebrows and the upper lip;[33]
- Eat bananas, coconuts, dates, garlic;[34]
- Do three minutes of Right Nostril Breathing (see below).

[31] Summer Solstice, 10th June 1974 (*www.libraryofteachings.com*)

[32] *The Aquarian Teacher*, p.248

[33] *The Aquarian Teacher*, p.248

[34] *The Aquarian Teacher*, p.255

Yoga Set for Boosting Your Energy

Breathing Exercise

Energy Boost[35]

Sit in Easy Pose with a straight spine. Gently block off your left nostril with the thumb of your left hand. Keep the other fingers straight and slightly separated. Begin Breath of Fire through the right nostril. Continue for 3 minutes. Then inhale and mentally circulate energy throughout your body and Aura.

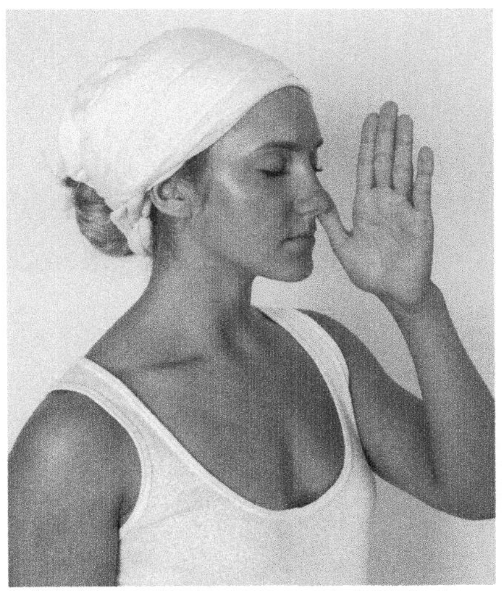

The right nostril is connected to the left side of the brain. As we saw in the previous chapter, one nostril is always dominant for a period of 90-150 minutes then the other nostril takes over. So this breathing practice can be challenging at first if the right nostril is not dominant at the time you begin. Isolating the breathing to the right nostril only is very energising and improves concentration.[36]

Kriya

Surya Kriya[37]

Right Nostril Breathing: sit in Easy Pose with a straight spine. Rest the right hand in Gyan Mudra on the right knee. Block the left nostril with the thumb of the left hand. The other fingers point straight up. Begin long, deep, powerful breaths in and out of the right nostril. Focus on the flow of the breath. Continue for 3 minutes. Inhale and relax.

Sat Kriya: sit on the heels with the arms overhead and the palms together. Interlace the fingers except for the index fingers, which point straight up. Men cross the right thumb over

[35] *Praana Praanee Pranayama*, p.108

[36] *The Aquarian Teacher*, p.96

[37] *The Aquarian Teacher*, p.352-353

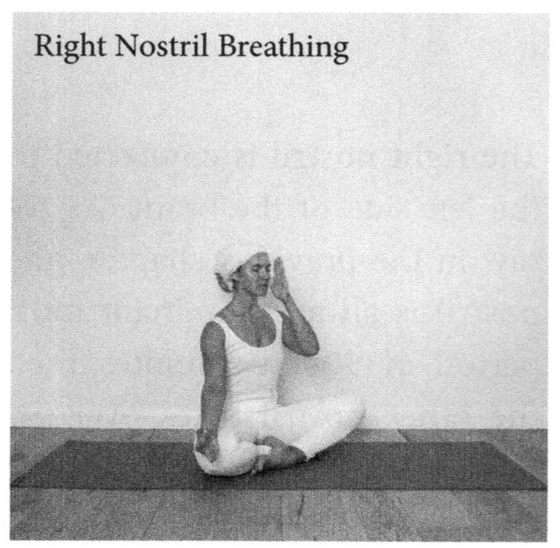
Right Nostril Breathing

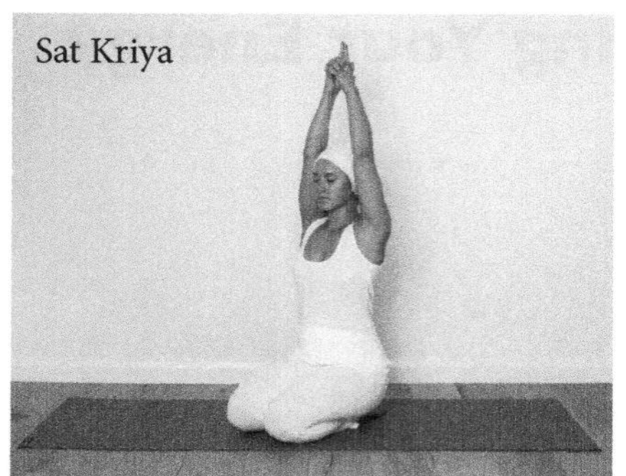
Sat Kriya

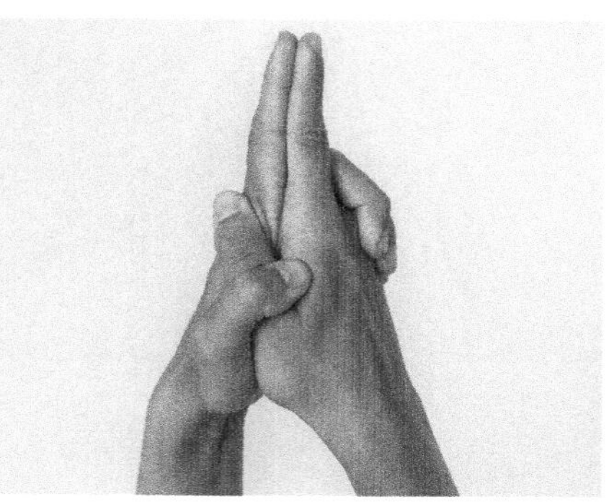

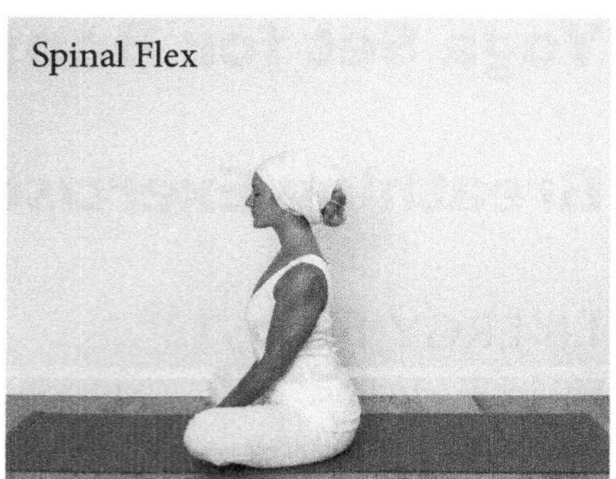
Spinal Flex

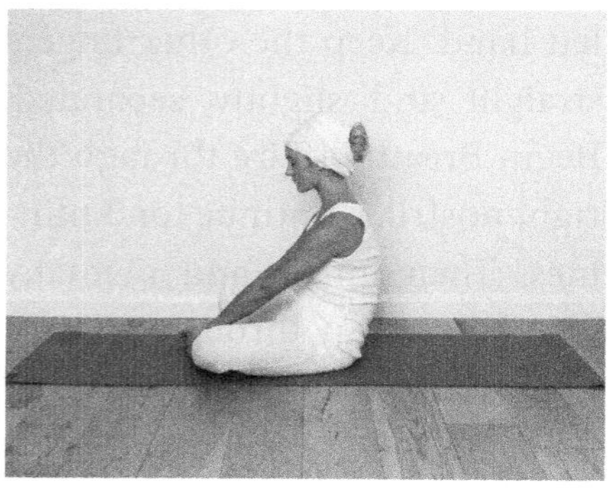

the left thumb; women cross the left thumb over the right. Begin rhythmically chanting *Sat Naam*, emphasizing *Sat* as you pull the navel in. On *Naam*, release it. Focus at the Brow Point. Continue for 3 minutes. Then inhale, suspend the breath, apply the Root Lock and imagine your energy radiating from the Navel Point and circulating throughout the body. Relax.

Repeat the exercise for a further 3 minutes. Then inhale, apply the Root Lock, and mentally draw all the energy to the top of the fingertips. Relax.

Spinal Flex: sit in Easy Pose. Grasp the shins with both hands. Inhale, stretch the spine forward and lift the chest. Exhale, let the spine flex backwards. Keep the head level during the movements. On each inhale, mentally vibrate the mantra *Sat*. On the exhale vibrate *Naam*. On each exhale apply the Root Lock. Continue rhythmically with deep breaths 108 times. Then inhale and hold briefly with the spine perfectly straight. Exhale. Relax.

Frog Pose: Place the toes on the ground, heels together off the ground, fingers on the ground between the knees, and lift the head up. Inhale, raise the buttocks high. Lower the forehead towards the knees and keep the

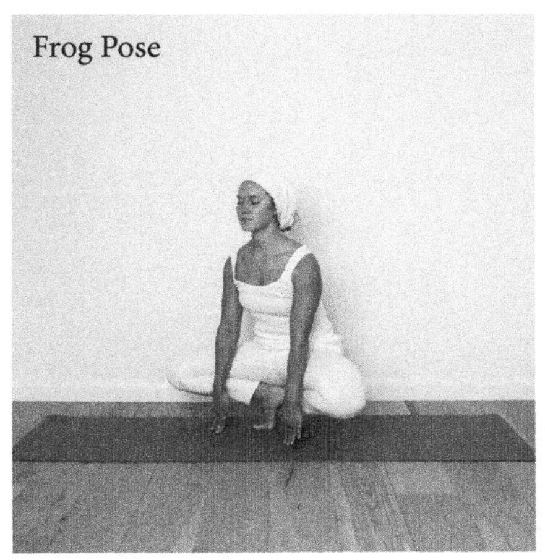
Frog Pose

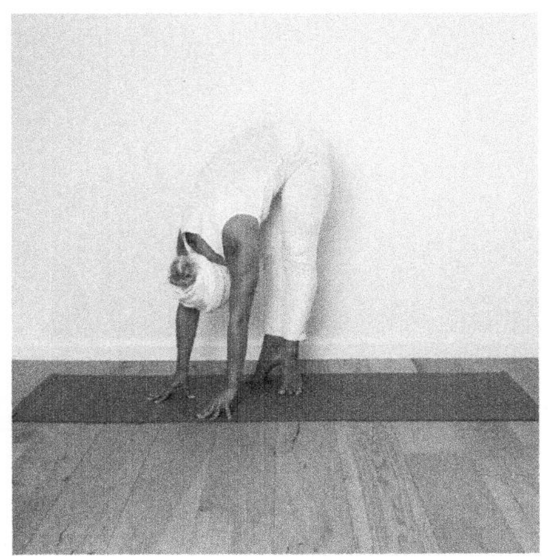

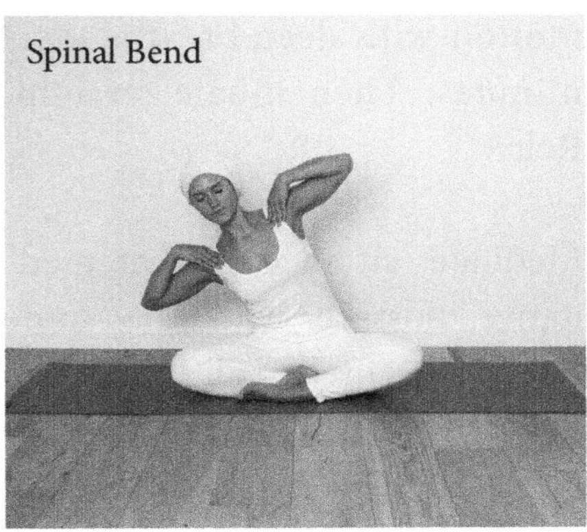
Spinal Bend

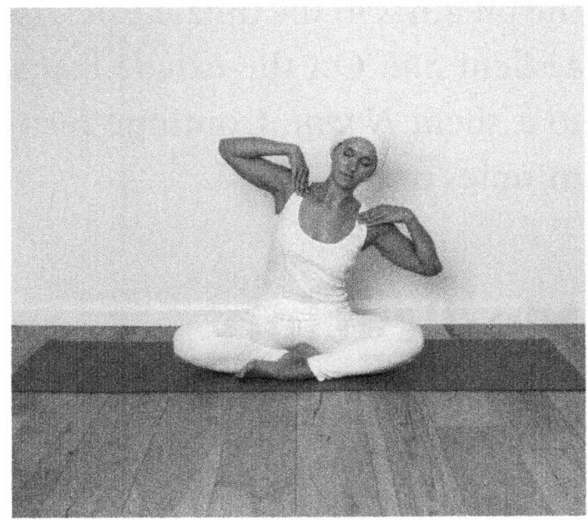

heels off the ground. Exhale, come back to the original squatting position and face forward. Continue with deep breaths 26 times. Inhale up, then relax down onto the heels.

Neck Turns: sitting on the heels, place the hands on the thighs. With the spine very straight, inhale deeply as you turn the head to the left. Mentally vibrate *Sat*. Exhale completely as you turn the head to the right. Mentally vibrate *Naam*. Continue inhaling and exhaling for 3 minutes. Inhale with the head straight forward. Relax.

Spinal Bend: sit in Easy Pose. Grab the shoulders with the fingers in front and the thumbs behind. The upper arms and elbows are parallel to the ground. Inhale as you bend to the left, exhale and bend to the right. Continue this swaying

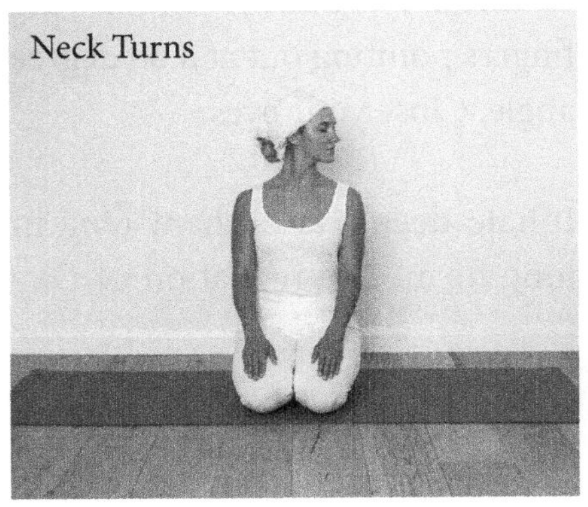
Neck Turns

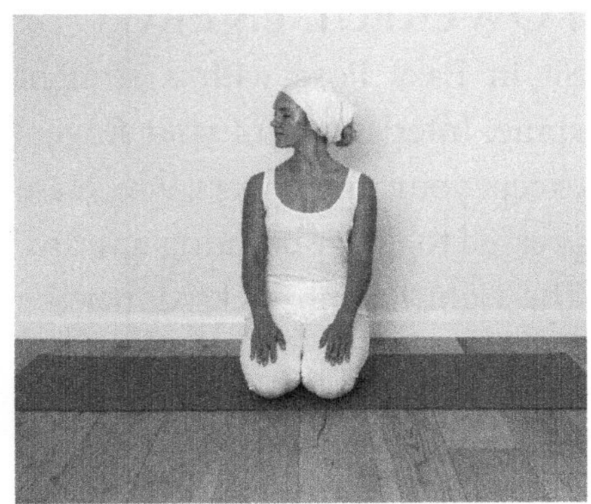

motion with deep breaths for 3 minutes. Then inhale straight. Relax.

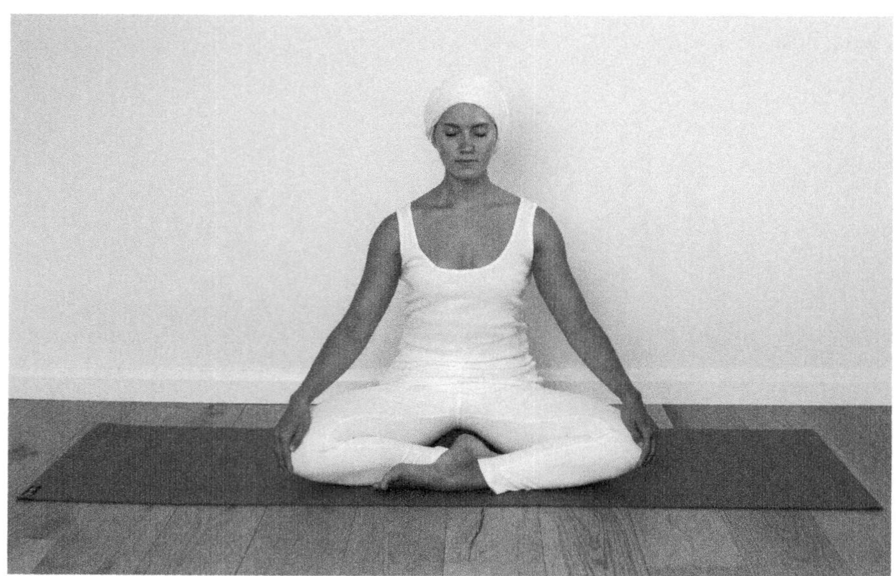

Meditate: sit in a perfect meditative posture with the spine straight. Direct all attention through the Brow Point. Pull the Navel Point in, hold it and apply the Root Lock. Watch the flow of the breath. On the inhale listen to a silent *Sat*. On the exhale listen to a silent *Naam*. Continue for 6 minutes or longer.

Meditation

Meditation for Absolutely Powerful Energy[38]

Sit in Easy Pose with a straight spine. Interlace all of your fingers except your ring fingers, which are pressed together pointing upward. The right thumb locks down the left thumb. The hands are level with the diaphragm, several inches out from the body, with the ring fingers pointing out at a 60 degree angle. Close your eyes.

Inhale deeply and chant *Ong* in long form, one recitation of *Ong* per exhalation (approximately 15 seconds). The sound is created through the nose; the mouth is held slightly open but no air comes out through the mouth. The sound comes from the nose by way of the back of the upper palate. Your upper palate will

[38] *Praana Praanee Praanayam* p. 42-43. First taught by Yogi Bhajan on 17th May 1976

vibrate. Concentrate to do it correctly. Continue for 8 minutes.

"It may make you cough or sneeze or there may be pressure in the ears, but it will give you bright eyes, better ears, and good nose—your E-N-T will be perfect. It will affect the thyroid. It will vibrate your whole brain and do a lot of good things. All the hot air will come out through the nose. The mouth is open, but the sound comes out only through the nose.

*"Ong is the sound of the Ajna chakra, the sixth center of consciousness. Vibrating the thalamus is a privilege. That's why 'Om, Om, Om', there is no such thing 'Om'. There is, however, the sound of the Infinite which comes through the central nervous system (**Shushmuna**) and touching the central nervous system. I have explained how to do it; it comes from the back of the nose but you have to keep the mouth open. It can go to any pitch. It requires practice but the practitioner enjoys it. It is very fruitful. It is so fruitful and so enjoyable that all you have to do is a maximum five times and by the third time you will be sitting like this... in bliss. Therefore it is very important, if you want to be in love with yourself, to practice this sound. That will give you a great essence and joy of life"*

~ Yogi Bhajan

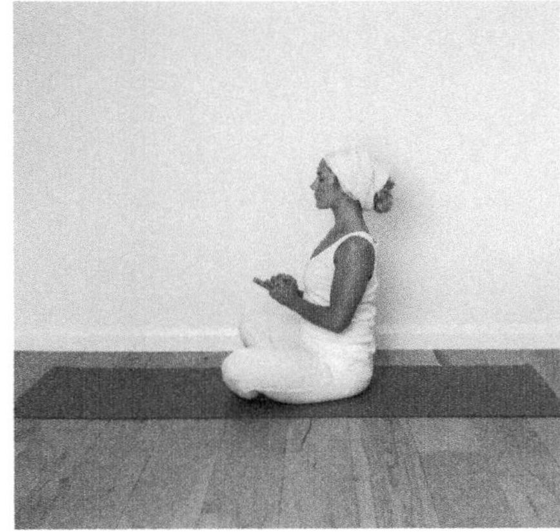

Chapter 5
Lightening the Load:
Managing Stress

"The main problem in the world is stress. It is not going to decrease – it is going to increase. If through pranayam the shock can be harnessed, the entire stress and disease can be eliminated."

~ Yogi Bhajan[39]

"Wherever there is stress, you will use up oxygen. You will not be in a position to be handicapped by lack of oxygen if you do Breath of Fire every day."

~ Yogi Bhajan[40]

We experience stress when we don't have the energy to meet the demands we face. Never have demands on parents been higher than they are today.

With so much choice available to us, we may have agonized for years over whether to have children at all, when to have them and how to even find the right partner for the job! In addition to the physical toll of pregnancy we may have had trouble conceiving, been through numerous bouts of IVF and suffered the heartbreak of miscarriage.

New parents, many of whom have had little or no experience of looking after children before, discover a whole world of stressors they could never have imagined. Looking after young children is utterly relentless. Some also have special needs (many of which we are only just beginning to recognise and understand) which may not be diagnosed until the parents have already lived with the consequences for several years. Some are born with physical or mental disabilities or life-limiting conditions.

Although we are accustomed to living in a society that exalts personal freedom, at home with a newborn baby we no longer have autonomy

[39] *The Aquarian Teacher*, p.89

[40] *Praana Praanee Praanayam*, p.77

over even the simplest things: we can't go out for a walk when we feel like it – and we certainly can't sleep when we choose to!

We soon become aware that mothers have very low social status. In paid work it is normal to occasionally receive some positive feedback, even thanks, for our efforts, as well as a salary. Yet despite doing a "job" that is literally 24/7, mothers get little credit – but plenty of criticism when things go wrong.

"She [the mother] gets a credit for raising a great child, once in a while, a great child happens, you know. It's not that bad, and mother gets the credit for it... womanhood is not being appreciated."

~ Yogi Bhajan[41]

There appear to be so many decisions to make. Should we work? What kind of childcare is best? Should we breastfeed? Are we feeding our children the right food? The pressure to buy baby products is incredible; the average spend in the UK on a child in its first year is now just over £9,000[42]. And too many people seem to use the impersonal nature of the Internet as a platform to validate their own parenting choices by spouting judgemental attitudes – making us feel more and more insecure and stressed.

Despite all of this pressure, media images of happy families (created by a huge advertising industry) tell us there is something wrong with us if we are not bursting with happiness! The idealisation of motherhood is more intense than it has ever been, even though a degree of ambivalence towards one's children and the experience of parenting has been shown to be normal for all parents.[43]

Partly because of this idealisation and partly because of all the social taboos surrounding parenthood (also arguably stronger than ever before), there is a pattern of dishonesty many parents slip into as soon as they have children. This includes lying (to themselves as much as to others) about their true feelings surrounding their children.[44] It seems it is almost impossible for most parents to talk about the pressures they feel and the

---

[41] From a lecture given on 1st July 1993 in Espanola, NM, reproduced in the Library of Teachings *http://www.libraryofteachings.com/lecture.xqy?q=meditationforsuddenstressandshocksort:relevance&id=69ceeb51-a2d7-eecb-1c0f-a8ae87fe93e7&title=KWTC-Class-#4*

[42] *Shattered: Modern Motherhood and the Illusion of Equality by Rebecca Asher* (Harvill Secker; 2011)

[43] See Barbara Almond's *The Monster Within* (The Regents of the University of California, 2010) for a detailed examination of this topic

[44] See Susan Mausart's *The Mask of Motherhood* (Penguin Books, 1999) for a detailed examination of this topic

toll those pressures take on their mental and physical health and their relationships with their children, their partner, their relatives and friends.

Stress not only causes all kinds of physical and emotional difficulties, it also makes parenting itself much harder. We can end up in a crazy situation in which we shout at the children because we are stressed about the cost of providing them with the perfect Christmas, or because we are so stressed about the psychological effects of being too stressed in front of them! Stress damages relationships and causes deep unhappiness.

Is this You?

- Do you get snappy and impatient?
- Do you suffer from disturbed sleep (over and above any disturbances caused by the children)?
- Do you feel your personality has changed? For example, have you become unusually verbally or physically aggressive (swearing a lot more than you normally would, for instance)?
- Are you often tearful?
- Have your sexual habits changed?
- Have you become withdrawn, indecisive or inflexible?
- Do you regularly experience anxiety, fear, anger, frustration or depression?
- Have you noticed you breathe more rapidly than you used to?
- Do you suffer from regular headaches, nausea or indigestion?

Reflection Points

- Can you minimise stress in the home? Being unable to find anything, toys getting lost or broken, dangerous situations with the children and feeling the house is out of control all increase stress. Set yourself the challenge of doing 15 minutes of decluttering a day for 30 days, rather than trying to tackle it all in one go;
- Misplacing things (which is very easy to do when you are tired) adds to stress; while you look for your keys, the children have got their shoes and socks off again and it seems as though you will never get everyone out of the house. Always put important things, like house and car keys, in the same place;
- Minimise housework so you can rest when you get the chance. Get the shopping

delivered to save time and avoid the stress of taking children to the supermarket. Cook enough for a couple of meals at a time and freeze half. Get a cleaner if you can possibly afford it, even if it's just once a fortnight – unless you find cleaning therapeutic!

- Spend five minutes jotting down the key points in the day when you feel particularly stressed (for example bath-time, getting yourself ready for work and children ready for nursery/school, running for the train, when you are preparing dinner and they are tired and grumpy) so you are aware of your stress triggers;
- Harness the power of (carefully chosen) music. Music can affect our mood and the memory of particular pieces rekindles emotions. A calming melody played regularly in the evening when the children are asleep anchors it as a trigger for relaxation. You can then play it when needed at times of stress (using headphones if necessary). Energising music can be too much when children are around, especially for the highly sensitive (see previous chapter);
- Is your diet exacerbating your stress by adding to your toxic overload? Avoid stimulants and especially refined sugar. Keep blood sugar levels steady by eating three balanced meals a day. Onions also help to keep blood sugar balanced.[45]
- Are you getting enough exercise? Exercise prevents some of the damaging effects stress has on the body;
- Can you incorporate some genuine relaxation into your day even if it's just for a few minutes (see Chapter 3)?

Yogic Viewpoint: Meditation

Meditation promotes a sense of inner peace, well-being, stability and calm. It promotes the ability to focus energy, enhancing effectiveness and efficiency. It resolves core issues of stress-producing patterns. It releases reactions and unconscious habits, subconscious fears and blocks, all of which can increase our stress response to particular events. It promotes clarity of mind and the

[45] *The Aquarian Teacher*, p.254

ability to be present. It develops the Neutral Mind, which enables us to be more objective in our outlook, impervious to the effects of stressful situations.

Meditation is the process of cleansing the mind. There are many different styles and approaches to meditation. The extraordinary range and variety of techniques used in the Kundalini Yoga tradition contain specific, practical tools that carefully and precisely support the mind and guide the body through the use of breath, mantra, mudra and focus. It is precise, effective and practical.

Mantras stimulate 84 **meridian points** on the upper palate of the mouth, which systematically call different parts of the brain into action.

The words used in the mantras of Kundalini Yoga come from many traditions and can be in many languages. Some are in English. Many are from Punjabi or Sanskrit. Many are from the Sikh scriptures. If this makes you wonder whether chanting words you don't understand means you are chanting to some god you don't understand, Yogi Bhajan explained why this is not the case:

"You are chanting in your mind to evoke a state or to feel your own sacredness or soul.There is no concept at all of "chanting to someone". It is an energetic act that changes your brain, stimulates hormone balance, and engages you in a special conversation with your own mind about vastness and truth."[46]

Only when we sit quietly and turn our focus inwards can we appreciate just how much is going on in the mind at any one time. When we begin to meditate, any hope of quietening it can seem hopeless as we are constantly distracted by thought after thought. In Kundalini meditation there are always focus points to help; every time you notice your concentration has wandered, gently bring the attention back to the mantra, breathing practice or other points of focus the meditation uses. Don't fall into the trap of trying to evaluate your mental patterns; you may find some very unpleasant thoughts coming up! This is a cleansing process. Allow the meditation to do its job and absorb the negativity that has been holding you back.

THE FIRST 40 DAYS

Minimising stress during the first 40 days of a child's life is critical, according to the Kundalini Yoga

46 *The Mind: Its Projections and Multiple Facets* by Yogi Bhajan, Ph.D. (Kundalini Research Institute; 1998), p.145

teachings. Yogi Bhajan taught that during this period the mother's body goes through an incredible adjustment and it is vital that she nurtures herself during this time. Ideally, she would have an assistant, or *sevadar*, on hand throughout this period so she can relax and bond with the child. The Kundalini Research Institute advises during this time:

"The child is learning how to be at home on the Earth. If you are relaxed, contained and content, the child will be able to move forward in fearlessness and strength. Take care of you and keep the child in a serene environment so that the essential bonding of mother and child can be created. Many traumas in a child's life can be avoided if you make the time for this precious union now, in the first few weeks."[47]

LETTING GO

Becoming parents teaches us, if we haven't learned it already, that we don't have as much control as we might think we do. Our children are their own selves, regardless of what we might like them to be. As they grow up they are learning to survive without us and at some point will make their own way in the world. There may be other things we have to let go of while they are still young: having as much time to invest in our careers, for example, the freedom to go on holiday wherever we like, or those weekend lie-ins.

In Yoga we practise letting go every time we lie down in Corpse Pose. The name of the pose reminds us we cannot control everything; at some unknown moment, we will die. Every time we exhale, we let go.

AVOIDING OVERWHELM

The last two thousand years of human history are known as the Piscean Age in the Kundalini Yoga teachings. It was a period in which women were exploited dreadfully and knowledge was used by a self-serving elite to control the masses. The Piscean Age ended on 11th November 1999 with the start of the Age of Aquarius. We have already been through a period of transition that ended in 2012[48] and we are now, through the global availability of information, able to see just what has been going on in this world of ours. People who have committed terrible crimes, sexual crimes against children for example, are being unmasked. Politicians who have lied to the people who voted for them have been found out. There

---

47 *I Am A Woman*, p.136

48 *The Aquarian Teacher*, p.7

is still a lot to be uncovered but now we have the opportunity to make information accessible to everyone, information is indeed power.

The downside of the Internet and all our rapidly evolving technology is that we are in danger of being swamped. It is easy to be distracted by information every time we switch on our phones and tablets. The news is on 24 hours a day. And there are people who would like us to be distracted from looking too closely at some of the things big corporations and influential people are doing. We need to learn how to filter the information with which we are bombarded, not just so we can use the opportunity that accessible information gives us, but also to keep ourselves mentally and physically healthy.

In a lecture entitled *Consciousness in the* ***Aquarian Age***, Yogi Bhajan explained:

"Now, as we enter the Aquarian Age, previously unknown challenges such as viral epidemics and psychological and spiritual ailments beset us, with more on the way. Depression and fatigue-related psychological illnesses are at epidemic proportions and rising at accelerating rates… even the most competent, productive, and intelligent people have lost their sense of balance to the inescapable pressure of information overload, the lack of time, and increased social and personal demands… Electronic technology will only bring us more information, more choices, more contacts, and more complexity… We do not need more choices. We are flooded with choices. We need an elevated capacity to make choices. We do not need more information. We need the wisdom to use all the information."[49]

Top Tips for Quick Stress Relief:

- Have a glass of cold water. This re-sets the nervous system and calms the emotions;
- Check your posture: straighten your spine, lift your head up. Are you slouching? Are you frowning? Are your teeth clenched? Are there obvious areas of tension in your body, especially in your shoulders or neck? Shake your arms and legs if possible to shake out some tension;
- Place your left hand on the centre of your chest at your **Heart Centre**. The palm is flat

[49] Excerpted from *The Quantum Technology of the Shabd Guru*, by Yogi Bhajan and Gurucharan Singh Khalsa (*The Aquarian Teacher*, p.5)

against the chest, fingers parallel to the ground, pointing to the right. This creates a deep stillness at the natural home of your prana and induces a feeling of calmness;[50]

- Sit in Easy Pose with a straight spine or lie on the back and do some Long Deep Breathing for 3 minutes or until you feel calmer. As well as having an immediate calming effect, Long Deep Breathing regulates the body's pH (acid-alkaline) balance, which affects our ability to handle stressful situations;[51]

- Sit in Easy Pose with a straight spine. Block off your right nostril with the thumb of your right hand. Keep the other fingers straight up like antennae. Take twenty-six long, deep and complete breaths through the left nostril. Then inhale and relax. This will soothe you and bring you into a calm state.[52]

Yoga Set for Reducing Stress

Breathing Exercise

Eight-Stroke Breath for Energy and Stress Release[53]

Sit in Easy Pose with a straight spine, chin in and chest lifted. Close your eyes and concentrate on the breath. Inhale through the nose in eight equal strokes or parts. Exhale through the nose in one deep and powerful stroke. Continue for 11 minutes.

To end: inhale deeply, hold the breath for 5-10 seconds then exhale. Inhale deeply, hold the breath for 15-20 seconds and roll the shoulders backwards. Exhale powerfully. Inhale deeply, hold

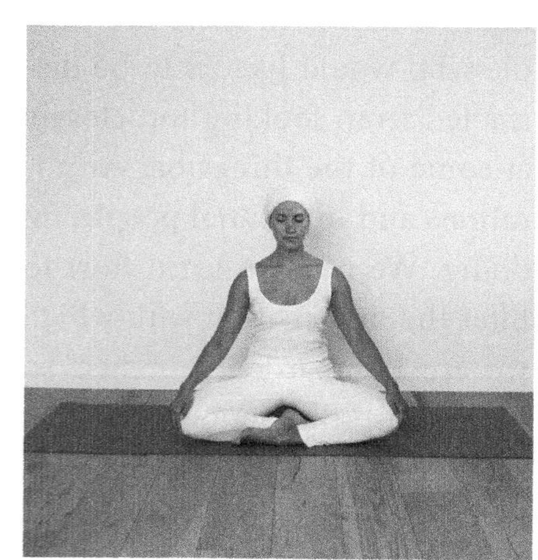

[50] *The Aquarian Teacher*, p.395

[51] *The Aquarian Teacher*, p.92

[52] *Praana Praanee Praanayam*, p.107

[53] *Praana Praanee Praanayam*, p.165. Originally taught by Yogi Bhajan on 8th August 1994

the breath for 15-20 seconds then roll your shoulders backwards as fast as you can. Exhale and relax.

"The eight strokes will make you watch and count the breath and that will force you to relate to your breath. Best procedure is that you do this exercise every evening. Eleven minutes a day of eight-stroke breathing can give you enough energy to balance your [daily] consumption of [praanic] life and take you out of stress. Is it possible? Do you have eleven minutes?"

~Yogi Bhajan

Kriya

STRESS SET FOR ADRENALS AND KIDNEYS[54]

Lotus Mudra: In Easy Pose, rub the palms together. Inhale and stretch the arms out to the sides, parallel to the ground, with palms facing out. Exhale and bring the hands together, hitting the bases together, fingers stretched in Lotus Mudra. Continue for 2 minutes. To end, inhale with palms together, exhale and relax.

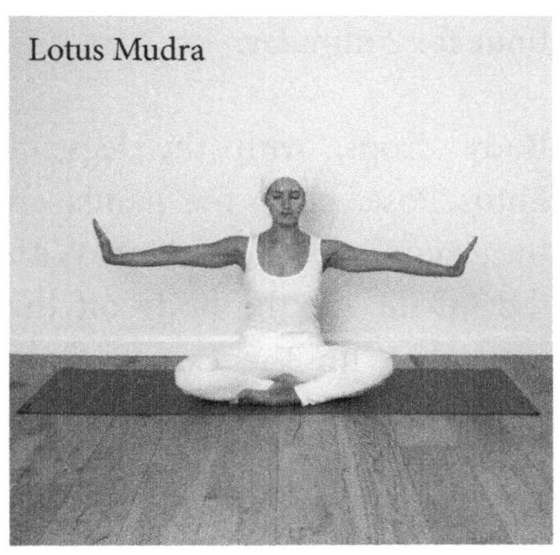

Lotus Mudra

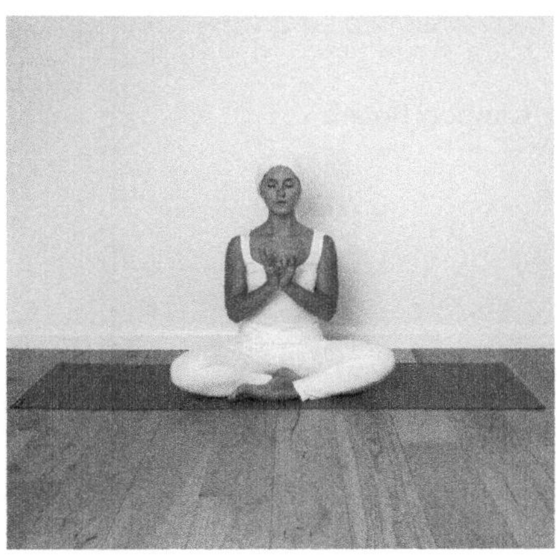

Link the little fingers in front of the Heart Centre, curling the other fingers into pads, with the thumbs sticking up. Lower the hands to the solar plexus. Pull on the little fingers and do Breath of Fire from below the navel. Feel a pull across the back. Continue for 2 minutes. Inhale, exhale and relax.

Cannon Breath: still in Easy Pose with a straight spine, begin Breath of Fire through an open mouth. Inhale and concentrate on the spine. Continue for 2 minutes.

[54] From *The Aquarian Teacher*, pp.350-351

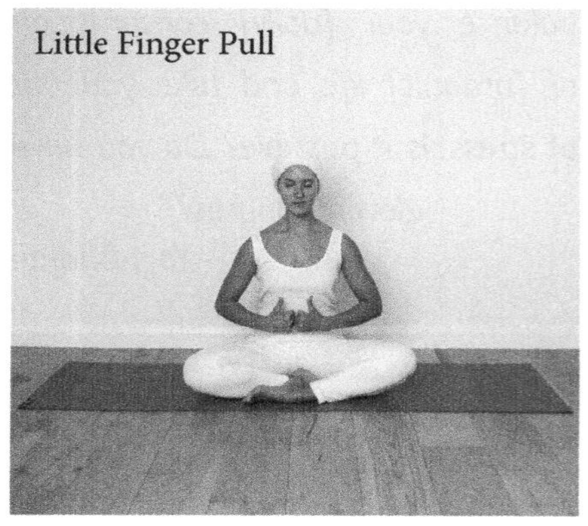
Little Finger Pull

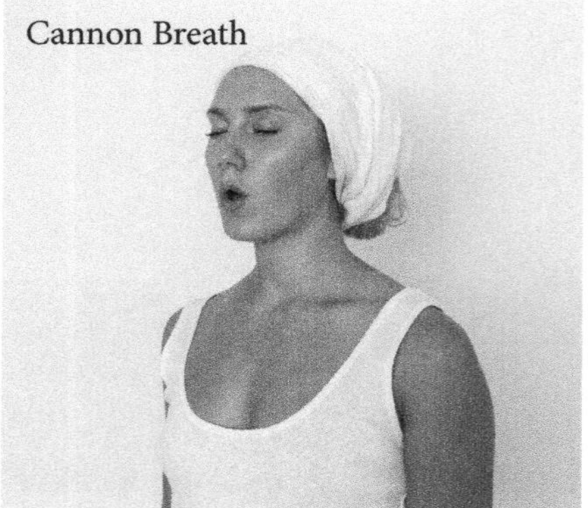
Cannon Breath

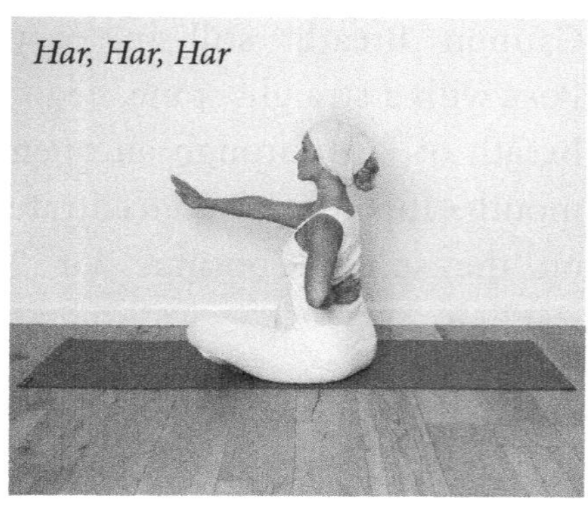
Har, Har, Har

In Easy Pose, place the left hand on the back at the bottom rib, with the palm facing out. The right arm is straight out in front with the palm forward and up at 60 degrees. Keeping the spine straight, stretch from the shoulder. With the eyes wide open, chant *Har, Har, Har* powerfully from the navel. Continue for 2 minutes.

Body drops: with the legs in Lotus Pose, place the hands on the ground next to the hips. With the inhale, lift the body off the ground. With the exhale, drop the body. Continue for 2 minutes.

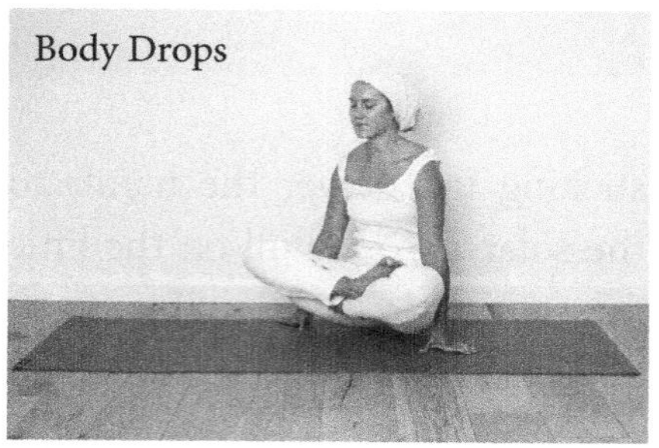
Body Drops

Author's suggestion: Alternatively the legs may be in Half-Lotus Pose. This is challenging; do your best and make sure you keep the back straight.

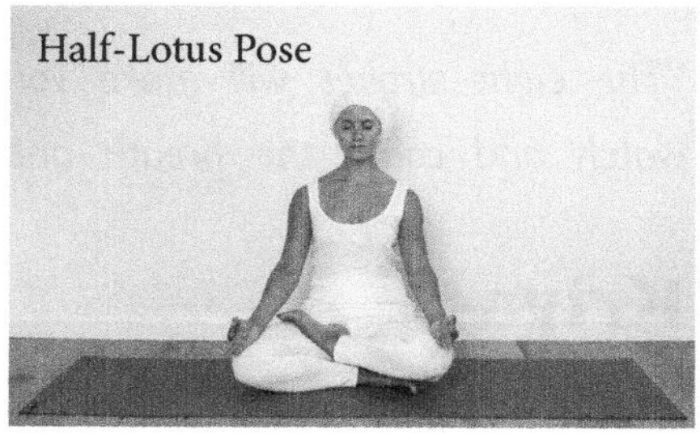
Half-Lotus Pose

In Easy Pose, place the hands in front of the solar plexus, left hand facing the body, right hand pressing the left wrist with the base of the palm. Look down with powerful, long deep breathing. The power of the breath is the depth to which you will cleanse. Continue for 2 minutes.

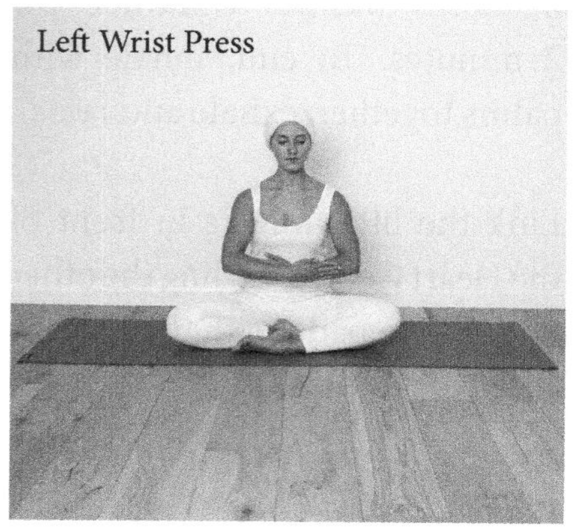
Left Wrist Press

Front Stretch with Spine Straight: sit with the legs stretched out in front, arms out parallel to the ground, hands in fists, thumbs pointing up. Inhale stretching forward, exhale leaning back. Keeping the arms parallel to the ground, breathe powerfully. Continue for 2 minutes. Inhale, exhale and relax.

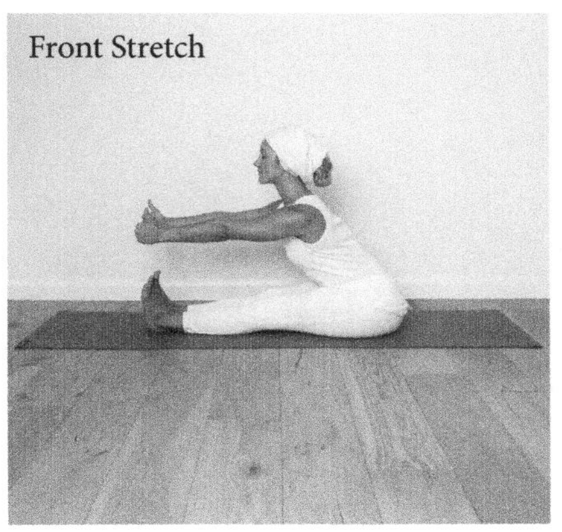
Front Stretch

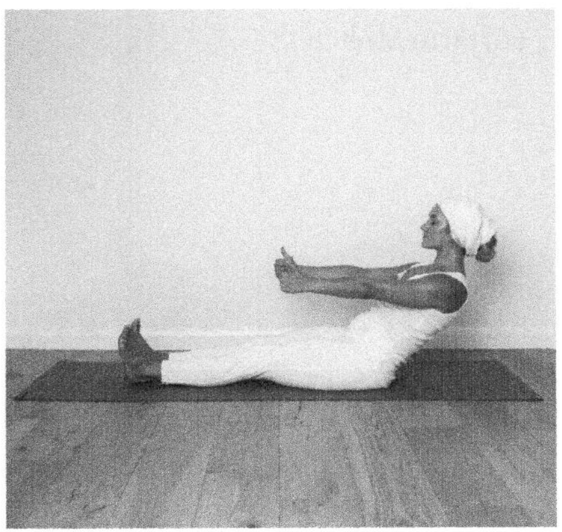

Pelvic Lift: lying on the back, bend the knees, bringing the soles of the feet flat onto the ground, heels at the buttocks. Hold the ankles. Inhale the pelvis up; exhale down. Continue for 2 minutes.

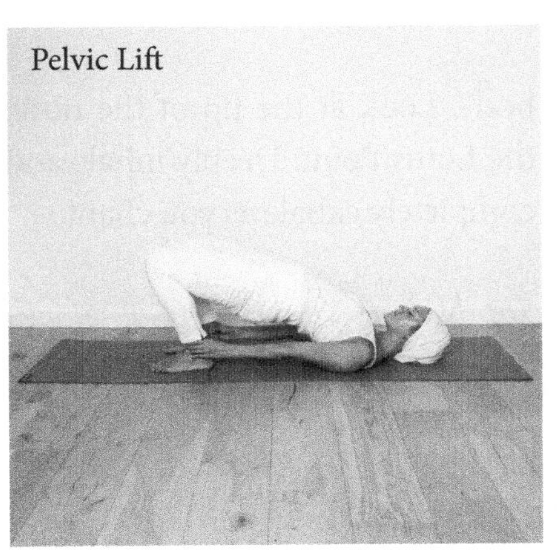
Pelvic Lift

Modified Cat-Cow: in Cat-Cow position, exhale as you bring the left knee to the forehead and inhale as you stretch the leg out and up behind. Caution: do not over-extend. Continue for 1 minute then switch legs for 1 more minute.

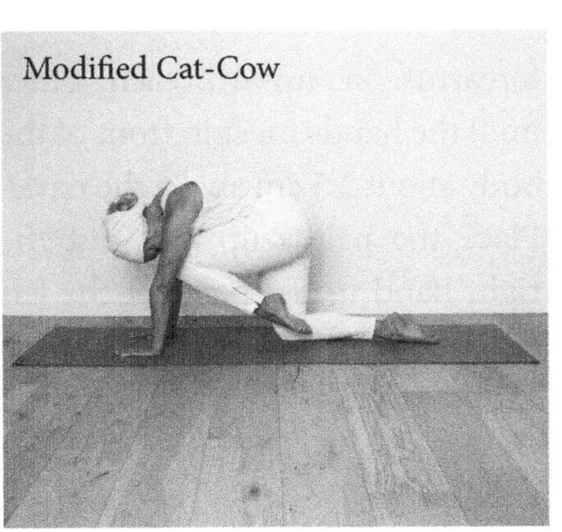
Modified Cat-Cow

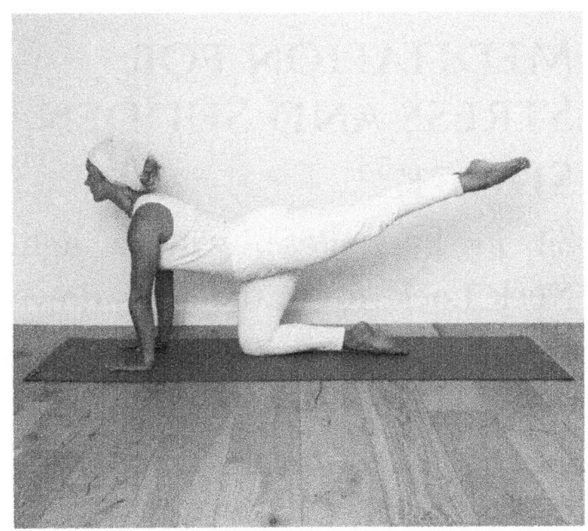

Sitting on the heels, bring the forearms to the ground in front of the knees, palms together, thumbs pointing up. Inhale as you stretch over the palms and exhale back. Keep the chin up to create pressure at the lower back. Continue for 2 minutes.

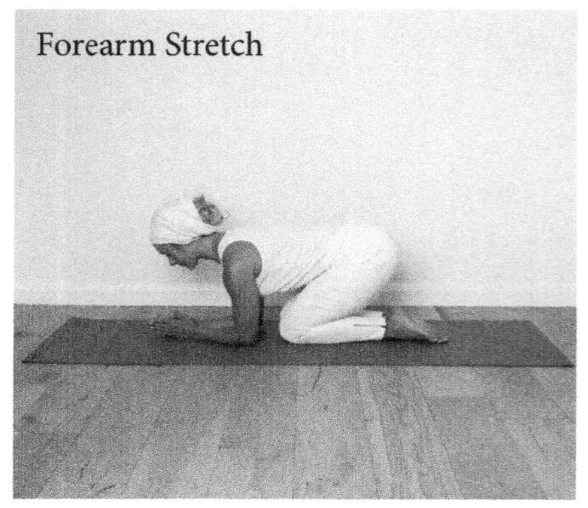
Forearm Stretch

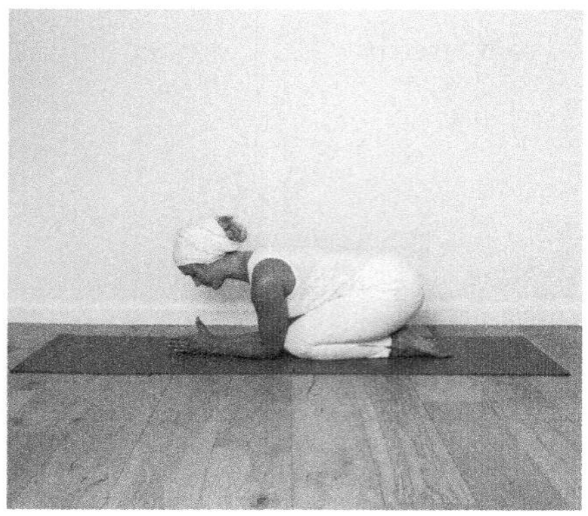

Back rolls: lie on the back, bring the knees to the chest, nose between the knees, breathing normally, and roll back and forth on the spine. Continue for 2 minutes.

Have a glass of water and totally relax in Corpse Pose for as long as possible.

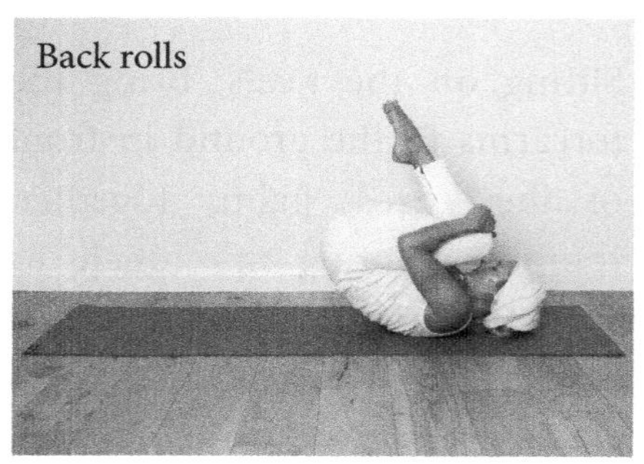
Back rolls

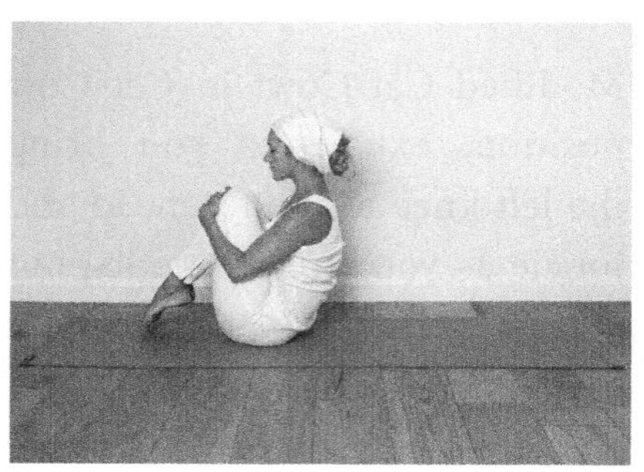

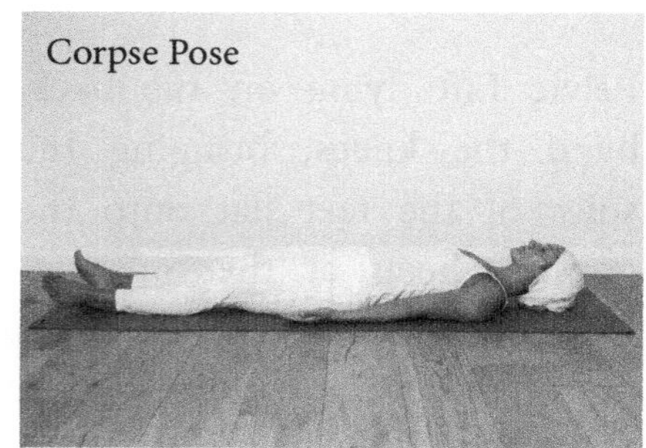
Corpse Pose

Meditation

MEDITATION FOR STRESS AND SUDDEN SHOCK[55]

Sit in Easy Pose, with a light **Neck Lock**. Relax the arms down with the elbows bent. Draw the forearms in toward each other until the hands meet in front of the body about 2.5 cm above the navel. Place the palms up and rest the right hand in the palm of the left hand. Place the thumbtips together and pull the thumbs toward the body. Look at the tip of the nose: the Lotus Point. Deeply inhale and completely exhale as you chant:

Sat Naam Sat Naam Sat Naam
Sat Naam Sat Naam Sat Naam
Wha-Hay Guroo

[55] The Library of Teachings

Chant the mantra 3 times. The entire mantra must be chanted on only one breath. Use the tip of the tongue to pronounce each word exactly and chant in a monotone. The rhythm must also be exact.

To end: inhale and completely exhale 5 times. Then deeply inhale, hold the breath and stretch the arms up over the head as high as possible. Stretch with all the strength you can muster. Exhale and relax down. Repeat twice.

Begin with 11 minutes. This meditation can be slowly built up to a maximum of 31 minutes.

This meditation balances the left hemisphere of the brain with the base of the right hemisphere. This enables the brain to maintain its equilibrium under stress or the weight of a sudden shock. It also keeps the nerves from being shattered under those circumstances.

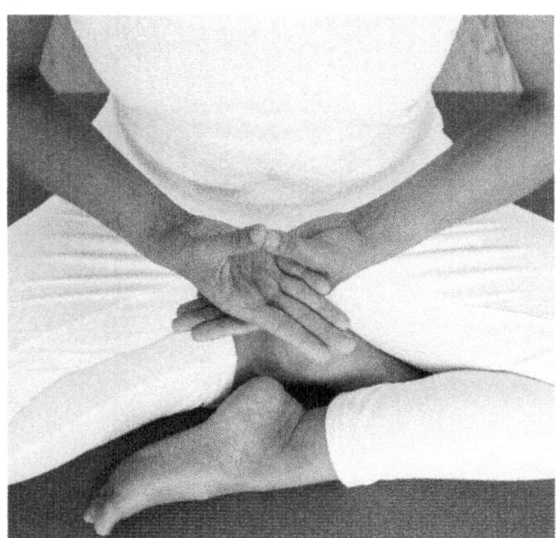

Chapter 6
Escaping the Shadow of Fear:
Freeing Yourself from Anxiety

"There are two forces which work in life – love and fear.

Love and fear are two sides of the same coin.

Therefore if you are afraid, remember, it's a moving force to be dealt with."

~ Yogi Bhajan[56]

The modern attitude to parenting is child-centred with the utmost importance now placed on keeping children safe. The advertising surrounding the massive baby-product market tells us our child could die if we don't buy the correct safety mattress or the correct car seat. The media reminds us about all the dreadful things that happen to children – from accidents to paedophiles – if we take our eye off them for a second. We are bombarded with articles about how to bring our children up correctly – and how doomed they are if we get it wrong. Buy a forward-facing buggy, for example, and your child could have such poor communication skills she could end up in prison.[57]

The arguments are conflicting. Apparently we should respond to a child's every need or he won't trust us – but if we don't encourage independence he will never be able to manage on his own. We should never let a baby cry – but if she doesn't sleep well it's our fault because we held her too much. Give older siblings lots of undivided attention – but don't forget to give the baby undivided attention at the same time. And don't give children too much attention or they will become too demanding! Keep children safe at all times – but don't forget they must take risks if they are to learn and grow!

---

56 *The 8 Human Talents*, p.99

57 Liz Attenborough of the Talk To Your Baby campaign in an article published in the *Guardian* on 22nd November 2008 (*Are modern buggies bad for babies?*) and quoted in *Shattered: Modern Motherhood and the Illusion of Equality* by Rebecca Asher

Being responsible for the safety and well-being of a very small, vulnerable person can be frightening enough but in such a fearful, critical world, surrounded by all these mixed messages, it is hardly surprising parents now seem to feel more anxious about their role than ever before.

There are lots of ways in which anxiety manifests itself. People may develop specific anxiety disorders such as Obsessive-Compulsive Disorder or phobias such as Agoraphobia (perceiving unfamiliar or wide-open spaces and places like shopping centres or bridges as uncomfortable or unsafe). Alternatively, they may feel anxious or worried all the time for no obvious reason, imagining all the worst things that could happen (Generalised Anxiety Disorder). They may suffer from health anxiety (for themselves or for a child) or panic disorder, suffering from panic attacks that come on suddenly and sometimes for no apparent reason.

Like all emotions, anxiety can serve a useful function. It is a safety mechanism and can save a life. It stimulates our "flight or fight" response – a natural and unavoidable reaction to a perceived threat. But when that perception is distorted and the person perceives the threat as worse than it actually is or underestimates their ability to deal with it, the anxiety is no longer appropriate. They may be tense, anxious and unhappy at a fairly constant level and eventually this will affect their health.

In an article entitled "Raising Successful Children",[58] clinician Madeline Levine argues parents must acknowledge their own anxiety if they are to help their child to thrive. "Overparenting" and, in particular, doing things for children that they are capable of doing for themselves, reduces their motivation and increases dependency. Levine refers to decades of psychological research in which it has been demonstrated that children thrive best in "an environment that is reliable, available, consistent and noninterfering". Levine argues parents who overprotect their children do so because of their own anxiety rather than because it is what is best for the child: "*Your child's job is to grow, yours is to control your anxiety so it doesn't get in the way of his reasonable moves toward autonomy.*"

Research also shows that parents with anxiety disorders tend to have children who develop

[58] Published in the *New York Times* on 4th August 2012

anxiety disorders. According to the NHS, you are estimated to be five times more likely to develop Generalised Anxiety Disorder if you have a close relative with the condition.[59]

Is this You?

- Do you regularly find yourself worrying about your child's health?
- Are you overly sensitive to criticism of your parenting? Do you dwell on it? Does the worry stay with you and, if anything, get worse?
- Do you suffer from a range of anxiety-provoking thoughts: are the children safe? Are they happy? How will we manage financially now we are down to one income? What if my partner loses his or her job? How will I manage the children on my own if I get ill or my partner leaves me? What will happen to the children if I die?
- Do you suffer from any of the following physical sensations: a sick feeling in your stomach like "butterflies", dizziness or a feeling you are going to fall, sweating or trembling, finding it difficult to breathe, finding it hard to swallow or to get your words out, panic attacks or a rapid heart rate that feels like a heart attack might be starting?
- Do you tend to pace around or feel you can't settle?
- Are you argumentative or short-tempered with others?
- Do you suffer from any of the following emotional patterns: feeling you are not good enough, dreading failure, foreseeing disaster, feeling vulnerable or unsafe, feeling responsible for others but never sure you can keep them safe enough, worrying you will let others down, worrying you will have a panic attack, feeling you are going to die or feeling things are unreal?
- Do you suffer from disturbed sleep (over and above any disturbances from the children)?
- Do you start finding fault in others for little reason? Or put people down to make yourself look good in comparison? Do you nag or blame other people unfairly? Do you regularly find fault with yourself? Or feel angry with yourself or even self-harm?
- Do you cry a lot?

[59] See the NHS website: http://www.nhs.uk/Conditions/Anxiety/Pages/Introduction.aspx

- Have you formed any unhealthy habits, or developed any strange fears, phobias or obsessions?

Reflection Points

- Can you identify which issues cause you the most anxiety?
- Are there any patterns you can identify? (For example, does the anxiety get worse when your children are at school or with someone other than yourself?)
- How does anxiety manifest in your body? Can you identify particular bodily sensations when it starts?
- Can you identify any specific methods you have developed for controlling your fears? For example, avoiding the thing that worries you, seeking repeated reassurance from friends or relatives, seeking reassurance from the medical profession over and over again for yourself or your children, developing safety behaviours such as checking on children repeatedly during the night, taking prescription drugs to keep calm, controlling something else such as having a particular and restricted way of eating or just eating lots and lots for comfort, or getting at someone else rather than focusing on the real cause of the anxiety?
- Can you identify any unhealthy forms of escapism you have developed as a way of avoiding or lessening anxiety? For example, drinking too much alcohol or going shopping and spending more than you can afford?
- Watch your mind as often as you can (see below). Do you notice any particular patterns of thought that tend to increase your anxiety?

Yogic Viewpoint: Watching our Thoughts

When we sit in meditation for the first time it is normal to find it difficult to concentrate; we notice our mind is wandering all over the place. When we commit to holding our arms in the air for a few minutes, as we do regularly in Kundalini Yoga, our thoughts are very hard to avoid! During our practice we can start to train ourselves to focus on the task in hand and to disregard the thoughts that don't serve us in that moment. This gives us the ability to become aware of our thoughts when we are off the mat too, busy with our daily lives.

It is a skill well worth the practice it takes to develop. We soon become aware the mind works like a muscle: it develops short cuts and repeats patterns so we don't have to re-think everything every time. Yogi Bhajan described the mind as the map we use on our journey through life. Sometimes these short cuts save us time and are useful, but often they are not. An anxious response might appear as if from nowhere: a pattern the mind has learned from previous experience.

The Negative Mind

According to the Kundalini Yoga teachings, every thought we have is filtered through three **Functional Minds** – the **Negative Mind**, the **Positive Mind** and the Neutral Mind.[60] Each has its own characteristics and each can be stronger or weaker depending upon the individual. In the enlightened mind all three are strong and in balance. The enlightened mind is flexible, creative and able to reflect the uniqueness of the soul.

The Negative Mind is the fastest to act and keeps us safe. It is what gives us the ability to determine whether there is danger in a particular situation. If we see a friend on the opposite side of the road, the Negative Mind reminds us to stop and look for cars before running across to greet them. But if it becomes too strong and out of balance with the Positive and Neutral Minds we lose our sense of perspective and worry about everything.

The Negative Mind is mastered with what are known in the Yogic tradition as **yamas** and **niyamas**. These are defined in **Patanjali**'s Eight Limbs of Yoga Practice, compiled between 200 and 600CE and describing the foundations upon which the philosophy of Yoga is based. The yamas are the qualities to which the Yogi should aspire in his or her external interactions: *ahimsa* (avoiding anything which causes harm to oneself or others), *satya* (truthfulness, forgiveness, letting go of masks), *asteya* (non-stealing, using resources properly, letting go of jealousy), *brachmacharya* (sensory control, channelling emotions and moderation) and *aparigraha* (non-possessiveness, fulfilling needs rather than wants).

The niyamas are the disciplines which the Yogi should observe: *shaucha* (purity of body, evenness of mind, thought and speech), *santosha* (contentment, acceptance), *tapas* (purification, determination), *svadhyaya* (study, meditation, reflection) and *ishvara pranidhana* (faith).

This may seem a long list of things to do in order to defeat anxiety!

60 *The Mind: Its Projections and Multiple Facets*, p.112

Mastering the yamas and the niyamas is indeed challenging and may involve reviewing many aspects of our lives, but there are many techniques in Kundalini Yoga that can help. Long Deep Breathing, for example, helps us with managing our emotions which in turn helps us to practise brachmacharya.

ANXIETY AND THE CHAKRAS

Anxiety is a sign of difficulties with several of the chakras. At our most earthly and basic level, feeling fearful is a sign we are insecure and our Root Chakra is not functioning well. We do not feel confident we have everything in place that we need to survive. At our most spiritual level, if our Crown Chakra is blocked or out of balance we may fear death and being separated from our children. Many mums worry about how their children would manage without them. Sitting in the middle between the upper and lower chakras is the Heart Chakra. When this is blocked or out of balance, we can experience fear and attachment.[61]

INTUITION

Anxiety also thrives when we do not trust our ability to make good decisions. Psychiatrist and mother of four Ann Dally has argued we need to learn to rely on our intuition more. The current generation of mothers who, she says, "buy baby books and magazines galore, thrive on the whole idea of techniques of baby and child care and are always searching for advice from outside rather than for their own feelings and intuition". This, she argues, only serves to make women feel more isolated and unsure of themselves, leading ultimately to increased anxiety and guilt.[62]

We have been conditioned to look outside of ourselves for the answers to our problems and it is easy for us to forget the inner resources we have. Yogi Bhajan taught that a woman's biological, physiological, sociological and mental capacity, which includes her powers of intuition, is 16 times greater than a man's, provided we explore it.[63]

We may become more aware of our intuition once we become mothers; we realise we know things about our own children, and they know things about us, that cannot be explained in any logical way. Developing faith in this intuitive bond reduces our susceptibility to anxiety. We don't always need to read lots of conflicting advice from "experts"; if we pay attention

---

61 *The Aquarian Teacher*, p.185-586

62 *The Mask of Motherhood*, p.34

63 *I Am a Woman*, p.72

to our hunches instead we may find we already know what is best for our children.

Developing our powers of intuition, particularly with practices that stimulate the **pituitary gland** by slowing down the breath (such as the One Minute Breath and the Meditation for Emotional Balance below), takes practice. But it opens us up to an internal guidance system with the capacity to serve us on a daily basis throughout our lives.

Top Tips for Defeating Anxiety

- Have a glass of cold water. A water imbalance in the system puts the kidneys under pressure and can cause worry and upset;[64]
- Eat celery, which soothes the nervous system and calms the nerves;[65]
- Avoid caffeine (tea, coffee, fizzy and "energy" drinks) which increases anxiety;[66]
- Avoid drinking alcohol and smoking, both of which have been shown to make feelings of anxiety worse;[67]
- Use Long Deep Breathing as often as possible. It influences the parasympathetic nervous system to produce an instant calming effect. Practised regularly, it gives the capacity to manage negativity and emotions, supporting clarity, cool-headedness and patience;[68]
- Regular exercise reduces tension. To help fight anxiety, the NHS recommends 150 minutes a week of exercise that increases your heart rate and makes you breathe faster.[69] Swimming, cycling, running or fast walking are all excellent forms of aerobic exercise. If you can't get out of the house, the Har Aerobic Kriya in Chapter 13 is a great alternative;
- Learn to relax (see Chapter 3).[70]

---

64 *The Aquarian Teacher*, p.399

65 *The Aquarian Teacher*, p.255

66 See the NHS website: http://www.nhs.uk/Conditions/Anxiety/Pages/self-help.aspx

67 See the NHS website: http://www.nhs.uk/Conditions/Anxiety/Pages/self-help.aspx

68 *The Aquarian Teacher*, p.92

69 See the NHS website: http://www.nhs.uk/Conditions/Anxiety/Pages/self-help.aspx

70 See the NHS website: http://www.nhs.uk/Conditions/Anxiety/Pages/self-help.aspx

Yoga Set for Reducing Anxiety

Breathing Exercise

ONE MINUTE BREATH

Sit in Easy Pose with the spine straight, chin in and chest lifted. Start by inhaling slowly for 10 seconds, holding the breath in for 10 seconds, and exhaling slowly for 10 seconds. Gradually build up the times (keeping them equal to each other) until the entire breath cycle takes one full minute. Continue for 5 minutes.

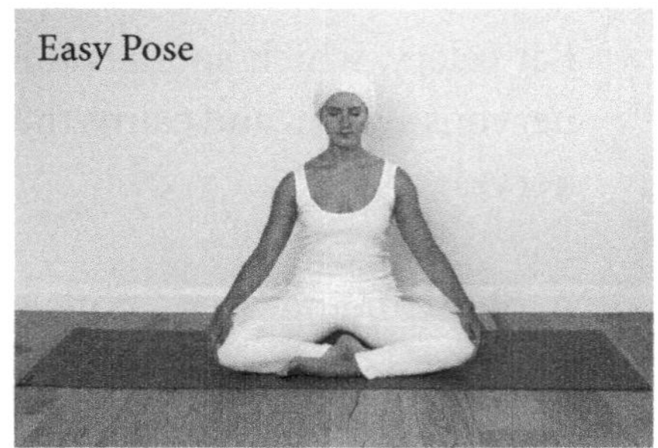

Easy Pose

Caution: it can be tempting when we hold the breath in to hold lots of tension in the body. Holding the neck and throat muscles tightly for more than 10 seconds can be dangerous. Instead, focus on *suspending* the breath by relaxing the muscles of the diaphragm, ribs and abdomen that are responsible for the constant motion of the breath.[71]

Once mastered, the One Minute Breath is a fantastic way to dramatically reduce anxiety, fear and worry.

Kriya

HEALTHY BOWEL SYSTEM[72]

Windmills: stand with the legs slightly wider than shoulder width apart. The arms are out to the sides, parallel to the ground and with the palms facing down.

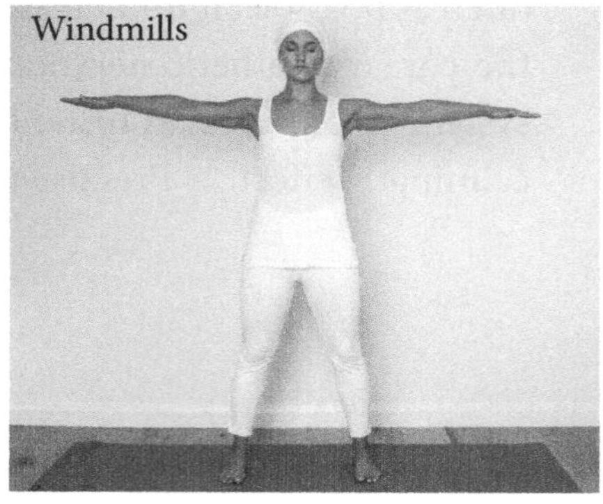

Windmills

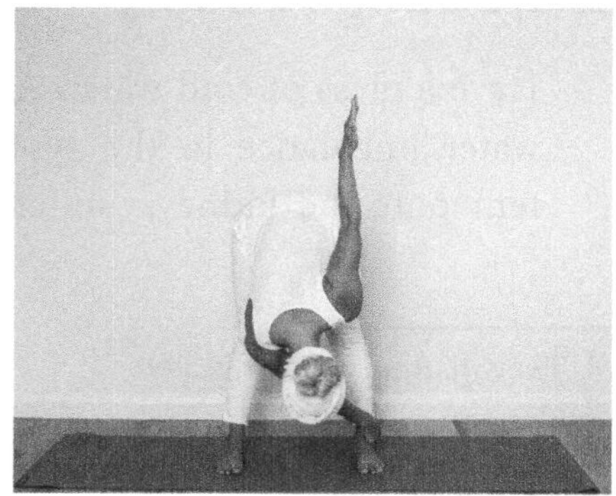

[71] *The Aquarian Teacher*, p.93

[72] *The Aquarian Teacher*, p.359. First taught by Yogi Bhajan on 4th July 1977

Exhale, bend from the hips and twist towards the left, bringing the right hand towards the left foot. The left arm rises up behind the body. Inhale and return to the starting position. Continue for 1 minute, in a rhythm of about 10 seconds per cycle. Then switch to the opposite hand and foot and repeat for 1 minute.

Continue the same motion but alternating sides and pausing for 5 seconds as the hand touches the foot. Continue for 3 minutes.

Continue the same alternating motion, but pause for 25 seconds as the hand touches the foot. Continue for 2 minutes.

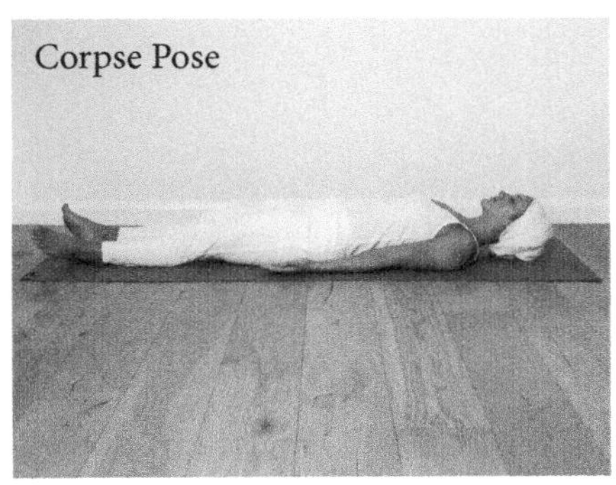
Corpse Pose

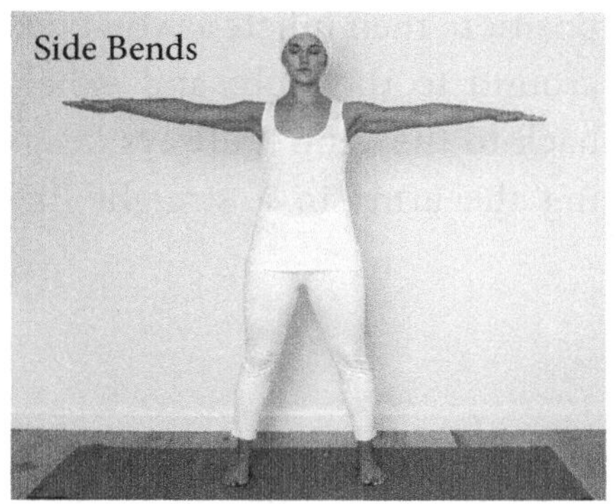
Side Bends

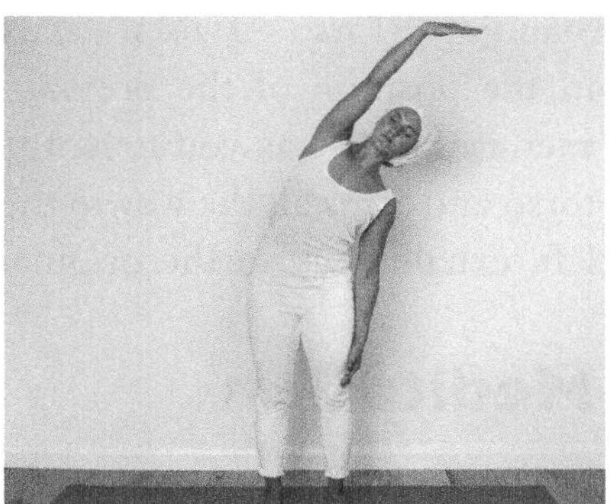

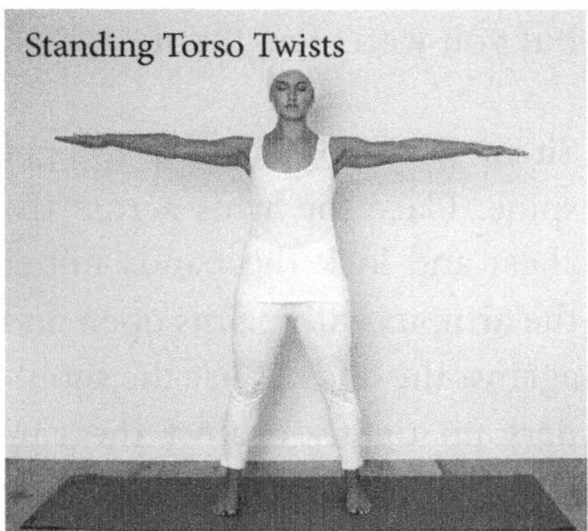
Standing Torso Twists

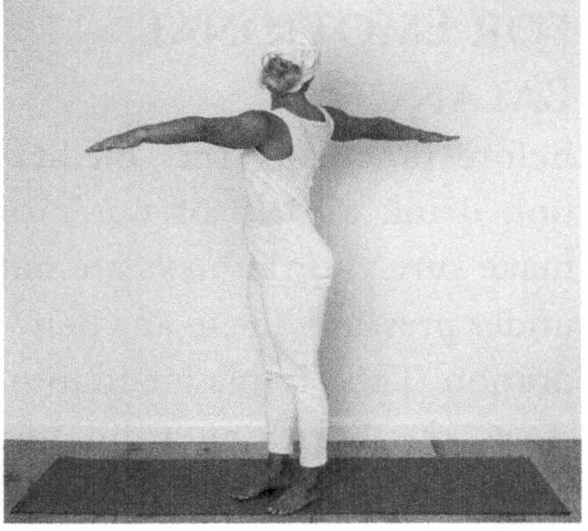

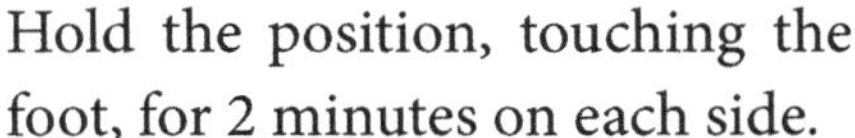

Hold the position, touching the foot, for 2 minutes on each side.

Relax on the back in Corpse Pose for 2-3 minutes.

Side Bends: stand with legs wide, arms parallel to the floor and palms down. Inhale and bend to the side from the waist, letting the left arm come down the left side as the right arm comes up. Keep the spine vertical. Exhale and come back to the original position, inhale as you stretch down the right side and exhale as you return to the original position. The movement should take 6 seconds per side. Continue for 1 minute.

Standing Torso Twists: start in the position of the previous exercise. Inhale as you twist the torso and arms all the way to the left, exhale back to the original position, then inhale as you twist around to the right and exhale back to the centre, always keeping the arms in a straight line with each other. Each complete cycle should take 2-3 seconds.

Relax for 10 minutes.

Meditation

Meditation for Emotional Balance[73]

Before practising this meditation drink a glass of water to make sure your kidneys are not under pressure due to any dehydration. This simple meditation slows the breathing from our usual rate of around 15 breaths a minute to 4 breaths a minute. This promotes a calm mind; your thoughts will still be there but you won't feel them.

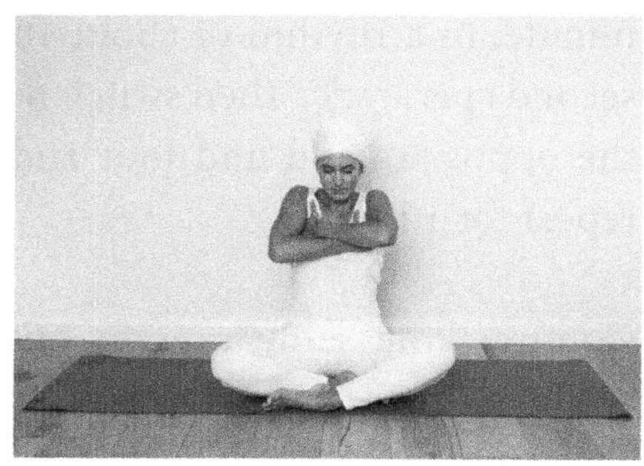

Sit in Easy Pose with a straight spine. Place the arms across the chest and lock the hands under the armpits with palms open and against the body. Raise the shoulders up tightly against the earlobes without cramping the neck muscles. Make sure the neck is not forward but in line with the spine. Close the eyes. The breath will automatically become slow.

Sit in this position for 3 minutes. With practice, you can gradually increase the time to 11 minutes.

[73] *The Aquarian Teacher*, p.399

Chapter 7
Clearing the Clouds of the Past:
Saying Goodbye to Guilt

"Feelings of guilt close us down and drive us deeper into dark patterns, making it very difficult to see the reality of a situation."

~ Yogi Bhajan[74]

Guilt is an emotion that almost goes hand-in-hand with being a mum. Here are just some of the issues about which women who responded to my recent survey (see Chapter 1), all of whom wished to remain anonymous, felt guilty:

"when I don't want to spend time playing with my daughter, as I chose not to go back to work and stay at home with her instead"

"if I'm spending time at home doing 'work' rather than 'being' with my children"

"for shouting and needing time to myself"

"about having a lower sex drive, particularly whilst breastfeeding at night"

"when my son is upset at nursery drop off (even though I know he loves it there)"

Getting the work/home balance right is a common source of guilt for modern women, fuelled by the constant barrage of social and media pressure about what is "right" for children, and the expectation that we should all want to be super-parents. Women who work part-time are constantly trying to fit everything in and may feel guilty that they don't spend enough quality time with their children. Women who work full-time may feel guilty about not spending enough time with their children full stop. Women who don't work may feel guilty they don't enjoy being at home with children as much as they anticipated, or they are not supporting the family financially, or they are not very good at their new role.

[74] *The Aquarian Teacher*, p.229

Like all emotional responses there is a reason why we experience guilt. It warns us we are compromising our core values. It is born of inner conflict about what we believe we should, or should not, have done. It is closely related to the concept of remorse and is often associated with anxiety. Psychopaths typically don't experience guilt or remorse about things they have done that have hurt other people but blame others or rationalize or even deny their actions.

Guilt is therefore an emotion that enables us (the non-psychopaths, at least) to judge whether something we are contemplating doing, or not doing, is acceptable. But the difficulty with many parenting decisions is we often do have to compromise our core values because we have so many different roles: as parents trying to raise healthy, happy and well-balanced children, as workers bringing money to the home, as professional people with obligations towards our clients, as homemakers trying to keep our homes running smoothly, as partners, as relatives to others (our own parents or siblings, for example), as neighbours, as friends. Once we have children (especially if we have more than one) we just can't do everything required to keep everyone happy. So our core values are inevitably compromised.

Like anxiety, guilt makes people unhappy and ill, impacting negatively on their children and other people around them.

Guilt serves a useful short-term purpose, a warning sign when something is wrong, but hanging on to it serves no purpose and can wear us down. It may be we have no choice but to return to work when we don't think it's the right thing for us or our children. But if we have to work in order to pay our mortgage then we have to work – it's no good staying at home with children if that means living on the streets with them. Yoga teaches us to accept the things we cannot change; this is the niyama known as *santosha* (see Chapter 6). Being compassionate towards ourselves by putting aside guilt that causes us suffering is an application of the principle of *ahmisa*.

It may be helpful to consider where the core value that is causing us such pain originated. Guilt is often the result of beliefs we hold of which we may not even be aware. For example, we may remember (possibly subconsciously) our own mother saying women should not go out to work if they have young children and that will have laid some kind of root in our psyche. We may not believe it in our conscious mind and we may have read every bit of research in existence demonstrating it isn't true, but it may still have created a negative thought pattern that throws up pangs of guilt every time we drop our child off at nursery. Releasing subconscious negative thought patterns is essential to relieving us of the layers of guilt we can find ourselves being pulled down by. Regular meditation (see Chapter 5) is an excellent way of releasing these thought patterns.

Psychotherapist and psychoanalyst Barbara Almond MD, author of *The Monster Within*, explains just how damaging maternal guilt can be:

"[T]he guilt produced by the pressure on women to be all-loving and all-giving towards their children takes a powerful toll on both mothers and their children… [Women] feel angry and disappointed in themselves and, in turn, angry and disappointed with their children. Anger and disappointment make them feel even guiltier, so they try harder and harder. It is a repetitive and exhausting cycle."[75]

[75] *The Monster Within*, p.11

Is this You?

- Do you feel guilty about things you can't do anything about? Do you dwell on past events, regretting decisions you made at the time?
- Do you find yourself mentally reciting negative thoughts such as "*It's all your fault. If only you were a better parent*" or "*That wouldn't have happened if you had been paying more attention*";
- Do you feel guilty about things that seem illogical if you step back and look at them objectively, like the mum who feels guilty about leaving her son at nursery when she knows he loves it there? If you find it hard to consider the situation objectively, imagine what you might advise a friend who tells you they felt guilty about the same thing;
- What core values do you hold about raising children? How might your own upbringing have affected these?
- Do you tend to suffer from anxiety?

Reflection Points

- Can you identify your core values in relation to parenting? How might your own upbringing have affected these? What did your parents tell you?
- Spend a few minutes thinking about the different roles you have. How do these overlap? How might they conflict with each other?
- What are the main triggers for your feelings of guilt?

- Are there any triggers you can change?
- If there is a trigger you can't change, is there a more positive framework you can find for it?

A positive mantra may help. For example, "*Every challenge I face is an opportunity to learn and grow. I always try to do my best for my family and if I slip up, I learn from my mistakes.*"

- Keep a note of any times in the month in which you feel particularly guilty, in case there is a link with your menstrual cycle (see Chapter 10).

Yogic Viewpoint: Watching the Mind

In the previous chapter we looked at the patterns the mind creates for us and how this can lead to anxiety. Guilt is another emotion which is tied up with thoughts about the past. Once we are used to watching the mind, it can be revealing to notice how often we lay the guilt on ourselves. "*Why did I do X?*" "*Why didn't I say something about Y?*" "*I can't believe I forgot Z!*" Yogi Bhajan called it "the game of self-belittlement".[76]

THE TEN BODIES

We have already looked at the Negative Mind and what happens when it is out of balance (see Chapter 6). As well as being one of the Functional Minds, the Negative Mind is also one of the **Ten Bodies**. We tend to think of ourselves as having one body, a physical one, but according to Yogi Bhajan we have ten: a **Soul Body**, the Negative Mind, the Positive Mind, the Neutral Mind, the Physical Body, the **Arcline**, the Aura, a **Pranic Body**, a **Subtle Body** and a **Radiant Body**. These Ten Bodies are powerful capacities of the psyche. It may seem challenging enough to have just one body to look after, so an extra nine may feel daunting! Fortunately, practising Kundalini Yoga regularly is a comprehensive way to work on all ten at the same time.

"If you understand that you are these Ten Bodies, and you are aware of those Ten Bodies, and you keep them in balance, the whole universe will be in balance with you."
~ Yogi Bhajan[77]

THE NEUTRAL MIND

One of these Ten Bodies is the Neutral Mind, which enables us to assess a situation objectively. If it is well balanced, we can

[76] *The Aquarian Teacher*, p.19

[77] *The Aquarian Teacher*, p.203

consider the dangers to which the Negative Mind is alerting us together with the opportunities spotted by the Positive Mind (see Chapter 8) and evaluate what our response should be in any particular situation.

The Neutral Mind is also known as the meditative mind and meditation is the key to balancing it. With the mind clear we can see the truth without being blinded by guilt.

The Sacral Chakra

According to Kundalini Yoga teachings, guilt is sometimes associated with poor functioning of the Sacral Chakra. This is the second of the major chakras, located in the sex organs. It is the chakra that governs our creativity, so feeding your creativity is an effective way of defeating guilt. This doesn't necessarily mean being an accomplished artist, but it does mean making time to do things you love, things that absorb you and lead you into a state of flow.

There are lots of ways of exploring our creativity when we have young children: colouring, painting, tracing... Even my little boys, who can barely sit still for long enough to eat a sandwich and have the joint attention span of a baby gnat, have always loved to scribble, make pictures with fuzzy felt and stickers, paint with stencils and build things with blocks. Some of our happiest moments when they were really young were when we were all absorbed in being creative together – little Jack scribbling with his crayons, Ben working on a Colour by Numbers picture, and me doing one of my colouring books for adults!

Living a creative life also means being imaginative in the way we think and the way we approach life. The times when I have felt I have helped my children the most have been when I have encouraged them to look at a problem in a different way and to think of an alternative way to deal with it. This gives them a new perspective and reminds them there is always a way through, even if it is not the way they initially anticipated.

"There is a way through every block"
~ one of Yogi Bhajan's 5 **Sutras**
for the Aquarian Age[78]

Being Present

Mindfulness is an important principle in Yoga; we practise being present, rather than dwelling on the past or the future. We learn to control our minds so they cannot keep going back over what has happened before; to free us to concentrate on where we are now and the roots we are putting down for the

[78] *The Aquarian Teacher*, p.6

future. This includes letting go of the past where the causes of our guilt lie. We cannot go back and change what happened or what we did, said or thought. Any decisions we made may look like the wrong ones with the benefit of hindsight. But if we genuinely practise *ahimsa* and take a compassionate look at those decisions, we can see they were the best ones we were able to make at the time. The only purpose the past serves is as a teacher; we can learn from the mistakes we made before and with every breath we have the opportunity to make a new start.

Top Tips to Eliminate Guilt

- Do a few Frogs (see pages 42-43) every day to stimulate the Sacral Chakra;
- To develop the Neutral Mind, put aside a few minutes every day for meditation;
- Create your own positive mantra and say it to yourself as often as possible. For example: "*by working, I am providing my children and myself with financial security. I have made the best decision for myself and my family*" or "*by being at home with my children I am giving my children as much time as I can. I have made the best decision for myself and my family*";
- Put aside some time every week to do something creative you really enjoy, whether it's something you do with the children, or when they are asleep;
- Consider that Yogi Bhajan described guilt as the opposite of love and true responsibility: "*This is real caring, not out of fear, but out of love and interdependence. Fear vs Love. It is from this perspective that we act with integrity.*"[79]

Yoga Set for Eliminating Guilt

Breathing Exercise

LONG DEEP BREATHING

Lie on the back with the left hand on the abdomen and the right hand on the chest. Inhale by relaxing and filling the abdomen. The hand on the abdomen will rise towards the ceiling. Continue

[79] *The Aquarian Teacher*, p.229

to inhale into the ribcage so the ribs expand out to the sides. Then lift the upper ribs and collarbones and inhale into the shoulders and upper chest. The lungs should feel fully inflated. Exhale completely, allowing the upper chest to deflate first, then the middle chest, then finally pull the abdomen in and up as the Navel Point pulls back toward the spine. Continue for 3 minutes.

Amongst other things, Long Deep Breathing helps to break subconscious habit patterns such as insecurities and fears that can lead to feelings of guilt. It gives us the capacity to manage our emotional responses and helps to speed up emotional healing.

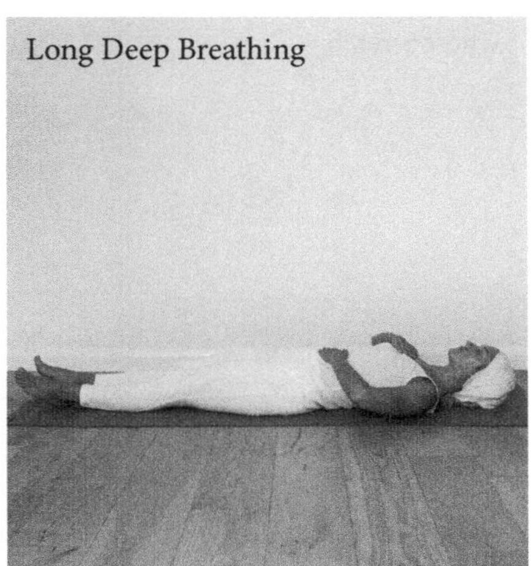
Long Deep Breathing

Kriya

Sat Kriya Workout[80]

Sat Kriya: sit on the heels with the arms overhead and the palms together. Interlace the fingers except for the index fingers, which point straight up. Men cross the right thumb over the left thumb, women cross the left thumb over the right. Begin rhythmically chanting *Sat Naam*, emphasising *Sat* as you pull the navel in. On *Naam*, relax the navel. Focus at

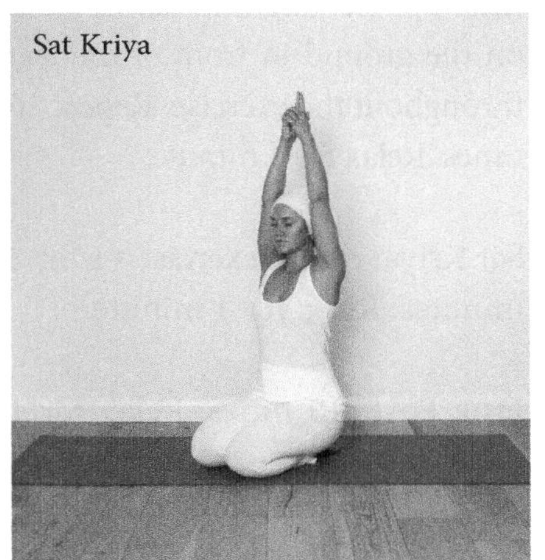
Sat Kriya

the Brow Point. Continue for 3 minutes. Then inhale, suspend the breath as long as you are able while applying the Root Lock and imagine your energy radiating from the Navel Point and circulating throughout the body. Relax for 5 minutes on your back.

Sat Kriya: repeat exercise #1.

Chest Stretch: sit in Easy Pose with a straight spine. Interlace the fingers and place the palms at the back of the neck. Spread the

[80] *The Aquarian Teacher*, p.379

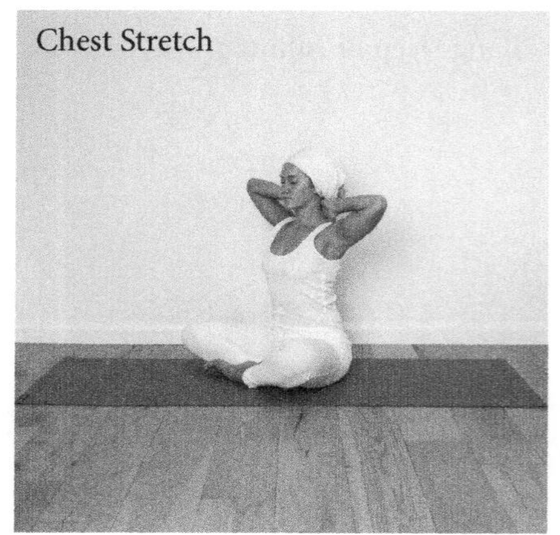
Chest Stretch

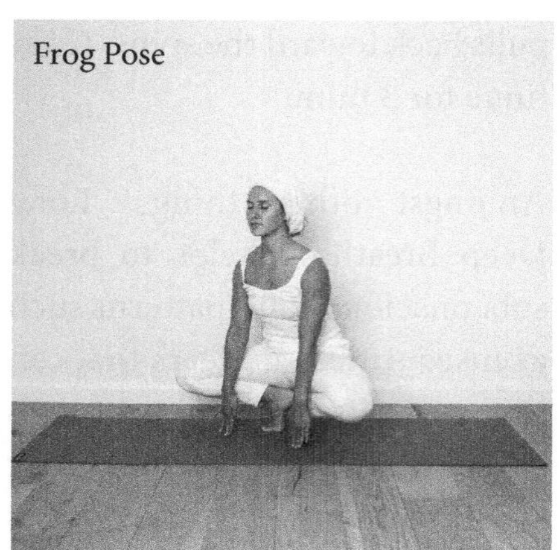
Frog Pose

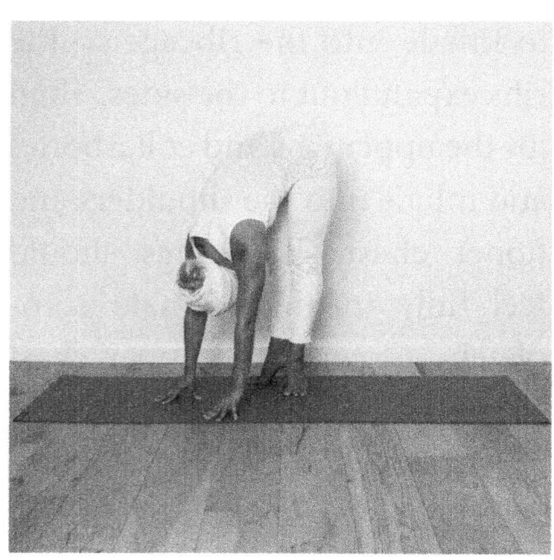

elbows open so they point away from the sides of the torso. Concentrate at the Brow Point. Begin long deep complete breaths. Continue for 3 minutes. Then inhale and hold the breath briefly. Exhale.

Sat Kriya: immediately repeat exercise #1 for 3 minutes. Relax for 2 minutes.

Frog Pose: stand up straight with the heels together. Squat down into the Frog Pose. Inhale as the buttocks go up and the head goes towards the knees. Exhale as you return to the squat position with the head up. The fingertips stay placed on the ground in front of the feet throughout the exercise. Repeat 26 times. Relax for 1 minute.

Sat Kriya: repeat exercise #1 for 3 minutes. Relax for 1 minute.

Frog Pose: 10 times. Relax for 1 minute.

Sat Kriya: repeat exercise #1 for 3 minutes. Relax for 1 minute.

Frog Pose: 15 times. Relax for 1 minute.

Sat Kriya: repeat exercise #1 for 3 minutes. Relax for 1 minute.

Frog Pose: 10 times. Relax for 1 minute.

Sat Kriya: repeat exercise #1 for 5 minutes. At the end inhale deeply and hold with the Root Lock engaged for 30 seconds. Then exhale completely and hold the breath out with the Root Lock engaged for as long as is comfortable. Repeat this breath-holding cycle 2 more times. Relax for 15 minutes.

Meditation

Meditation to Conquer Self-Animosity[81]

Sit in Easy Pose with a light Neck Lock. Maintain an alert attitude. Relax the arms at the sides and raise the forearms up and in towards the chest at the heart level. Draw the hands into fists and point the thumbs straight up toward the sky. Press the fists together in such a manner that the thumbs and fists are touching. The palms are toward each other. Hold the upper torso straight without rocking back and forth. Fix the eyes at the tip of the nose.

Breath pattern:

> Inhale through the nose;
>
> Exhale completely through the mouth;
>
> Inhale deeply and smoothly through the mouth;
>
> Exhale through the nose.

Continue for 3 minutes. The time can be gradually built up to 11 minutes.

To end: inhale and stretch the arms up over the head. Keep the stretched position as you take 3 more deep breaths. Relax.

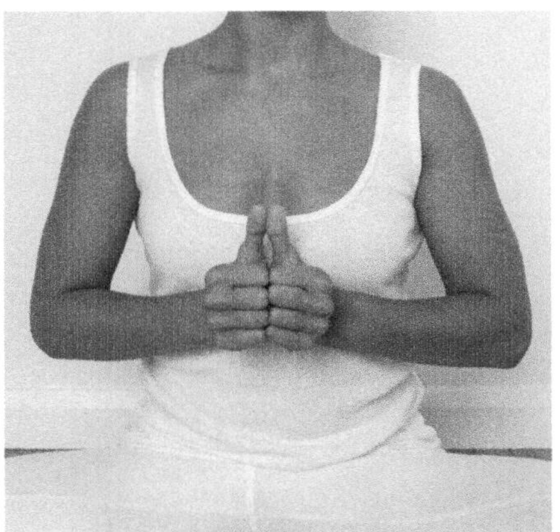

[81] *The Aquarian Teacher*, p.397

Chapter 8
From Darkness to Light:
Fighting Depression

"Without control of those many facets [of the mind], the undirected mind will create depressions, delusions, identity splits, and a deep core feeling of emptiness."
~ Yogi Bhajan[82]

"In this changing world, humans are being eaten inside by deep depression. It is an urgent need of the time to reverse this process."
~ Yogi Bhajan[83]

Once you become a parent you significantly increase your risk of depression throughout the remainder of your life. This was the (somewhat depressing) conclusion drawn by Florida State University professor Robin Simon and Vanderbilt University's Ranae Evenson in a recent parenting stress study.[84] They found parents have significantly higher levels of depression than adults who do not have children, both mothers and fathers are equally affected (which contradicted previous indications that parenthood affects women more) and the effects are lifelong. The researchers believe this is not because parents don't find any pleasure in their roles, but because they have more to worry about than non-parents, so the emotional toll of parenting can be very high.

It is important to note the term "depression" is often used informally in relation to a particular emotional state (see my example in the first line of this chapter), but what I am actually referring to in this chapter is depression as a medical condition.

---

82 *The Mind: Its Projections and Multiple Facets*, p.9

83 Foreword to *The 8 Human Talents*, p.ix

84 Evenson RJ, Simon RW, "Clarifying the Relationship Between Parenthood and Depression" in *Journal of Health and Social Behaviour*, December 2005

Having children is one of the biggest life changes and although it is something people often choose and do regard as positive in itself, there can nevertheless be many associated losses, especially for women. We are a generation accustomed to being out in the world, socialising, travelling and interacting with other adults all the time. Yet we parent in probably the most isolated way in human history; we are virtually trapped in our homes with a young baby and, as childcare is no longer shared by the community and extended family, we are emotionally and intellectually isolated by being removed from company with other adults. After being brought up to believe we had the career opportunities and the potential for financial independence previous generations of women had never had, we suddenly find those opportunities compromised when we become mothers.

Two types of depression are linked specifically with pregnancy and childbirth. According to Dr Vivette Glover, Director of the Fetal and Neonatal Stress and Research Centre, one in every ten pregnant women will suffer from Antenatal Depression (AND) and around one in every thirty will be depressed in both the antenatal and postnatal period.[85] AND is commonly associated with guilt and anxiety, for example about whether you will be able to cope with the demands of parenting. Postnatal Depression (PND), which can start at any time in the first year after the birth, is known to affect 10-15 per cent[86] of new mothers but the true figure is estimated to be much higher. It commonly includes a sense of feeling guilty about not coping with the demands of a baby, or about not loving the baby enough, being hostile or indifferent to the baby or your partner, having panic attacks, experiencing an overpowering anxiety (often about things that wouldn't normally bother you such as being alone in the house) and experiencing obsessive fears about the baby's health or well-being, or about yourself and other members of the family.

Looking after young children is very challenging for someone suffering from depression. They may become even more socially isolated, not asking for help or support, and distancing themselves from others. Going out for a walk with the baby in the pram may seem like a tremendous effort.

[85] PANDAS website: http://www.pandasfoundation.org.uk/help-and-information/pre-ante-and-postnatal-illnesses/pre-antenatal-depression.html#.VhO8ocuFPIU

[86] Mind: www.mind.org.uk

They may suffer from disturbed sleep, on top of being sleep-deprived because of the children. They may feel helpless and lack self-confidence and self-esteem, which impacts on their parenting decisions.

Depression is also a very dangerous condition. The person may experience a sense of unreality, self-harm, or even become suicidal. Suicide is still a leading cause of death amongst new mothers; according to the latest Saving Mothers' Lives report,[87] 29 of the 261 maternal deaths (i.e. during pregnancy or within the following six months) that occurred in the UK between 2006 and 2008 were suicides. The report highlights that all mothers are at risk regardless of their age, ethnicity, financial, employment and marital status. Contributing factors are a family or personal history of mental illness, traumatic childbirth experiences and lack of support before or after the birth.

Is this You?

- Do you tend not to eat properly, feeling it's too much effort?
- Do you suffer from disturbed sleep (over and above any disturbances from the children)?
- Do you lack energy and find yourself doing less and less?
- Do you use more tobacco, alcohol or drugs than you usually would?
- Are you unusually irritable or impatient?
- Do you feel helpless and lack self-confidence and self-esteem? Do you feel sensitive to how other people see your parenting?
- Have you lost interest in sex?
- Do you find it hard to remember things, to concentrate or make decisions?
- Do you tend to blame yourself and feel unnecessarily guilty about things?

Reflection Points

- Make a note of any days when you feel particularly low and any days when you feel better. You may notice patterns that tie in with your menstrual cycle (see Chapter 10);

[87] Centre for Maternal and Child Enquiries (CMACE). *Saving Mothers' Lives: reviewing maternal deaths to make motherhood safer: 2006–2008: The Eighth Report on Confidential Enquiries into Maternal Deaths in the United Kingdom.* BJOG; vol.118, Suppl. 1, March 2011.

- Spend some time thinking about anything that may be bringing you down that you could avoid, such as watching the news. Are there any relatives or friends who tend to make you feel low after speaking to them? Can you avoid them for a while or speak to them less often?
- Consider whether there are any people or things that tend to make you feel better. Does uplifting music help?
- Keep a journal and use it to make a note at the end of each day of 5 things for which you are grateful, even if they seem quite small;
- Create your own positive mantra to repeat as often as possible. For example: *"I am a calm and confident parent."* Alternatively Yogi Bhajan's *"There is a way through every block"* (see earlier in this chapter) may be helpful;
- Are you getting enough exercise? Exercise produces endorphins which make you feel happier. Use the Har Aerobic Kriya in Chapter 13 if you can't get out of the house.

Yogic Viewpoint: Overcoming Depression

Yoga enhances a personal sense of well-being. Improving the function of the glandular system, one of the known benefits of regularly practising Kundalini Yoga, also creates a sense of well-being. Specific practices such as Long Deep Breathing stimulate the production of endorphins that relieve depression. It has also been speculated by researchers that depression comes in part from a slow-down in the production of much-needed cells as we age. Yoga increases the generation of new cells.

The Positive Mind

Whereas the Negative Mind alerts us to danger, the Positive Mind alerts us to opportunity. The Positive Mind is optimistic, so strengthening it reduces depression. Like the Negative Mind, it can also get out of balance, leading the person to dash from one opportunity to another, never settling on anything and seeing it through.

Yogi Bhajan taught that we can bolster the Positive Mind by strengthening our Navel Point and using positive **affirmations** (see the Reflection Points above for a couple of examples). Positive affirmations have been used for many years and in various traditions. In *Kundalini Yoga: The Flow of Eternal Power*, Shakti

Parwha Kaur Khalsa explains how they work:

"Through the use of words vibrating in the form of mantra, positive affirmations and positive thinking, we can heal. Every word is a sound current (even if inaudible) which sets energy in motion. This energy goes out in ripples or waves and (to switch analogies in mid-ocean) the vibrations eventually return to us like a boomerang, bringing more of the same. There is power in positive thinking and positive affirmations! That power can work to expedite the healing process for ourselves and others… We create whatever situation we affirm… By mentally creating health, we set up favourable circumstances for that condition to manifest physically."[88]

Mantra

The use of mantra is particularly effective in fighting depression. The movement of the tongue on meridian points in the upper palate stimulates the **hypothalamus** and changes the brain chemistry. Amongst other things, the hypothalamus triggers the regulation of moods, emotional behaviour and sexuality. It is well known that listening to music affects our mood. Many positive states of mind, including the relief of depression, can be created through the use of mantra and the science of sound. See Chapter 11 for more information about mantra.

The Third Eye

According to the Yogic teachings, depression can be an indication that the sixth chakra is sluggish. This can be stimulated by practising Kirtan Kriya (see Chapter 12), meditating on the Third Eye and any exercises in which the forehead rests on the floor.[89]

The Pituitary Gland

Also associated with the Third Eye, the pituitary gland is responsible for the production of the "feel-good hormone" serotonin. Pranayam, such as Long Deep Breathing, is particularly helpful in stimulating the pituitary gland.

Sat Kriya

Sat Kriya is explained in Chapter 9 as one of several exercises in a kriya. It can, however, also be practised as a stand-alone kriya and is considered to be one of the most important exercises in the Kundalini Yoga canon. Particularly if you are very short of

[88] *Kundalini Yoga: The Flow of Eternal Power*, p.69-70

[89] *The Aquarian Teacher*, p.186

time, Sat Kriya (for a minimum of 3 minutes and no longer than 31 minutes) is excellent as a daily practice. It balances the energies of the lower chakras and stimulates the Kundalini energy directly. It tones the nervous system, calms the emotions, and channels the creative and sexual energies of the body. It is a practice that relaxes and releases many phobias about sexual behaviour, potency and capacity. It is a kriya that works on all levels of your being.

"Sat Kriya is to purify your being. Disease, ailment, weakness, impotency, laziness and negativity – all improper things will leave you."
~ Yogi Bhajan[90]

Top Tips for Defeating Depression

"When you are totally depressed and negative, do the following experiment: take a shower, rub yourself thoroughly with a soft towel, and then dress yourself from top to bottom in white. This will change your temperament, consciousness, and energy"
~ Yogi Bhajan;[91]

- Eat a banana first thing in the morning and a tablespoon of raisins at 4pm. This maintains daily levels of potassium which prevents depression;[92]
- Avoid sugar and alcohol; the "high" each creates is always followed by a low!
- Long Deep Breathing helps to break subconscious habit patterns that can lead to a negative response. It also stimulates the endorphins that fight depression;[93]
- The mantra Sat Narayan gives inner peace and happiness:[94] "*Sat Narayan Wahe Guru, Haree Naryan Sat Naam*". There are some beautiful musical versions available;
- Whistle Breath is said to be an effective way of strengthening and balancing the sixth chakra: pucker the mouth, concentrate at the Third Eye point, inhale making a high-pitched whistle, and exhale through the nose;[95]

---

90 *The Aquarian Teacher*, p.113
91 *The Aquarian Teacher*, p.245
92 *Kundalini Yoga: The Flow of Eternal Power*, p.276
93 *The Aquarian Teacher*, p.92
94 *The Aquarian Teacher*, p.87
95 *The Aquarian Teacher*, p.97

- Consider changing your hair style! Yogi Bhajan taught that cutting a fringe into the hair leads to sickness and that when the Mongolians conquered China, they ordered people to cover their foreheads which caused them to be depressed and fearful.[96]

Yoga Set for Depression

Breathing Exercise

Two-Stroke Breath to Stimulate the Pituitary[97]

Sit in Easy Pose with a straight spine. Put your thumbs on the **mounds of Mercury**. Keep the index fingers extended and close the other three fingers over the thumb, holding it in place. With the right palm facing out and the left palm facing in, touch the pads of the two index fingers together, making a connection between them. They will form a "V" in front of you. Place the mudra so that the tip of the "V" is about the level of the bridge of your nose.

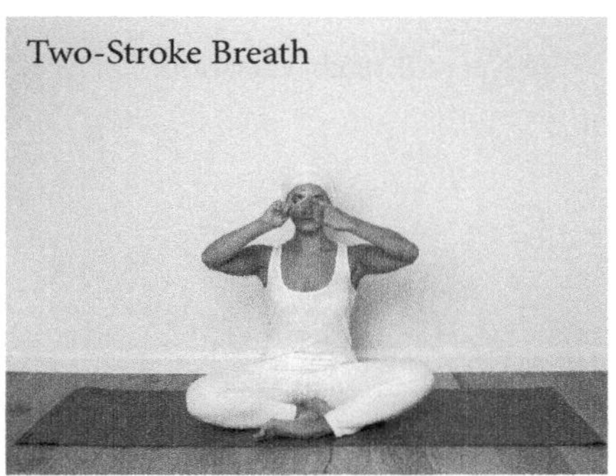
Two-Stroke Breath

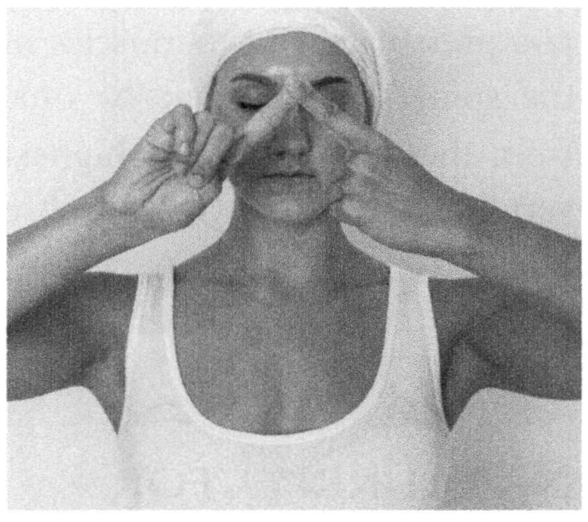

Slowly close your eyes so they are nine-tenths closed and look at the "V" with your "inner eye". Inhale powerfully through the mouth in two strokes or parts (1 second per stroke = 2 second inhale). Exhale powerfully through the nose in two strokes (1 second per stroke = 2 second exhale). Breathe with your full strength. Continue for 11 minutes.

To end: inhale deeply; hold the breath for 20 seconds as you squeeze your body inwardly from fibre to fibre. Exhale like cannon fire: powerfully out through

[96] KWTC lecture given on 31st July 1984 in Espanola (*www.libraryofteachings.com*)

[97] *Praana Praanee Praanayam*, p.155. First taught by Yogi Bhajan on 3rd June 1998

the mouth. Inhale deeply; hold the breath for 20 seconds as you put all the strength of the body into pressing the two index fingers together. "*Press it to bring out a balance and central nerve strength*". Exhale. Inhale deeply; hold the breath for 20 seconds as you pressurize all the muscles of the spinal column, one by one, from the tailbone to the highest vertebra of the neck (the vertebra called "C1", where the neck connects to the skull). Exhale and relax.

NABHI KRIYA FOR PRANA-APANA[98]

Life Nerve Stretch Variation: sit with the right leg straight out and the left foot on the right thigh. Hold the big toe of the right foot with both thumbs pressing against the toenail and the first two fingers of both hands applying a pressure against the soft part of the toe. Pull back on the big toe. Stretch the spine straight. Tuck the chin into the cavity above the chest. Begin Breath of Fire. Continue for 1 minute. Then inhale, change legs and continue for 1 minute more. Inhale and relax.

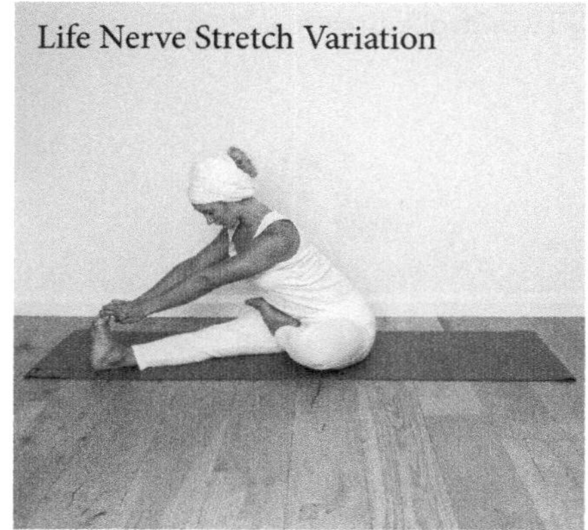
Life Nerve Stretch Variation

Kicking buttocks: lie on your back with your arms at your sides. Bring the knees into the chest and begin alternately kicking the buttocks with the heels. Inhale as you raise each leg, exhale as you strike the buttocks. Continue for 2 minutes. Inhale and relax.

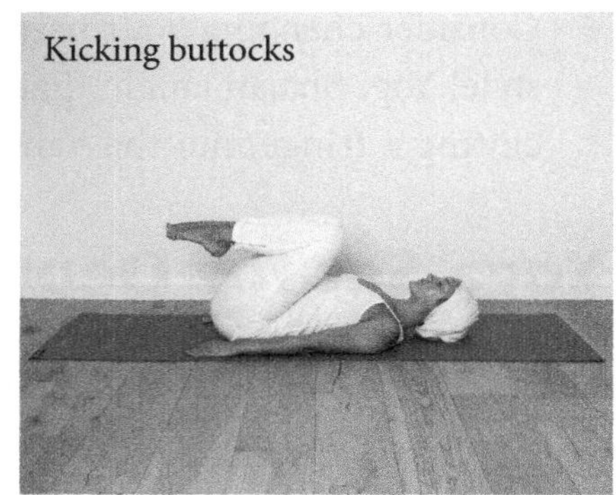
Kicking buttocks

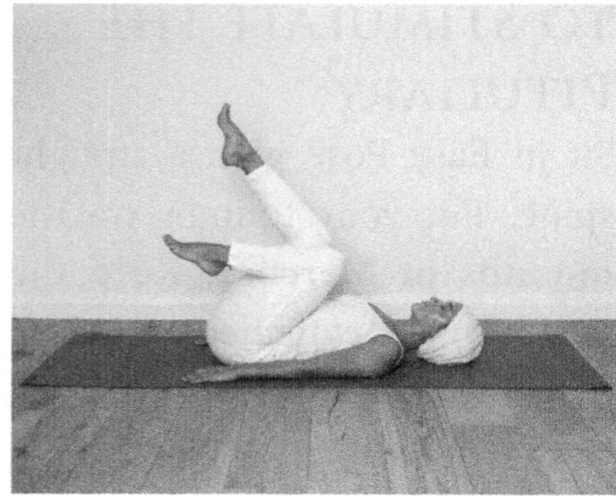

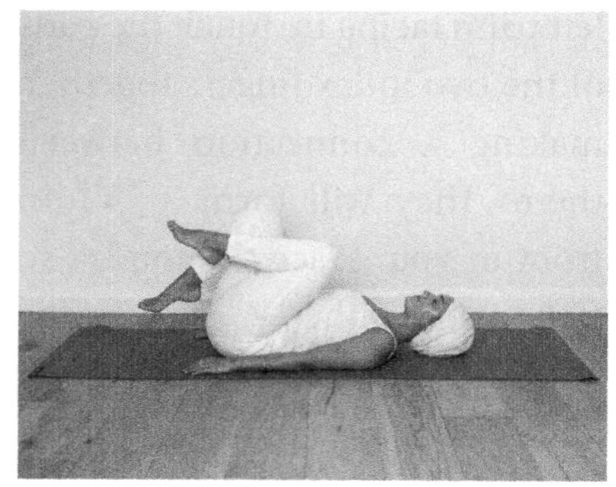

[98] *The Aquarian Teacher*, pp.346-347

Leg push-pull: remaining on the back, raise both legs to a height of 18 inches, inhale and draw the left knee to the chest. Exhale as you extend the left leg and simultaneously draw the right knee to the chest, keeping the lower legs parallel to the floor. Continue this push-pull motion with powerful breathing for 2 minutes. Inhale and extend both legs out. Exhale and relax.

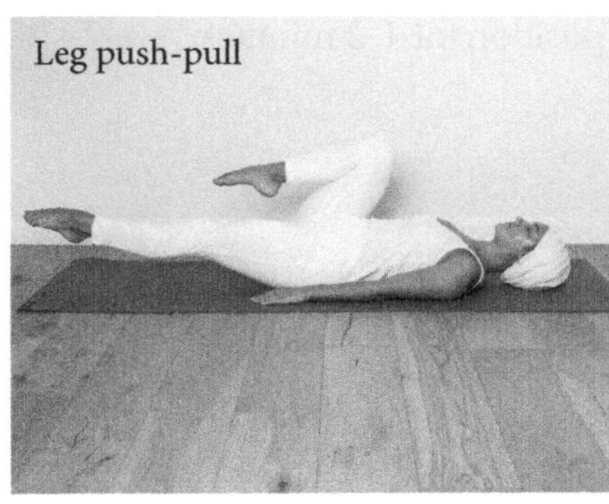
Leg push-pull

Front Platform: lie on the stomach. Place the hands under the shoulders and raise the body until the elbows lock. The weight of the body is supported by either the palms or the fingertips and the tops of the feet. The body, from the head to the toes, forms a straight line. Begin Breath of Fire. Continue for 2 minutes. Inhale and hold the breath briefly. Exhale. Inhale. Then exhale completely and hold the breath out briefly. Inhale and relax.

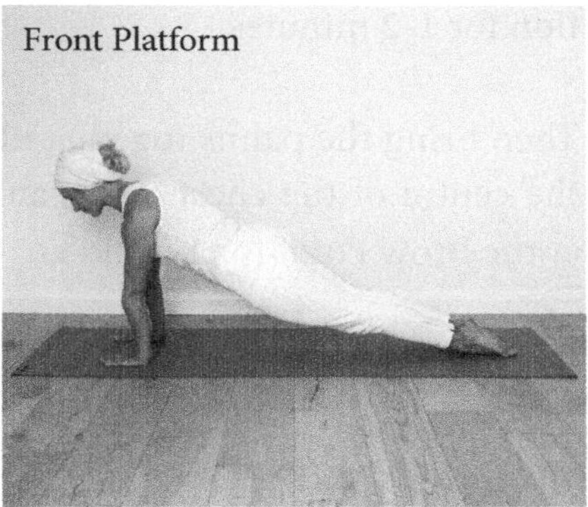
Front Platform

Stretch Pose: lie on the back, push the base of the spine into the ground, bring the feet together and raise the heels 6 inches. Raise the head and shoulders 6 inches and stare at your toes with the arms stretched out, pointing at the toes. In this position inhale and hold briefly. Exhale. Inhale. Exhale completely and apply the Root Lock. Inhale and relax.

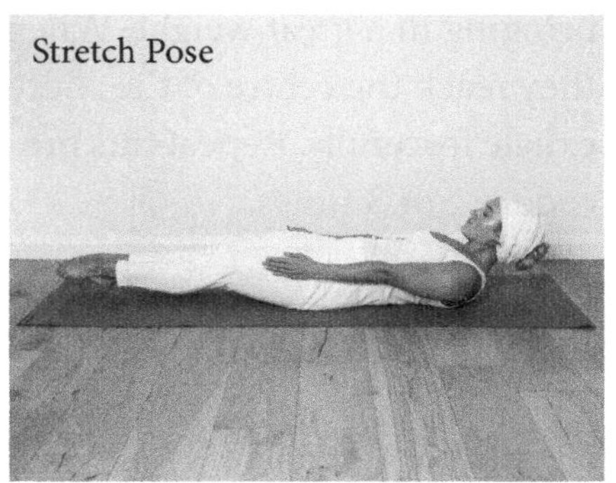
Stretch Pose

Heart Centre Stretch for Healing: sit in Easy Pose. Spread the arms at an angle of 60 degrees, parallel to the ground, as if to receive someone. Spread and tense all the fingers. Take a few long, deep breaths.

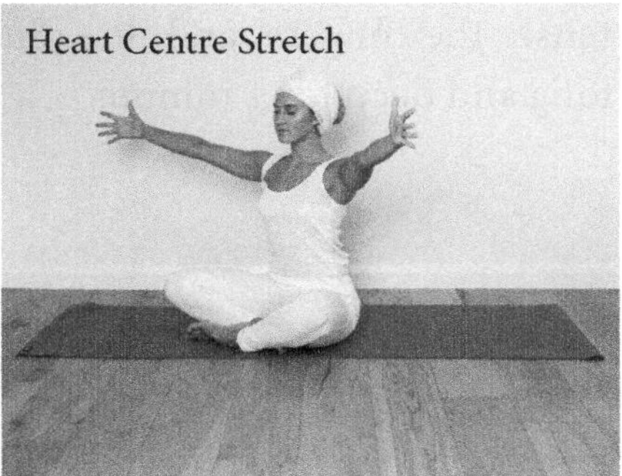
Heart Centre Stretch

Inhale and bring the fingers into tight fists. Slowly bring the fists to the centre of the chest as if bringing in a great weight. When they reach the centre of the chest, exhale forcefully. Repeat this procedure 2 or 3 times.

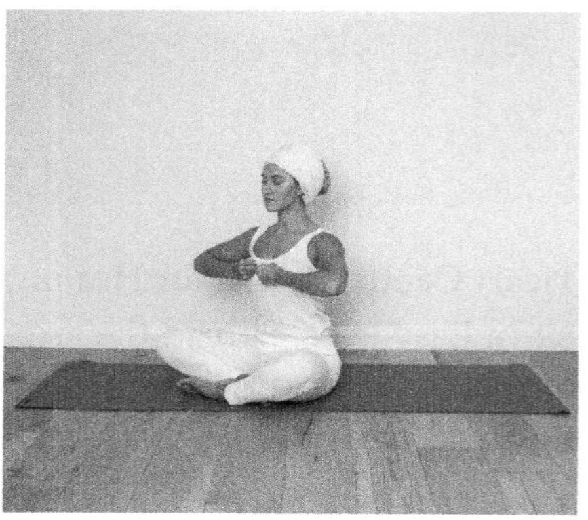

Then, spreading the arms at an angle of 60 degrees or more, tense the fingers and breathe long and deep for 1 minute.

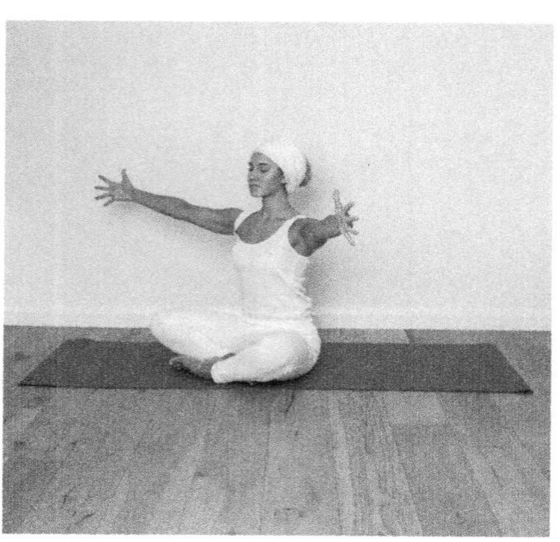

Then slowly bring the hands to a position 4 inches apart in front of the chest with the palms facing each other, fingers pointing up. Staring at the space between the palms, feel the energy flow between the hands. Continue long deep breathing in this position for 1-2 minutes.

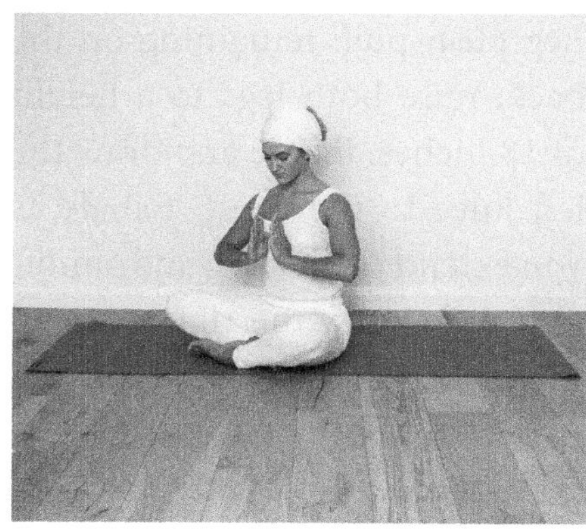

Then bring the palms together at the centre of the chest. Meditate at the Brow Point for 1 minute.

Then bending forward from the waist, bring the forehead and the palms to the floor. Relax in this position for 1-2 minutes.

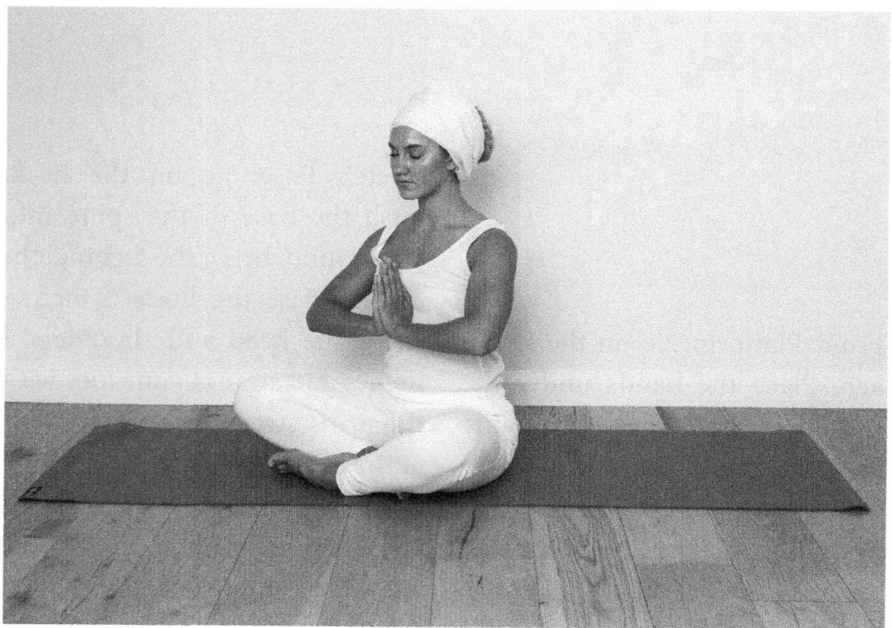

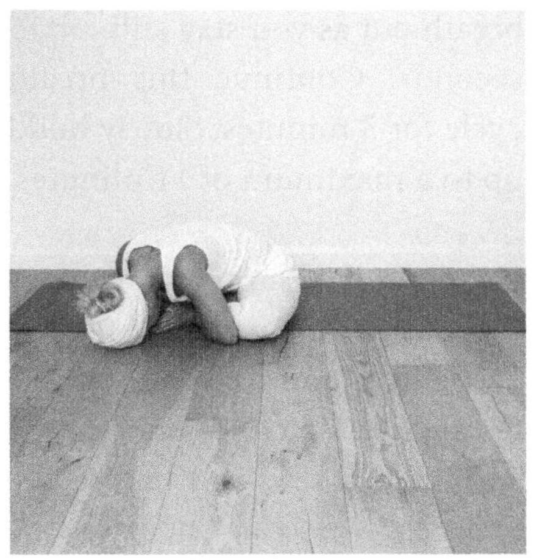

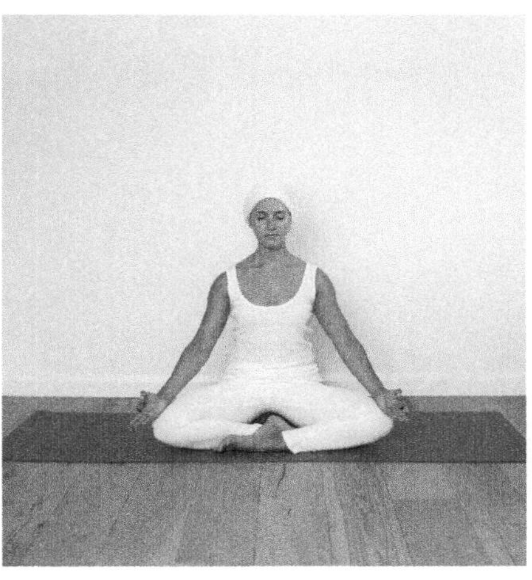

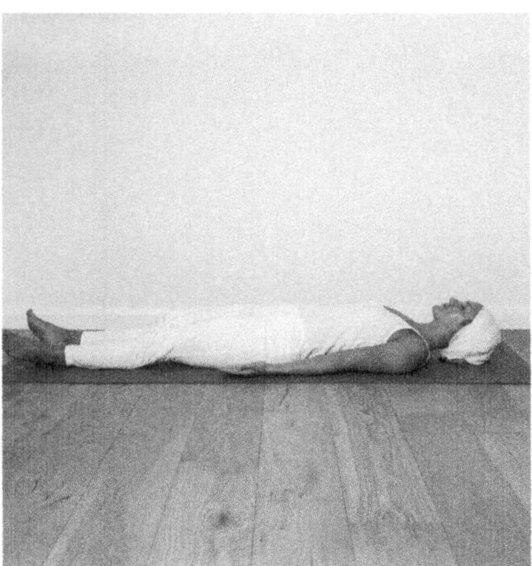

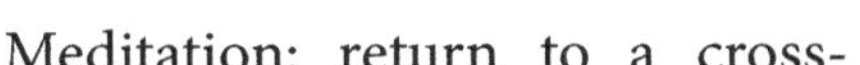

Meditation: return to a cross-legged sitting position. Meditate.

Deeply relax.

Meditation

THE CALIBER OF LIFE MEDITATION[99]

This meditation is known to conquer mild depression and discouragement.

Sit in Easy Pose with a light Neck Lock. Extend both arms straight forward, parallel to the ground. Curl the fingers of the right hand into a fist. Extend the thumb straight up. Keep the elbow straight and move the fist to the centre of the body. Move the left arm to the centre and wrap the fingers of the left hand around the right hand's fist. Extend the left thumb straight up. Adjust the grip of the hands so that the thumbs can touch along their sides as they point up. The tips of the thumbs will form a little "V". Focus the eyes on the thumbnails and through the V. Look through the V like a gunsight, seeing far away and seeing the V. Inhale deeply and fill the lungs for 5 seconds. Exhale completely and empty the lungs for 5 seconds. Then suspend the

[99] *The Aquarian Teacher*, p.389. First taught by Yogi Bhajan in October 1979

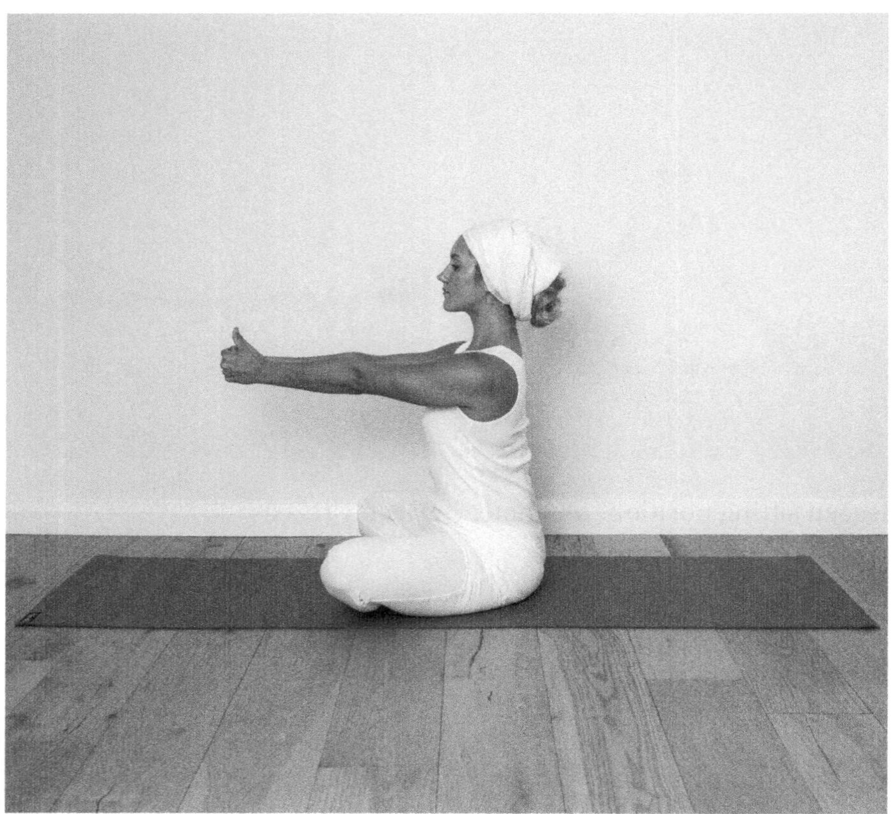

breath out as you stay still for 15 seconds. Continue this breath cycle for 3 minutes. Slowly build up to a maximum of 11 minutes.

Cautions: be sure you can do the meditation perfectly for the entire length of time you choose to practise. If not, lessen the time and build up. As you master the practice, you can increase the time you hold the breath out from 15 seconds up to 60 seconds. Pick a time that is realistic for you. Remember to keep the elbows straight. If you feel dizzy or disoriented in this practice, be sure you are doing the suspension of the breath properly and holding the Neck Lock.

Chapter 9
Lengthening the Fuse:
Reducing Irritability and Anger

"You normally breathe 15 breaths a minute. If you can train yourself to breathe 8 breaths per minute, you can have your temper and your projection under control."
~ Yogi Bhajan[100]

A toddler asks for a drink of water over and over again while we are trying to feed his baby sister and have already explained five times we will get it for him in a minute. We feel the irritability physically: it rises up inside us and eventually we snap at him. Our response is illogical because previous experience has taught us it will make no difference to his incessant demands, other than to provoke an angry response from him, but it happens anyway. If we then add a big helping of guilt to the mix, sadly we have only compounded the problem.

Irritability is a form of anger but many people – especially women – find it very difficult to admit they experience it, especially if it is directed at their children. Anger manifests in different ways: bursts of temper, irritability, hostility and bitterness, to name a few examples. Is there any parent who can truthfully say they have never felt irritated by their children? Children learn social rules and boundaries by seeing how far they will stretch.

People don't usually feel angry all the time; anger has to be triggered by something. Triggers can be something irritating such as the relentless child asking for something repeatedly. Alternatively, the trigger could threaten some kind of cost. For example, we may risk loss of face in front of other parents if our child misbehaves. Or the trigger may be a transgression of some kind: the breaking of a rule the parent holds. People all have different basic beliefs

[100] *Sadhana Guidelines*, p.20

about themselves and others which stem from their upbringing and experience, including beliefs about what behaviour is and is not acceptable from children (and what kind of response is and is not acceptable from the parent). Examples of rules parents might hold include "children should do as they are told" and "children should not interrupt when adults are speaking".

Mood also affects how we react to a particular trigger. Mood is affected by factors such as our hormones, our state of health, what we eat and how tired and stressed we are.

Even when we experience anger, inhibitions frequently leap into action and prevent us giving vent to it as fully as we otherwise might. For example if other parents are present, we may be less likely to shout at our child than we would at home alone with him.

Like all our emotional responses, anger serves a purpose, reminding us about something that feels wrong. There are times when anger is justified. Without it, we would not have made the leaps forward we have made in relation to women's rights over the last hundred years, for example, such as the right to have parental responsibility for our own children. Anger can warn us we need more support, we are exhausted, we are depressed, we are stressed, we are experiencing other problems such as relationship or money worries that need resolving, we need professional help with identifying and managing special needs, and so on. Anger may relate to unresolved issues relating to the way we were brought up ourselves even if we have suppressed the original memories. Or we may feel anger because we know what the problem is but feel unable to do anything about it: we need more support with the childcare demands we currently manage, for example, but that support is not available to us.

Parents may feel angry with the children themselves: due to panic and fear when they do things that are dangerous or when we do not know how else to deal with a difficult situation, or frustration when they seem to make things much harder than they need to be. When we deal with family, friends and colleagues many of us have learned to mask our anger behind passive aggressive behaviour which is more socially acceptable than giving full vent to it. With children, we don't need to put on the mask and it would probably be too subtle for them anyway; venting our anger (or trying desperately hard to contain it) can therefore seem like a new experience for us. I remember one of my ex-husband's relatives saying when he became a parent he was shocked by how angry he could feel towards his daughter sometimes. It can be an uncomfortable thing to admit because however demanding and aggressive they can be towards us in return, children are smaller than us and they are vulnerable.

Anger has a habit of making things worse. In the Buddhist tradition it is even regarded as the root of all problems. Snapping at the toddler doesn't prevent his incessant demands, it just makes us feel bad. Anger can affect our relationships with our children and our self-confidence about our parenting abilities. It has a habit of feeding on itself and spiralling out of control. It provides a temporary release in a stressful situation which can become addictive: how many times have you got angry with your children simply out of habit?

Having identified the problem, we will feel better about ourselves and run less risk of damaging our relationships with our children if we can manage our anger better.

Is this You?

- Do you regularly feel irritable, either with the children, your partner or anyone else close to you? Do you feel unable to deal with challenging situations with equanimity?
- Do you find yourself snapping at people inadvertently?
- Do you regularly have angry thoughts? Do you find your mind regularly goes over things in the past that have made you feel angry?
- Have you said or done things in the heat of the moment you regret afterwards?
- Do you regularly complain to others about someone in your life who makes you feel angry?
- Do you feel bitter about your circumstances?
- Do you feel anger rising in your body, like your blood is boiling?

Reflection Points

- Do you know what kinds of things tend to trigger an angry response in you?
- Make a note in your diary of any days when you have found it particularly difficult to keep your anger under control and any days when it has seemed easier. You may notice patterns that tie in with your menstrual cycle (see Chapter 10 on Balancing Hormones);
- What beliefs do you hold about what behaviour is and is not acceptable from children, and what kind of response is and is not acceptable from the parent?
- Can any of your triggers be avoided? For example, if you

tend to snap at the children when they won't get ready to go out and you are running late, can you get them ready five minutes earlier?

- How does your mood tend to affect how you react to the particular trigger? Are you more likely to snap on the school run if you haven't eaten breakfast beforehand, for example, or at bedtime when you are tired?

- Are there any inhibitions that help you keep your anger under control? Can you spend more time with other adults around?

- Watch your physical and emotional response carefully. How do you feel shortly before you snap at the children? Like you are going to explode? A serious sense of humour failure? Being aware of your typical response can help you to keep the anger in check before it becomes unstoppable;

- What thought processes tend to accompany an angry response in you? For example: "he's doing it deliberately to get my attention because I am giving the baby some attention." If we practise watching our thoughts, we start to notice patterns and warning signs;

- Are there more positive thoughts you could substitute for the negative ones that have become engrained through habit? For example: "children don't annoy you deliberately, but they are naturally selfish and only lose that when they get older." This may take some practice!

- Are there any alternative responses you can try? Can you remove yourself from the situation for a minute or two? Can you think of any times when you have successfully kept your anger in check? What did you do differently then?

- Keep reminding yourself that unfuelled anger simply dissipates. Yogi Bhajan taught us: "just don't react". This can seem impossible at first but the more you train your mind and rehearse alternative scenarios, the easier it becomes;

- Despite our best intentions, there are probably still going to be times when our anger gets the better of us. Say sorry and move on – re-reading Chapter 7 on ditching the guilt if necessary!

Yogic Viewpoint: Managing Anger

Regular practice of Kundalini Yoga gives us the space to choose how we react to a particular situation. When we practise Yoga, we are investing in our future: building up the bank account for when we need reserves to fall back on. Yoga also teaches us to approach problems with a neutral mind.

Long Deep Breathing helps to break those unconscious habit patterns that can lead to an irritable or angry response. It also balances the parasympathetic and the sympathetic nervous system, which can be particularly helpful if we find ourselves (or more specifically, our sympathetic nervous systems) getting fired up too often.

The Physical Body

As we saw in Chapter 7, the Physical Body is one of the Ten Bodies. When it is weak, we may feel angry, greedy, jealous, competitive or ungrateful. As you might imagine, regular exercise is the key to strengthening the Physical Body.

Agni Tattva

This is the tattva, or element, of fire. It is said we are made, like everything else in the universe, from five elements: earth, water, fire, air and ether (or space). When we have too much fire, we feel and act angry. Yogi Bhajan taught that we cannot get rid of this anger because it is a projection of one of the essential elements, but we can train ourselves to channel our anger positively.[101]

The Navel Point

If you feel irritable you may have a displaced or weak Navel Point, especially if you also feel bloated or have other digestive problems. The Navel Point is an area in the body through which thousands of energy channels converge. The exact location was described in **The Upanishads** more than 2,500 years ago: in the centre of the stomach, between the navel and the last bone of the spinal column. Shaped like a bird's egg, the Navel Point can easily become displaced from its correct position by eating too much sugar and meat, taking drugs (including birth control pills) and tranquilisers, and lifting heavy objects (e.g. children!) especially during your Moon Cycle. Fortunately, it is relatively easy to reset the Navel Point to its correct position with dietary changes and yogic exercises that strengthen the area in which it is located.

[101] *The Aquarian Teacher*, p.210

How to test your Navel Point

The position, strength and rhythm of the abdominal heart or navel pulse correlate physically with the Navel Point. On an empty, or nearly empty, stomach:

1. Lie on the back. Completely tense and relax the entire body two or three times. This allows the abdominal muscles to totally relax and stimulates the navel pulse for easy location.

2. Do Stretch Pose (see page 89) for two or three minutes. This exercise is even better for relaxation and bringing out the navel pulse.

Next, make the tips of your fingers into a little circle. Press the tips down on the belly button toward the spine. Press firmly but with gentleness. You will be able to feel one point with your fingertips that beats strongly. If this beat is exactly in the centre of the navel, then the Navel Point is centred and in place. If it is displaced, many hard-to-diagnose maladies can exist in the person's body.

Top Tips for Reducing Irritability and Anger

- Avoid sugar and alcohol that create extra stress in the body;[102]

- Do Stretch Pose regularly to bring the Navel Point into alignment;

- Long Deep Breathing helps to release subconscious negative thoughts that may be fuelling our angry response. Lie on the back and do Long Deep Breathing for 3 minutes every day if possible;[103]

- Use a practice known as "Gatga" which helps to break habits: repeat the mantra *Ek Ong Kar Sat Gur Prasaad, Sat Gur Prasaad Ek Ong Kar* five times every time you feel angry.[104]

---

102 *The Aquarian Teacher*, p.254

103 *The Aquarian Teacher*, p.92

104 *Kundalini Yoga: The Flow of Eternal Power*, p.221

Yoga Set for Reducing Irritability and Anger

Breathing Exercise

Burn Inner Anger[105]

Sit in Easy Pose with a straight spine, chin in, chest lifted. Extend the index and middle fingers of your right hand and use your thumb to hold down the other fingers. Raise your right arm in front and up to 60 degrees. Keep your elbow straight. Place your left hand at the heart centre. Close your eyes. Make an "O" of your mouth and inhale and exhale powerfully through your mouth (2-second inhalation and 2-second exhalation). Continue for 11 minutes.

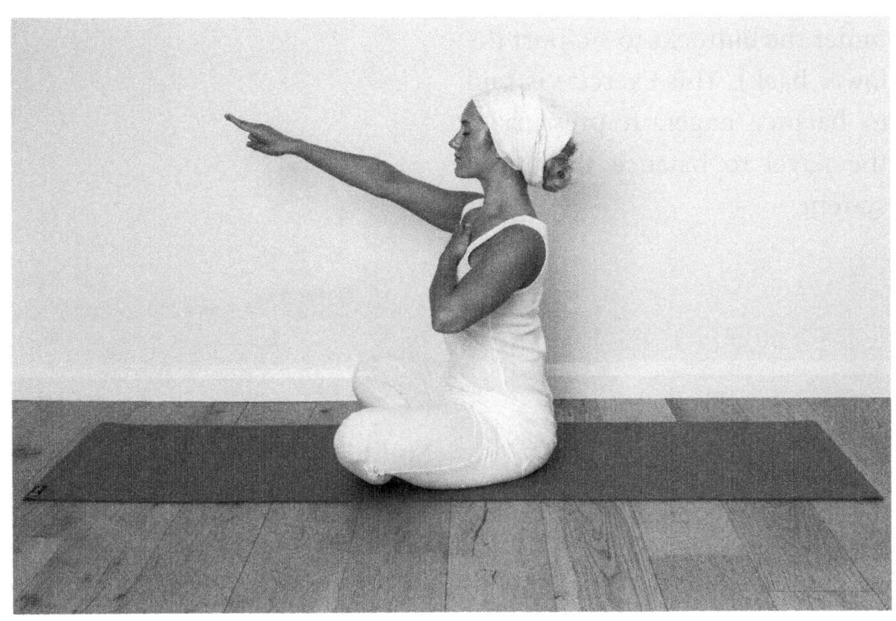

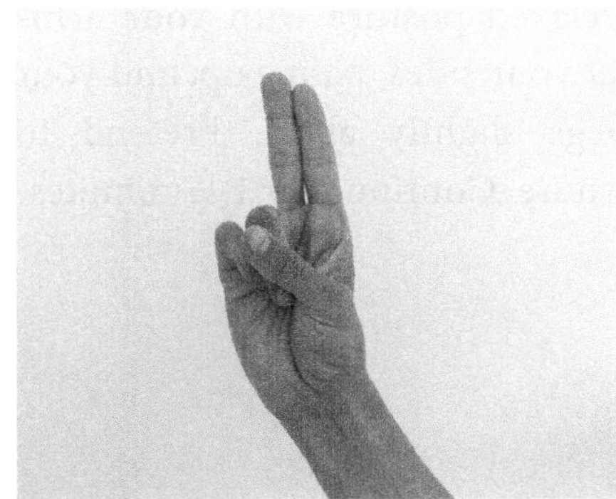

To end: inhale deeply, hold the breath in for 10 seconds, stretch both arms up above your head and stretch your spine as much as you can. Stretch the discs between your vertebrae. Exhale like cannon fire: forcefully

105 *Praana Praanee Praanayam*, p.147. First taught by Yogi Bhajan on 19th February, 2000

through the mouth. Repeat this breath sequence two more times.

"Breathe strongly and powerfully with emotion. Burn your inner anger and get rid of it. Take the help of the breath to get rid of the body's weaknesses and impurities."

~Yogi Bhajan

Kriya

KRIYA FOR RELIEVING INNER ANGER[106]

Lie down flat on your back in a relaxed posture with your arms at your sides, palms up, and your legs slightly apart. Pretend to snore. Continue for 1 ½ minutes.

Still lying on your back, keep your legs out straight and raise both legs up 6 inches from the floor and hold for 2 minutes (if necessary, place your hands under the buttocks to support the lower back). This exercise is said to balance anger. It pressurizes the navel to balance the entire system.

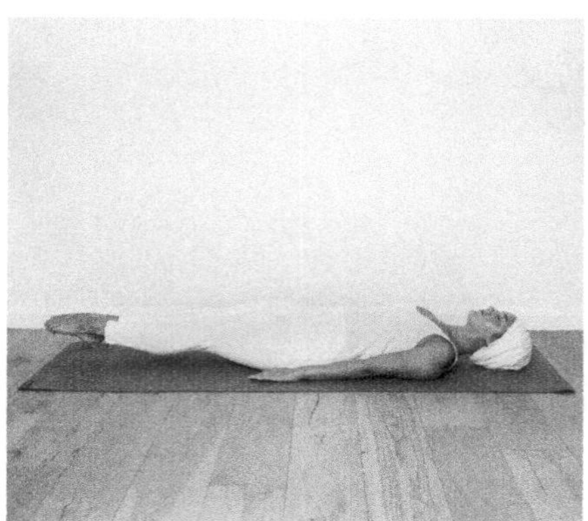

Remaining in the posture with your legs up at 6 inches, stick out your tongue and do Breath of Fire through your mouth. Continue for 1 ½ minutes.

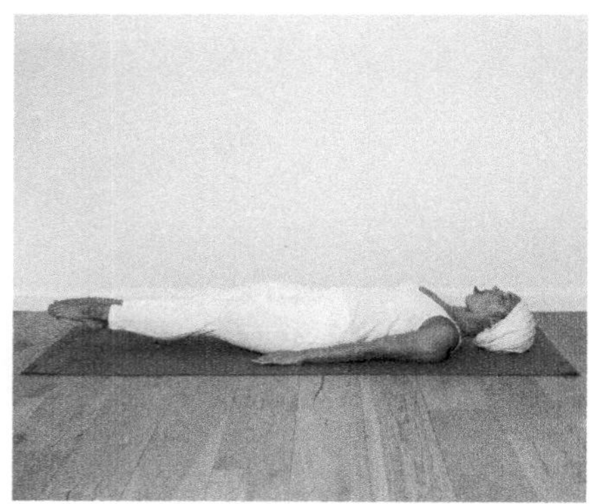

Still lying on your back, lift your legs up to 90 degrees with your arms on the ground by your sides. Begin to beat the ground with

[106] From the Library of Teachings, originally taught by Yogi Bhajan on 21st September 1988 (*www.libraryofteachings.com*)

your hands with all the anger you can achieve. Beat hard and fast. Continue for 2 ½ minutes.

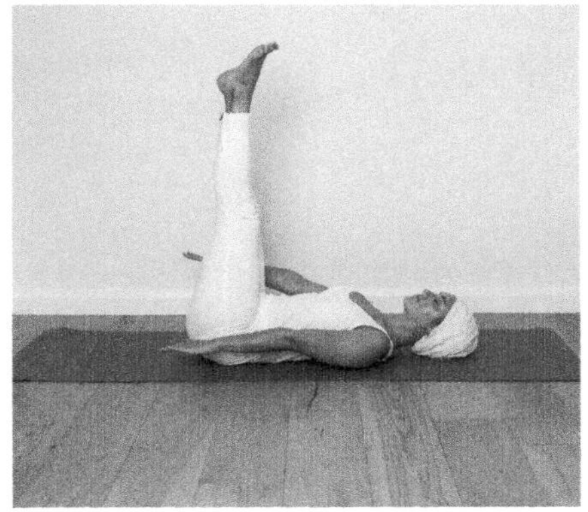

Still on your back, bring your knees to your chest and wrap your arms around them. Stick your tongue out. Inhale through your open mouth and exhale through your nose. Continue for 2 minutes.

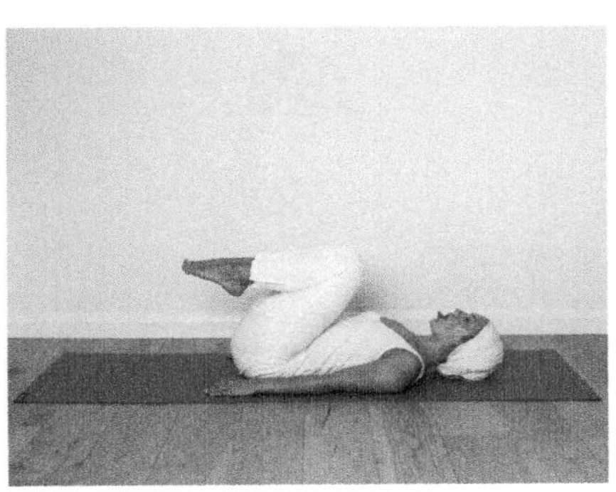

Sit in Celibate Pose: begin by sitting on the heels then spread the feet far enough apart so your hips will fit between them. Moving slowly, sit down on the floor with your feet on either side of your hips. Cross your arms over your chest and press them hard against your ribcage. Bend forward and touch your forehead to the floor as if you are bowing and then come back up. For 2 ½ minutes move at a pace of approximately

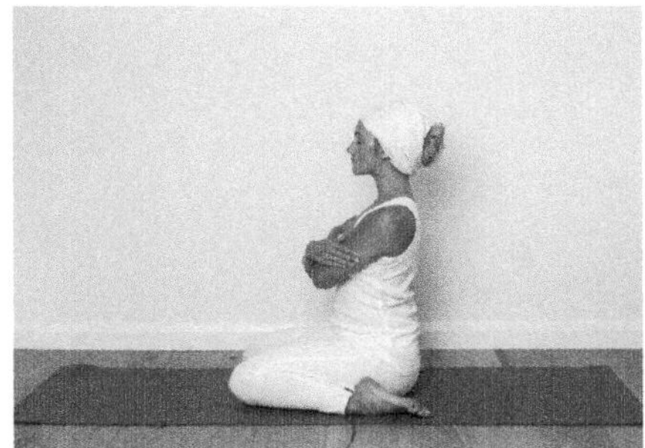

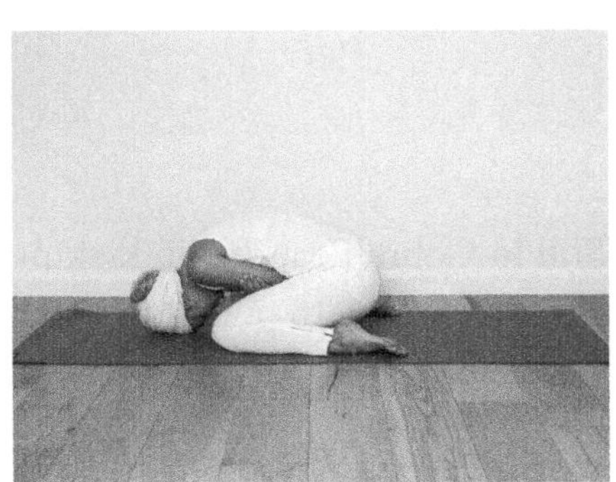

30 bows per minute, then for another 30 seconds speed up and move as fast as you can.

Sit with your legs straight out in front of you. Begin to beat all parts of your body with open palms. Move fast. Continue for 2 minutes.

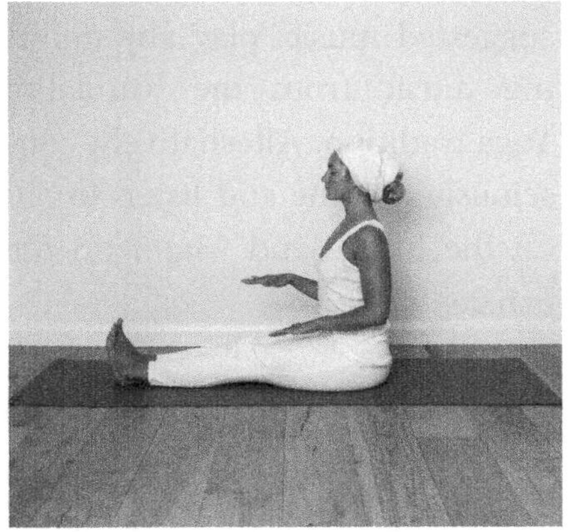

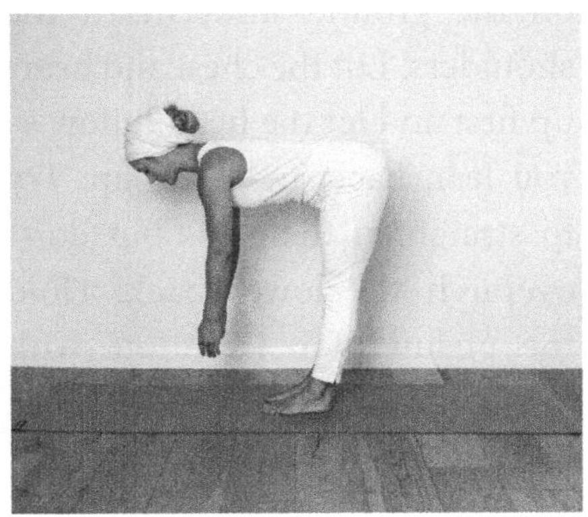

Stand up and bend forward, keeping your back parallel to the ground. Let your arms and hands hang down loosely. Remain in this posture and sing for 3 minutes (in class, Yogi Bhajan played a tape of *Guru, Guru, Wahe Guru, Guru Ram Das Guru*).

Author's note: if you don't have the suggested music, play any uplifting music from the Kundalini Yoga tradition. Alternatively, consciously breathe and listen to *Sat* on the inhale and *Naam* on the exhale.

Continue singing and come into Cobra Pose. Lie down on the stomach, placing the hands on the ground underneath the shoulders. Lift the chest and heart up first and let the head follow as you lean back and arch up. Try to straighten the arms but don't overarch the lower back. Hold the posture for 1 minute with normal breath.

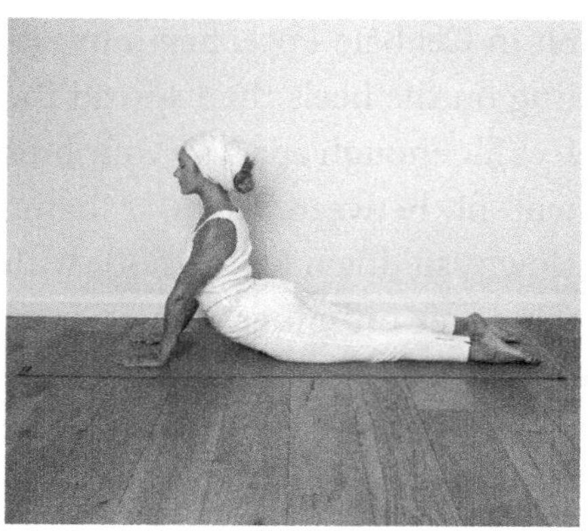

Still in Cobra Pose, begin circling your neck, as you continue singing. Continue for 30 seconds.

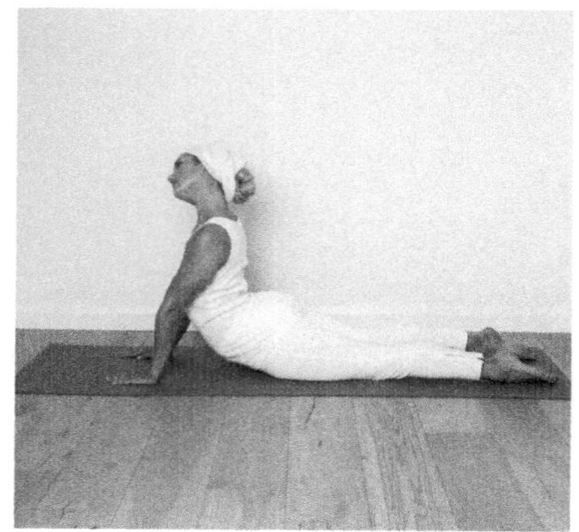

Still in Cobra Pose, begin kicking the ground with alternate feet. Continue for 30 seconds.

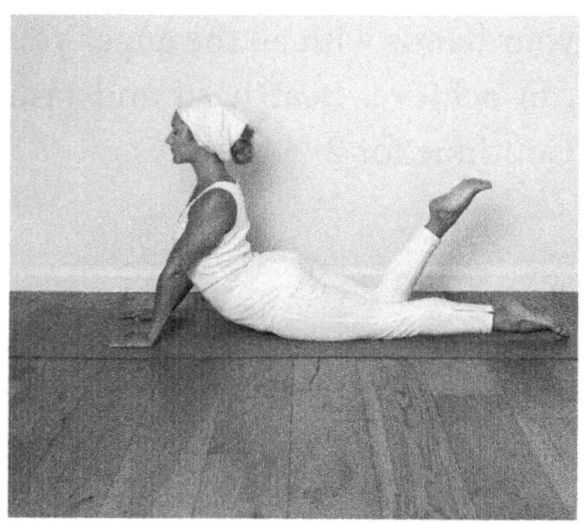

Sit in Easy Pose and close your eyes. Stretch your arms over your head, keeping the elbows straight and the palms together. Interlock your fingers except the index fingers, which are pointing straight up. Begin Sat Kriya in Easy Pose: chant *Sat* as you squeeze the

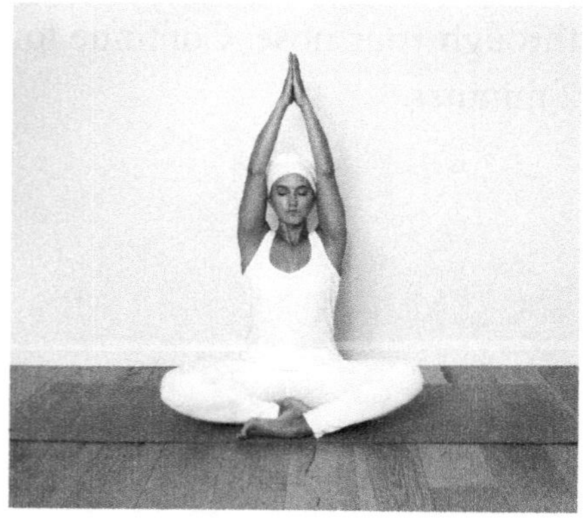

Navel Point in and up. Chant *Naam* as you release it. Continue for 1 minute 15 seconds.

Lie down in Corpse Pose (on your back with arms by your sides, palms face up) and nap for 5 minutes.

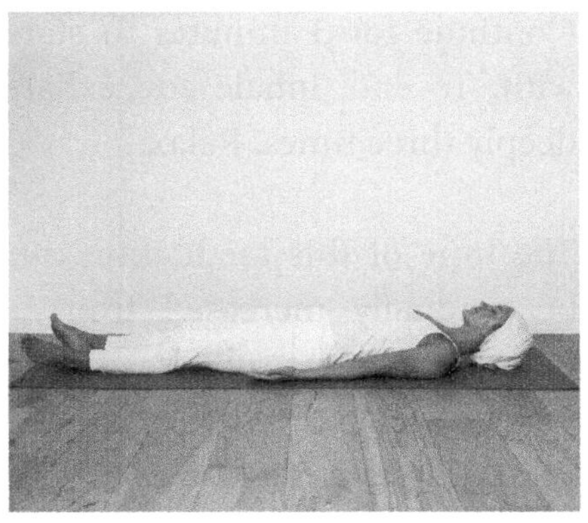

Meditation

Meditation for a Calm Heart[107]

This meditation is very calming and gives clarity to our relationship with ourselves as well as with others. Sit in Easy Pose with a light Neck Lock. Either close the eyes or look straight ahead with the eyes 1/10th open. Place the left hand on the centre of the chest at the Heart Centre. The palm is flat against the chest and the fingers are parallel to the ground, pointing to the right. Make Gyan Mudra with the right hand and raise the right hand up to the right side as if giving a pledge. The palm faces forward, the middle, ring and little fingers point up. The elbow is relaxed near the side with the forearm perpendicular to the ground (see next page).

Concentrate on the flow of the breath. Regulate each bit of the breath consciously. Inhale slowly and deeply through both nostrils. Then suspend the breath in and raise the chest. Retain it in as long as possible. Then exhale smoothly, gradually and completely.

When you hold the breath in or out "for as long as possible", you should not gasp or be under strain when you let the breath move again. Pull the chin in and become still and calm. To suspend the breath on the inhale, bring the attention to the clavicle and upper ribs, lifting the upper ribs slightly and holding them in place. Relax the shoulders, throat and face. To suspend the breath on the exhale, pull the Navel Point back toward the spine, lift the lower chest and diaphragm, and let the upper ribs relax and compress. Do not bend the spine and ribs.[108]

---

[107] *The Aquarian Teacher*, p.395. First taught by Yogi Bhajan in September 1981

[108] *The Aquarian Teacher*, p.93

Continue for 3 minutes to start with. To end, inhale and exhale deeply three times. Relax.

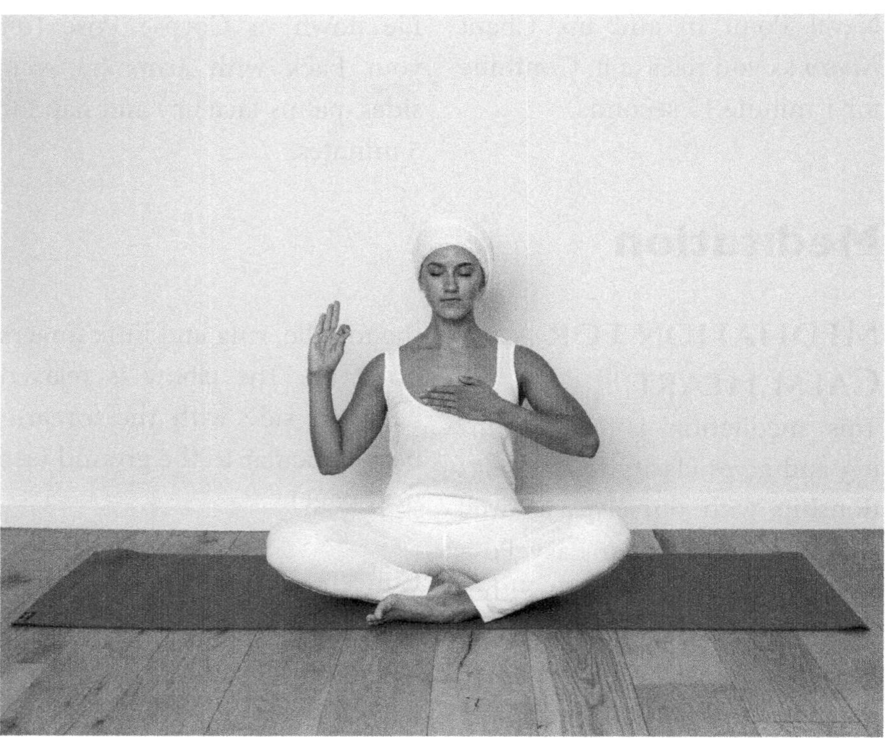

The time of this meditation can be gradually increased from 3 up to 31 minutes, which will give you an advanced practice of concentration and rejuvenation.

Caution: holding the breath in and out affects the blood pressure. If you have high blood pressure, take extra care not to hold the breath in for too long. If you have low blood pressure, take extra care not to hold the breath out for too long.

Chapter 10
Sunshine through the Clouds:
Balancing Hormones

"When you are upset, when you are not contained and you are feeling very bad, just take a long deep breath. Then begin to measure your breath so that you breathe five times per minute. It will not take longer than a minute and a half and you will be content."

~ Yogi Bhajan[109]

The importance of hormones in the human body cannot be understated; they are messengers that govern every aspect of how we function. Yogi Bhajan described the glands, which secrete hormones, as the guardians of our physical health and our stability in infinite consciousness. Hormones determine the chemistry of the blood, which in turn determines the composition of the personality. If, for example, we lack proper iodine in the thyroid gland or produce too much thyroxin we will lack patience and seldom succeed in staying calm and cool.

For women the role of hormones in the body is particularly complicated because we have a monthly cycle between puberty and menopause, during which our hormones fluctuate. Many women are sensitive to these changes.

Whether or not a woman has children, hormones will also play a significant role at different stages of her life: during puberty and adolescence, during perimenopause and during menopause. Many women report feeling more balanced after the menopause.

For women who have children there are additional hormonal upheavals to contend with during pregnancy, childbirth and breastfeeding. Within these cycles and upheavals is each woman's

[109] *Praana Praanee Praanayam*, p.69

individual response to her hormones and changes to them.

Premenstrual Syndrome

Hormonal imbalances can magnify parental exhaustion; a lack of energy is just one symptom of Premenstrual Syndrome (PMS). PMS can manifest in a wide range of physical and emotional symptoms, including some we have already considered: anger and irritability (see Chapter 9), depression (see Chapter 8), feelings of guilt and low self-worth (see Chapter 7) and feeling anxious and insecure (see Chapter 6).

Once you have had children you are more likely to suffer from PMS even if you didn't when you were younger; Marilyn Glenville PhD has argued[110] that women who fall into the following categories may be more likely to develop PMS, and the risk appears to increase if you fall into more than one category:

- You are in your 30s or 40s;
- You have two or more children;
- Your mother suffered from it;
- You have recently experienced a hormonal upheaval (for example, had a baby, a termination, a miscarriage or sterilisation, or have stopped taking birth control pills);
- You have experienced several pregnancies in quick succession.

Premenopause Syndrome

The premenopause period can start from age 30 and last for up to 20 years. It has been described as "a phenomenon that all women know about, but very few have a name for."[111] Now women are generally having children later they are very likely to already be in the premenopause stages when hormones are fluctuating more than they did earlier in their adult lives.

Dr Lee and Dr Hanley describe the symptoms of Premenopause Syndrome as follows:[112]

- Sore, lumpy breasts, especially premenstrually;
- Irregular periods;

---

[110] *Overcoming PMS The Natural Way* by Marilyn Glenville, PhD (Piatkus Books Ltd, 2002), p.17

[111] *What your Doctor may* not *tell you about Premenopause* by John R. Lee, MD, Jesse Hanley, MD and Virginia Hopkins (Grand Central Publishing, 1999), p.4

[112] *What your Doctor may* not *tell you about Premenopause*

- Loss of sex drive;
- Skin is dry, or not as smooth as it once was;
- Irritable and snappish;
- Difficulty getting out of bed in the morning;
- Infertility, uterine fibroids and/or PMS (even if you haven't had it before).

Birth Control Pills

Scientific research into links between oral contraceptives and mental health has produced some conflicting results. A study by researchers at Australia's Monash University in 2005, for example, found women who take birth control pills are twice as likely to be depressed as those who don't.[113] On the other hand a study of 6,654 sexually active women carried out by the *American Journal of Epidemiology* found women taking oral contraceptives displayed lower levels of depressive symptoms and were much less likely to report a suicide attempt in the previous year.[114]

One thing that is certain however is the contraceptive pill keeps us ignorant about the reality of our individual hormonal cycles. Many of us spent the earlier years of our adult lives on birth control pills. Whilst this was an effective method of preventing unwanted pregnancies for most, it did also mask the fluctuations of our regular hormonal cycles, presenting us with a whole new learning curve once we came off the pills to have our children.

Is this You?

- Do you feel more irritable at certain times in the month, especially in the run-up to your Moon Cycle?
- Do you experience sugar and food cravings, changes in sex drive, noise intolerance, changes in sleep pattern (including insomnia, restlessness and heavy or prolonged sleeping), restlessness, headaches or migraines and clumsiness when you are premenstrual?
- Do you experience mood swings, anger and irritability, depression and tearfulness, feeling unable to cope, feelings of guilt, insecurity and low self-worth, irrational thoughts, loneliness, forgetfulness and

---

113 Reported by Monash University on 1st March 2005 (http://monash.edu/news/releases/show/240)

114 *American Journal of Epidemiology*, 2013; 178(9): 1378-1388l; reported by Medscape (http://www.medscape.com/viewarticle/813583_4)

poor concentration or suicidal tendencies in the days leading up to your period?

- Do you have problems with your skin that seem worse at certain times in the month?

Reflection Points:

- How do your hormones tend to affect you? If you are unsure, keep a diary of how you feel and track how this coincides with your monthly cycle;
- Is your diet wreaking havoc on your hormonal system? Sugar, alcohol and caffeine can be particularly troublesome, throwing the blood sugar levels up and down chaotically. The yogic diet is very effective in balancing hormones and blood sugar levels;
- Are you looking after yourself enough? Getting as much good-quality sleep as you can (see Chapter 3), giving up smoking (see Chapter 12), exercising and stretching regularly, avoiding contact with synthetic xenoestrogens[115] (for example by only using BPA-free water bottles and food containers), minimising stress (see Chapter 4) and prioritising calm time for yourself (a hot bath with Epsom Salts in the evening or some time set aside for meditation before bed) can all help to balance your hormones.

Yogic Viewpoint: The Pituitary Gland

Known as the "master gland", the pituitary gland coordinates and regulates all the glands in the endocrine, or hormonal, system. The glands are known to become stronger through regularly practising Kundalini Yoga, which balances out the production of all our hormones including those relating to our menstrual cycle.

The pituitary gland is associated with the Third Eye and is responsible for the production of serotonin, which plays a major role in our emotional balance. We can stimulate the excretions of the pituitary gland through the sixth chakra.

The Arcline

For women the Arcline extends from earlobe to earlobe across the hairline and brow, like a halo,

[115] Chemical compounds that imitate the hormone oestrogen

and also from nipple to nipple. The Arcline is known as the sixth of the Ten Bodies and is associated with the pituitary gland. It regulates the nervous system and glandular balance so if the Arcline is weak your hormones may be out of balance. Stimulating the pituitary gland is the key to strengthening the Arcline.

THE BREATH

Controlling the breath is absolutely essential to balancing the hormones as it empowers us to control our moods and our reactions. There are many pranayama that can be used to support hormonal balance. Left Nostril Breathing, Long Deep Breathing and One Minute Breath are all very calming, stimulate the pituitary gland and can be used any time you feel your hormones are throwing your emotions out of balance. Twenty-five repetitions of Sitali Pranayam every morning and every evening is recommended to balance the hormonal body especially during the major transitions of the menstrual cycle and menopause.[116] Sitali Pranayam is performed as follows:

- Closing the eyes and concentrating on the Brow Point;
- Rolling the tongue into a "U" with the tip just outside the lips (if you cannot roll the tongue, stick the tip outside the mouth and curve it);
- Inhale, breathing through the rolled tongue;
- Exhale through the nose.

"May you never be afraid of your own excellence. Know that with every breath you have the chance, the opportunity to change, to transform. Use the breath to elevate yourself to that highest destiny, and allow the breath to carry you across any and every obstacle."[117]

~ Deva Kaur Khalsa and Sat Purkh Kaur Khalsa

Top Tips for Hormonal Balance

- Eat aubergines and mangoes;[118]
- Avoid refined sugar and alcohol to avoid adding extra stress to the body;[119]
- Ginger helps to relieve menstrual cramps;[120]

---

116 *I Am A Woman*, p.148

117 *I Am A Woman*, p.149

118 *The Aquarian Teacher*, p.254-255

119 *The Aquarian Teacher*, p.254

120 *The Aquarian Teacher*, p.255

- Do a couple of minutes of Long Deep Breathing at any time you feel your hormones are controlling your emotions.

Yoga Routine for Balancing Hormones

Breathing Exercise

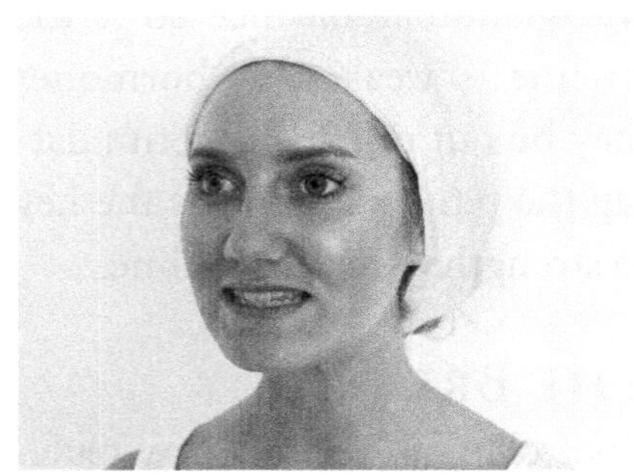

Sitkari Pranayam[121]

Sit in Easy Pose with the spine straight and the chin tucked in slightly. Inhale through the teeth, exhale through the nose. Continue for up to 3 minutes.

Sitkari breath boosts glandular function so helps to balance the hormones. It is also very cleansing.

Kriya

Sahibi Kriya to Master Your Domain[122]

1. Leg Lifts with Breath of Fire through an open mouth. Continue for 2 ½ minutes.

2. Alternate Leg Lifts: lying on the back, lift the left leg up

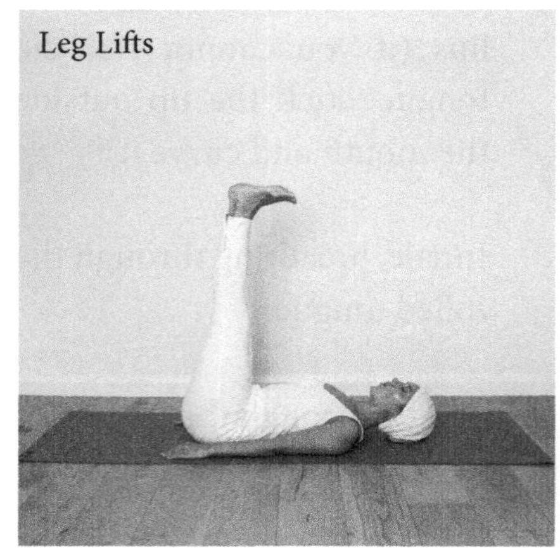

Leg Lifts

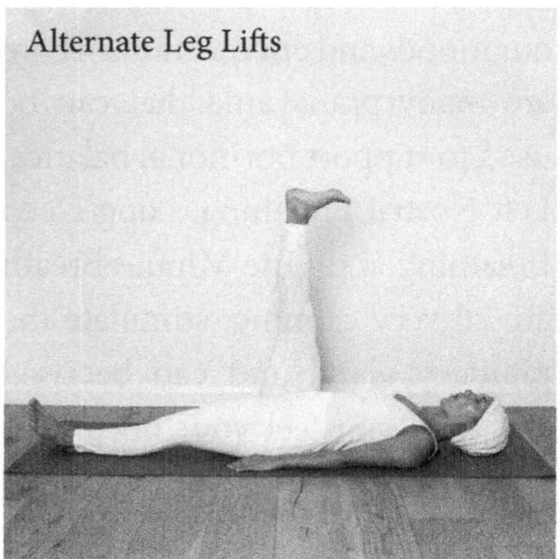

Alternate Leg Lifts

[121] *The Aquarian Teacher*, p.97

[122] The Library of Teachings: www.libraryofteachings.com

on the inhale, so the leg is perpendicular to the ground, then slowly lower it back down on the exhale. Lift the right leg on the inhale and slowly lower it back down on the exhale. Continue with these alternate leg lifts for 2 minutes.

3. On all fours, with the hands underneath the shoulders and the knees underneath the hips (Cow Pose), extend alternate legs up and back as high as possible. Begin Breath of Fire through a circled mouth, raising and lowering the legs rapidly in rhythm with the breath. Continue for 2 minutes.

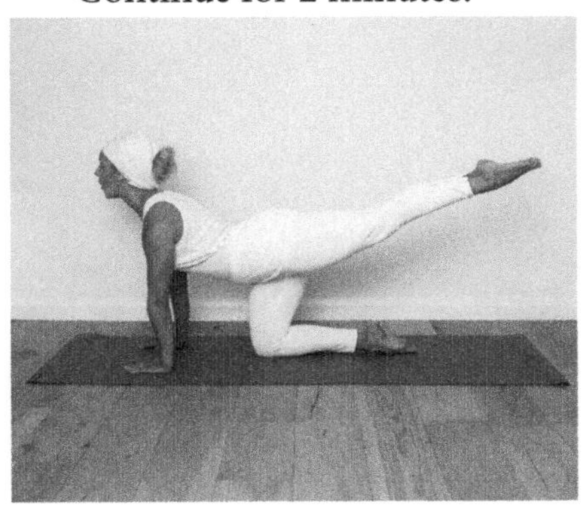

4. Then as you lift the right leg up and back, simultaneously lift the left arm straight out in front of the body. Lower them and raise the opposite arm and leg. Continue alternating the arms and legs, with Breath of Fire through the circled mouth, for 1 minute. To end: inhale, exhale and relax on the heels.

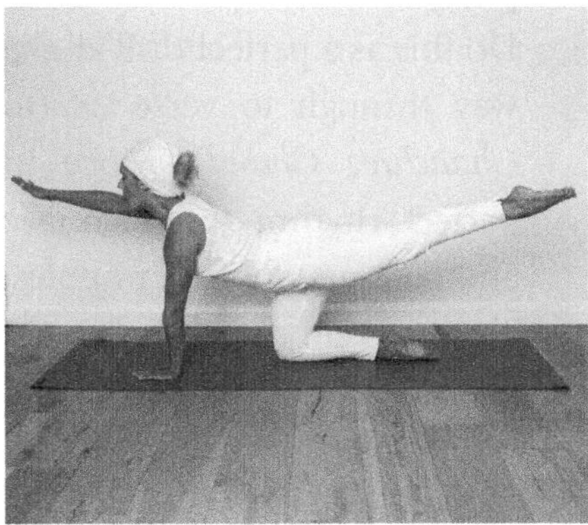

5. Frogs: Squat on the toes with the heels raised and touching each other, fingertips on the ground, and the face forward. Inhale as you lift the hips up, lock the knees, and draw the Navel Point in. The head moves last. Exhale as you bend the knees to return to the starting position. 26 repetitions.

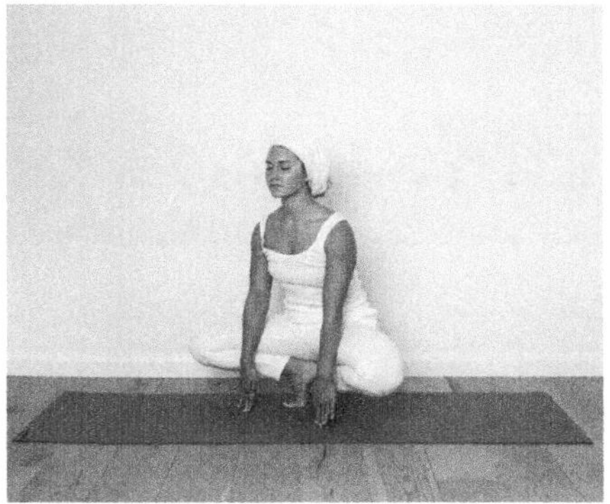

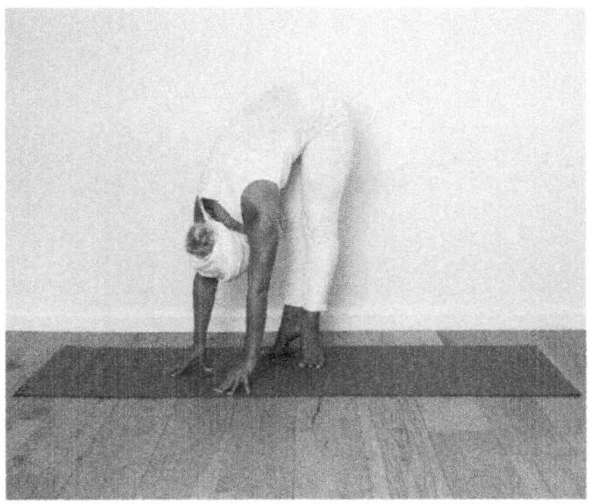

6. Sahibi Kriya: The recording of *Japp Sahib* is used in this exercise. Sit in Easy Pose with the navel pulled in and the

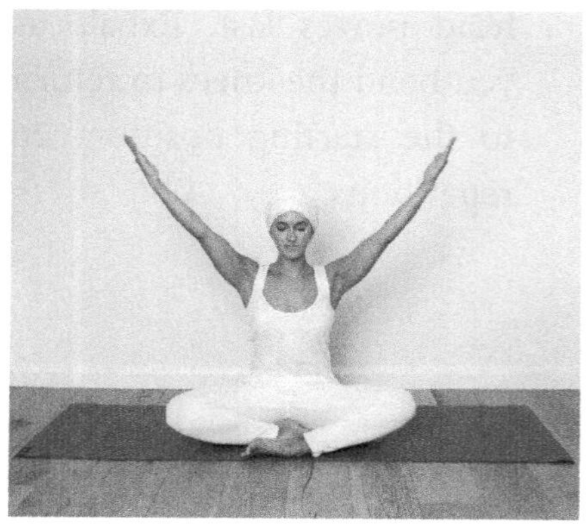

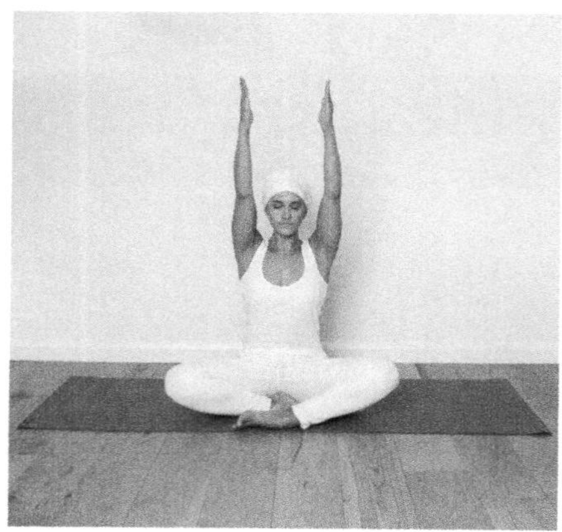

chest out. Tuck the chin in to form a straight line from the base of the spine to the top of the head. Lock yourself in this posture. Extend your arms up to 60 degrees with the palms facing each other. Keep the arms straight with no bend in the elbows. Inhale and extend the arms up to 90 degrees then exhale and lower the arms to 60 degrees. Extend the arms straight up to 90 degrees on the first accented beat (Namastang or Namo) then back down to 60 degrees on the second beat. Do not move at all during musical phrases. Continue movement, taking one complete breath every two seconds. Do this as a perfect drill all the way through to verse 28 (to *Chaachree Chand*). Move in perfect rhythm to the music and continue for 2 ½ minutes. To end: inhale, exhale and relax.

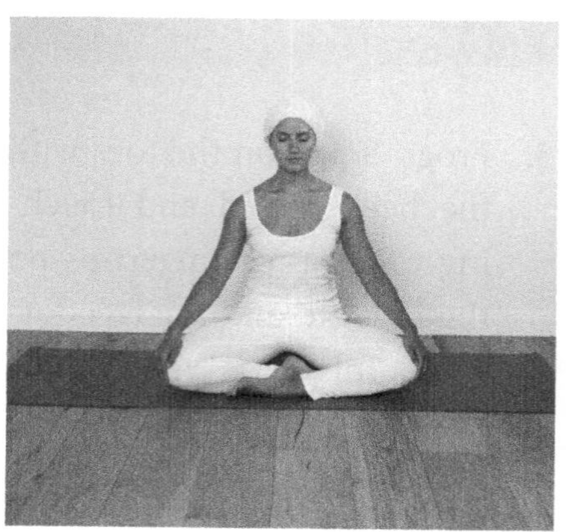

7. Sitting in Easy Pose, breathe long and deep and meditate to music. The song *Himalaya* by Sat Peter Singh was played in the original class taught by Yogi Bhajan. Select any uplifting and relaxing 3HO[123] music. Continue for 2 ½ minutes.

8. Lie down on the back with the legs crossed at the ankles and the hands crossed at the heart. Relax in this position and breathe long and deep. The song *Promises* by Sat Peter Singh was played in the original class. Select any uplifting and relaxing 3HO music. Continue for 2 ½ minutes.

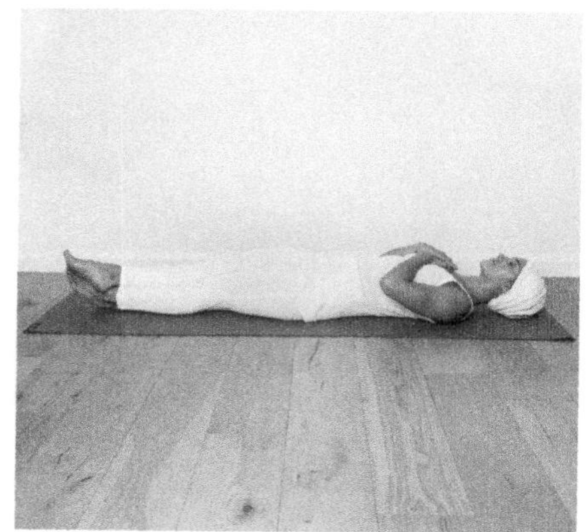

Meditation

BREATH MEDITATION SERIES FOR GLANDULAR BALANCE[124]

1. Sit in Easy Pose: break your inhale and exhale into 16 segments or short "sniffs". With each segment of the breath, both the inhale and the exhale, mentally vibrate *Sat Naam* and pull the Navel Point slightly. Continue for 5 minutes. Then add 1 minute each day to a maximum of 31 minutes per day.

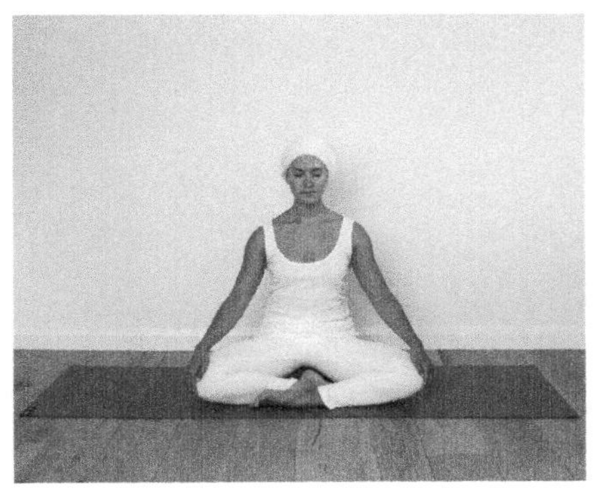

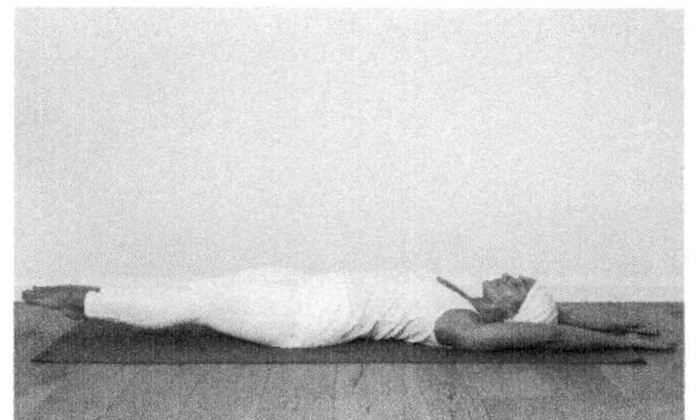

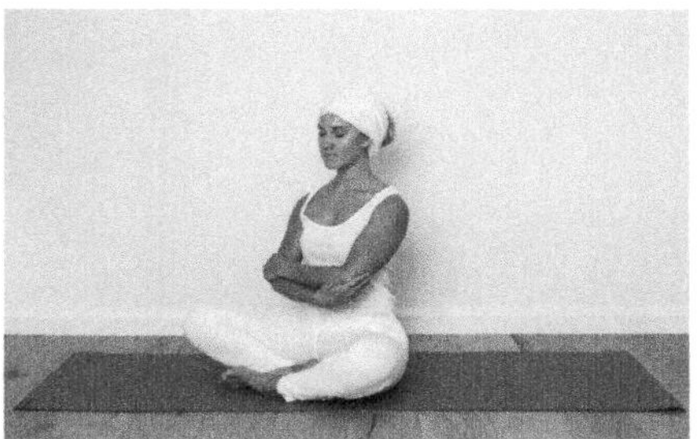

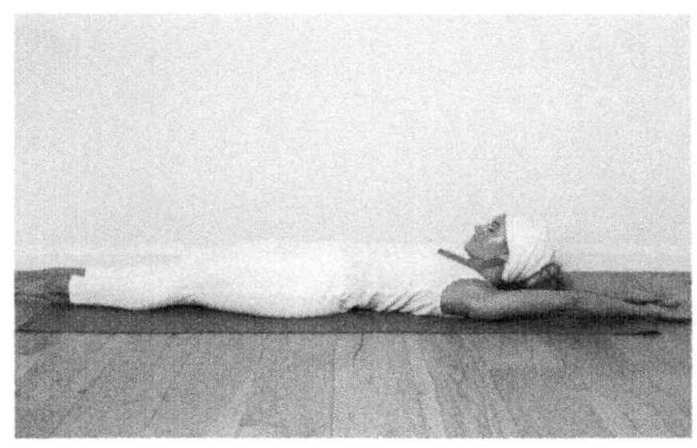

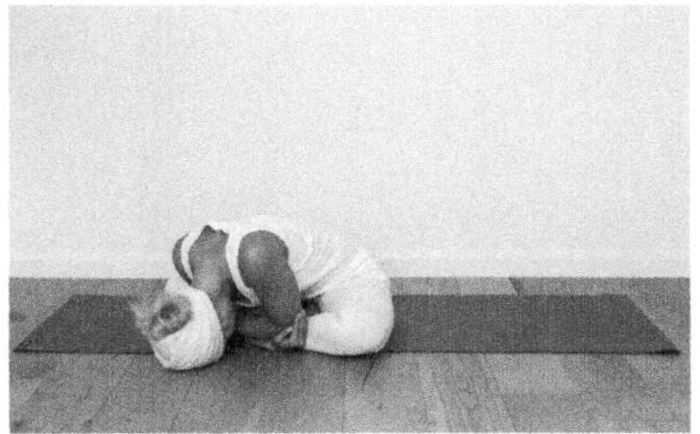

2. Lie on your back. Put the arms straight overhead on the ground with the palms up. Inhale and raise both legs 6 inches. Exhale and lower the legs, bringing the chin to the chest. Continue with Long Deep Breathing for 3 minutes. Rest for 2 minutes.

3. Sit in Easy Pose: grab opposite elbows, with your arms across the chest. Inhale in the upright position. Exhale and bend forward, placing the forehead on the ground. Continue for 3 minutes with Long Deep Breathing.

For a thorough glandular workout, keep the first exercise to 5 minutes then repeat the whole set 3 times.

[124] *Sadhana Guidelines*, p.119

Chapter 11
Strengthening the Inner Light:
Boosting the Immune System

"Kundalini Yoga teaches you the techniques and awareness to stay healthy. You gain a strong immune system, vital glands, a strong nervous system, good circulation, and an awareness of the impact of your habits."

~ Yogi Bhajan[125]

The human body has several layers of defence against bacteria, viruses, fungi, malignant cells and other harmful substances, starting with the Aura (or electromagnetic field), the skin and the mucous membranes. Any invading pathogens that get past those then face a generalised response from the immune system, followed by a specific response from the lymphocytes (a type of white blood cell).

Many things can weaken the immune system including stress, being rundown, not getting enough sleep, not getting enough exercise and not eating properly. There are also various auto-immune disorders that prevent the immune system from being able to distinguish between parts of the self and invading pathogens. As a result, the body attacks and destroys healthy body tissue by mistake. These disorders include systemic lupus erythematosus (SLE, or simply lupus), coeliac disease (gluten-sensitive enteropathy) and type I diabetes. Various other illnesses, drugs and chemotherapy also affect the function of the immune system.

It is common for young children to get ill fairly frequently: their immune system is battling lots of invading pathogens for the first time and is naturally weaker than an adult's immune system in any case. Unless, that is, the adult is a stressed, sleep-deprived mum!

Being frequently ill is not only miserable but also makes looking after children really difficult – there are no sick days! And it is much more difficult to recover

125 From a lecture called *What is Yoga?* published in *The Aquarian Teacher*, p.18

from illness when there is little chance of a good night's sleep.

Is this you?

- Are you susceptible to infection? Do you get colds, flu or fungal infections frequently?
- Do the severity of your symptoms seem worse and last longer than they should?
- Do you get recurrent infections such as kidney, sinus and ear infections or tonsillitis?
- Have you found a regular course of antibiotics is insufficient to kill a bacterial infection?
- Do you have raised brown rough skin patches, particularly on the abdomen and back (Actinic keratosis)?
- Are you suffering from stress?
- Do you drink alcohol or smoke frequently?
- Are you sleep-deprived?

Reflection points

- Note in your diary when you are ill to identify any patterns that may be developing. Are the children bringing infections home from preschool or school regularly? Are you more susceptible to infection during the winter months?
- Can you enlist any help with the children when you are ill?
- Are you nurturing yourself as much as possible during any child-free and work-free time you have available? Can you find any time to have a break, even if it's just a couple of hours once a week? Are there any responsibilities you could step down from for a while?
- Are you, and everyone in your home, washing your hands as effectively as possible, including the backs of the hands, the wrists and between the fingers, to reduce the risk of any infection spreading?
- Are you all strictly using your own towels and not sharing with anyone else?
- Can you open all the windows in your home for 10 minutes a day to allow the air to circulate?

Yogic Viewpoint

Yoga has a powerful cleansing effect. It stimulates blood circulation and the lymphatic system in particular (which carries the lymphocytes mentioned above). It massages the spleen (which purifies the blood by removing damaged and old red and white blood cells) and the **thymus gland** (which is involved in maturing white blood cells).

All pranayam supports the immune system because it oxygenates the blood.

Mantra and the Science of Sound

One of the things that differentiates Kundalini Yoga from many other forms of Yoga is the use of mantra as an integral part of the practice. This is not to say other forms of Yoga do not use mantra – many do – but you are unlikely to come across it used routinely in most non-Kundalini Yoga classes in the UK. Kundalini Yoga uses the ancient science of **Naad Yoga** which is based on the experience of how sound vibrations affect the body, mind and spirit through the movement of the tongue and the mouth and changes in the brain chemistry. Many of the mantras used in Kundalini Yoga come from **Japji Sahib**, the beginning section of **Siri Guru Granth Sahib**.

The power of mantra comes from the vibration of a specific, repeated sound in the body. We use mantras to alter and elevate our consciousness through repetition and the meaning of the specific words being chanted.

The movement of the tongue stimulates meridian points on the roof of the mouth. Repeated patterns of the same movement (i.e. chanting the same mantra over and over again) send messages to the hypothalamus in the brain. The hypothalamus, which carries out a variety of functions and is connected by blood vessels to the pituitary gland, translates these messages into instructions. These instructions regulate chemical messengers, or hormones, that go to all areas of the body.

In particular, stimulating the hypothalamus with sound and rhythm has a powerful effect on the immune system. It improves the use of cells like natural killer cells that fight viruses and cancer, and helps remove toxins.

It is clear there is a complex relationship between sound, the brain and many other facets of the human experience. A new field of study, known as Psychoneuroimmunology, is currently researching the connection between psychology, chemistry, neurology and the immune functions. In time, no doubt we will have a greater understanding of this relationship.

"Vibrate the Cosmos, the Cosmos shall clear the path."
~ one of Yogi Bhajan's 5 Sutras for the Aquarian Age[126]

[126] *The Aquarian Teacher*, p.6

THE AURA

The body's electro-magnetic field, or Aura, protects it from illness. So if the Aura is strong, illness cannot penetrate into the Physical Body. Meditation and wearing white clothing made of natural fibres strengthen the Aura,[127] as do arm exercises and postures such as Triangle Pose (see page 122).[128]

PRANIC BODY

All disease starts with the **Pranic Body**, one of the **Ten Bodies**, being out of balance. Pranayam brings the Pranic Body into balance.[129]

Top tips for boosting the immune system

- For the spleen: yellow vegetables, bananas, honey, sunflower seeds, yoghurt, okra, citrus fruit, buckwheat, olives, cabbage, vitamins C, D, F and B complex, iron, copper and manganese;[130]
- Garlic has many healing properties;[131]
- Onions are said to stimulate the production of blood and to keep the blood purified;[132]
- Avoid alcohol which poisons the body and increases stress, making us more vulnerable to lowered immunity;[133]
- Avoid acidic foods such as meat, eggs, starches, sweets and butter products. An acidic environment is susceptible to the development of cancer and other illnesses. According to the yogic tradition, for maximum health the blood should be 75% alkaline and 25% acidic;[134]
- Do as much pranayam as possible to balance the Pranic Body.

127 *The Aquarian Teacher*, p.202
128 *The Aquarian Teacher*, p.186
129 *The Aquarian Teacher*, p.202
130 *The Aquarian Teacher*, p.171
131 *The Aquarian Teacher*, p.254
132 *The Aquarian Teacher*, p.254
133 *The Aquarian Teacher*, p.254
134 *The Aquarian Teacher*, p.253

Yoga Set to Boost the Immune System

Breathing Exercise

Boost Your Immune System[135]

Sit in Easy Pose with your chin in and your chest lifted. Stick your tongue (the central vagus nerve) all the way out and keep it out as you rapidly breathe in and out through your mouth. Continue this panting diaphragmatic breath for 3-5 minutes.

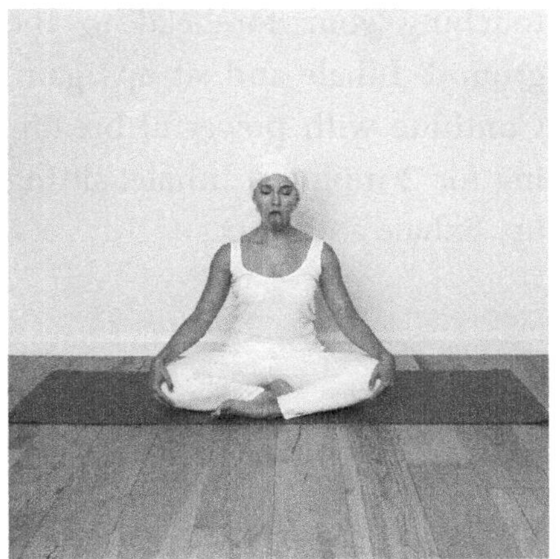

To end: inhale, hold the breath in for 15 seconds and press the tongue against the upper palate. Exhale. Repeat this sequence 2 more times.

This breathing technique is known as Dog Breath. It is a detoxifying breath that also strengthens the throat chakra and thyroid.

Kriya

Kriya for Disease Resistance[136]

Pumping the Stomach: sit on the heels. Stretch the arms straight up over the head with the palms pressed together. Inhale. Pump the stomach by forcefully drawing the navel in toward the spine and then

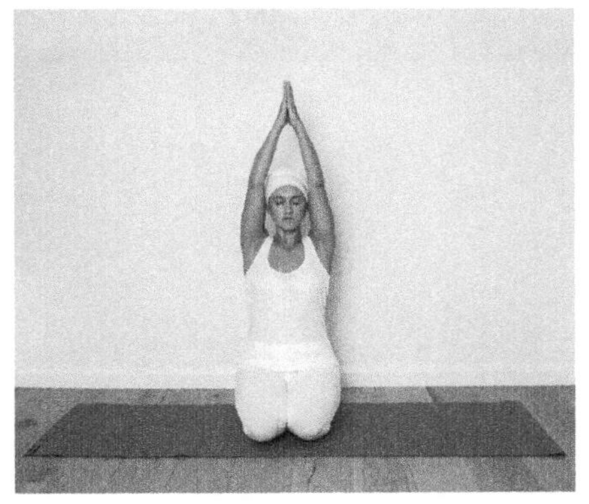

relaxing it again. Continue rhythmically until you feel the need to exhale. Then exhale. Inhale and begin again. Continue for 2 minutes. Then inhale, exhale and relax.

Bear Grip: still sitting on the heels, place the hands in Bear

---

[135] *Praana Praanee Praanayam*, p.187. First taught by Yogi Bhajan on 31st January 1996

[136] *The Aquarian Teacher*, pp.360-361

Grip (right palm facing the chest, left palm facing out, with the fingers gripping each other) at chest level with the forearms parallel to the ground. Inhale. Hold the breath and without separating the hands, try to pull them apart. Apply maximum force. Exhale. Inhale and pull again. Continue for 2 minutes. Inhale, exhale and relax.

Bear Grip

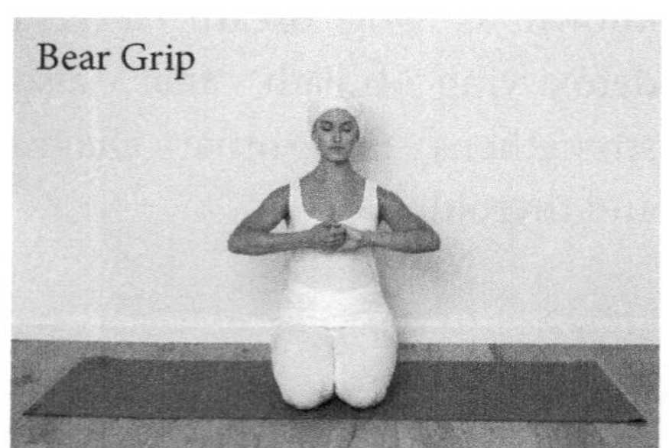

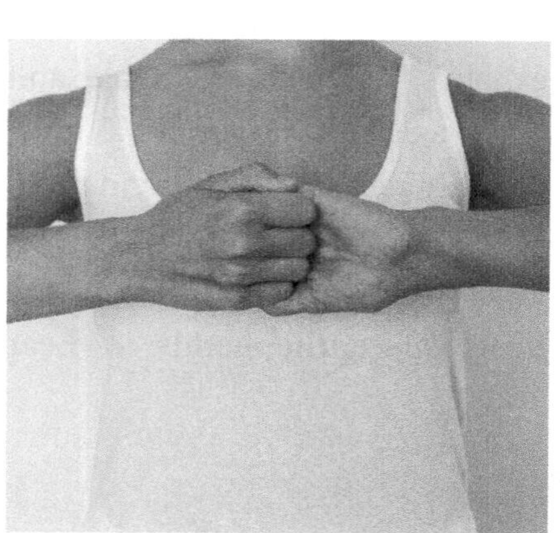

Sitting Bends: still sitting on the heels, interlock the fingers in **Venus Lock** behind the neck. Inhale. Exhale and bend forward, touching your forehead to the ground. Inhale and sit up again. Continue with powerful breathing for 2 minutes. Inhale, sitting up. Exhale and relax.

Sitting Bends

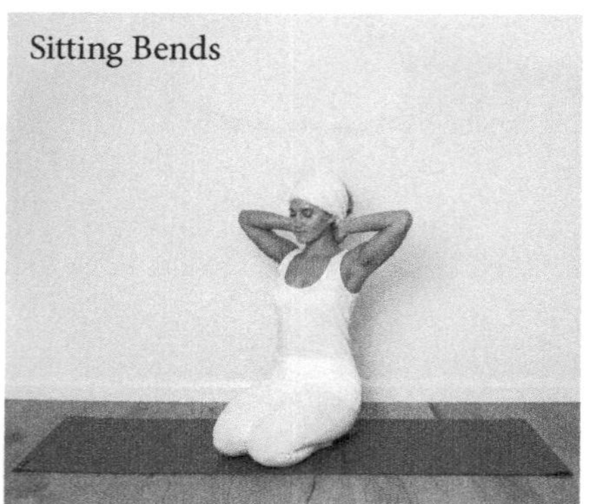

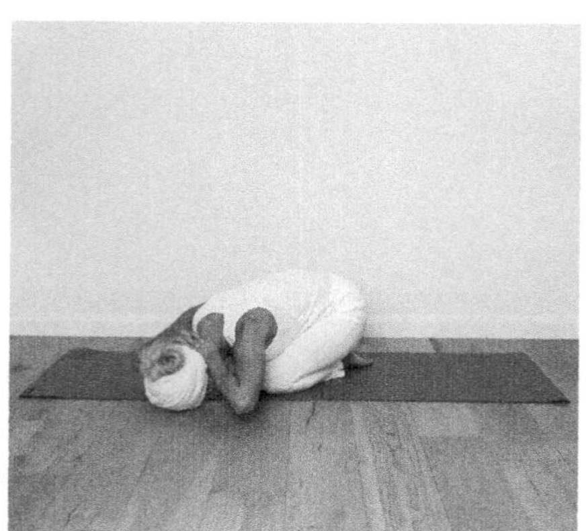

Front Stretch: sit with the legs stretched out in front. Hold the toes in finger lock (index finger and middle finger pulling the toe, and the thumb pressing the nail of the big toe). Exhale and lengthen the core of the spine, bending forward from the navel and continuing to lengthen the spine. The head follows last. Remain in this position breathing normally for 2 minutes. Then inhale, exhale and relax.

Front Stretch

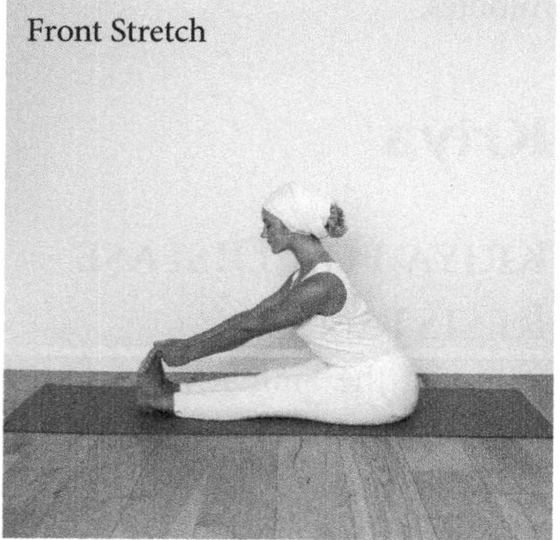

Neck rolls: sit in Easy Pose. Begin rolling the neck clockwise in a circular motion, bringing the right ear toward the right shoulder, the back of the head toward the back of the neck, the left ear toward the left shoulder and the chin toward the chest. The shoulders remain relaxed and motionless and the neck should be allowed to gently stretch as the head circles round. Continue for 1 minute then reverse the direction and continue for 1 more minute. Bring the head to a central position and relax.

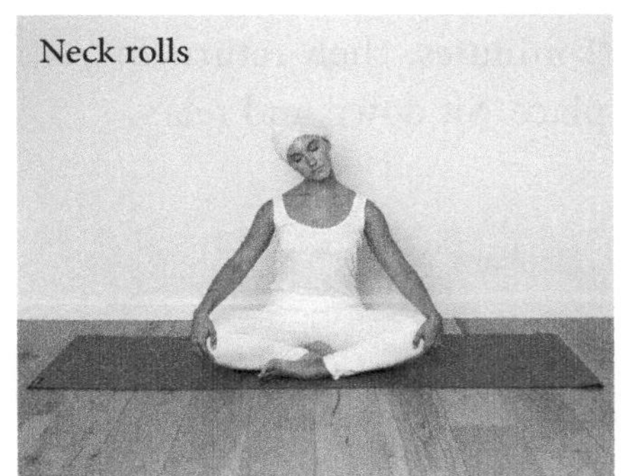
Neck rolls

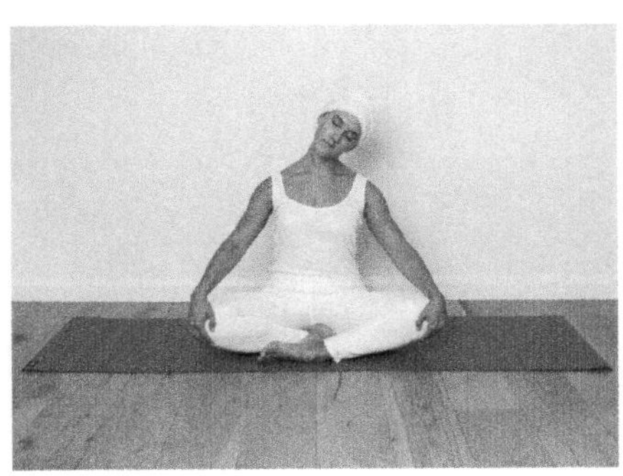

Author's suggestion: If you have any problems with the neck, or if this exercise does not feel right for any reason, you can move the head in small circles instead, as if you had a pencil extended from the top, so there is no movement in the neck. Alternatively, simply sit and picture the head moving.

Cat-Cow: come onto on all fours, with the hands underneath the shoulders and the knees shoulder-width apart, underneath the hips. The arms are straight. Inhale and flex the spine downwards as if someone were sitting on your back. Stretch the neck and head back. Then exhale and round the spine, bringing the chin towards the chest. Continue rhythmically with powerful breathing for 2 minutes. Gradually increase your speed as you feel the spine becoming more flexible. Inhale in the original, flat-back position. Exhale and relax.

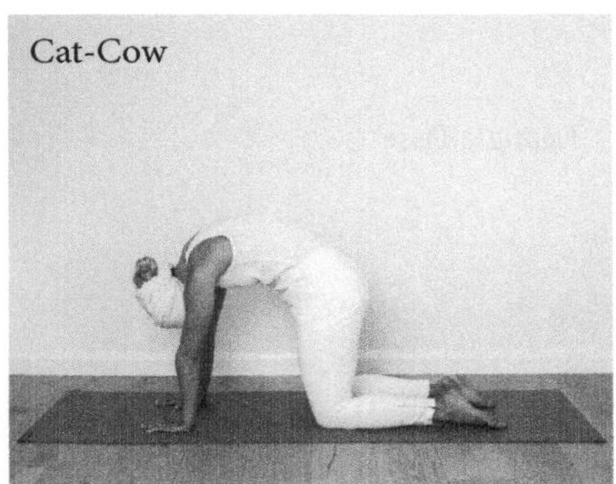
Cat-Cow

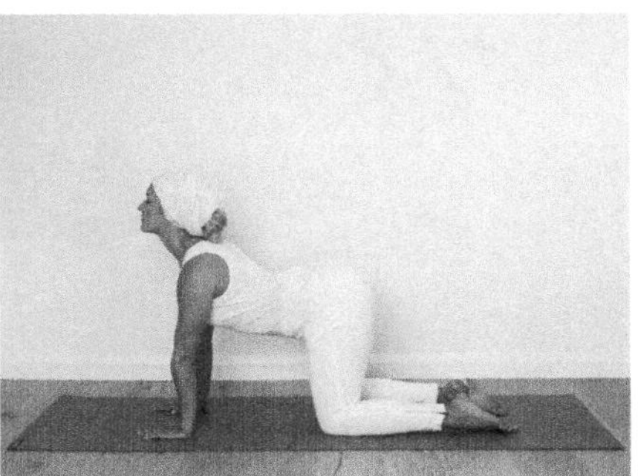

Author's suggestion: Keep the eyes closed.

Alternate Shoulder Shrugs: sit on the heels. Alternately shrug your shoulders as high as possible, keeping the head still. On the inhale, lift the left shoulder as the right shoulder goes down. On the exhale, lift the right shoulder up and the left down. Continue rhythmically with powerful breathing for 2 minutes. Inhale, raising both shoulders up. Exhale and relax.

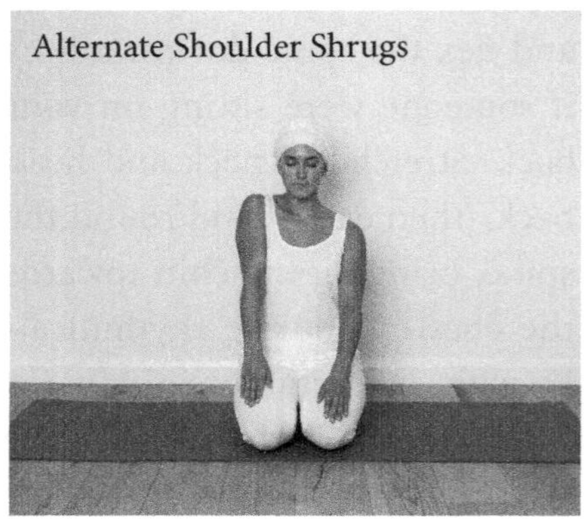
Alternate Shoulder Shrugs

Corpse Pose: lie on the back with the arms at the sides, palms facing up, and deeply relax for 5-7 minutes.

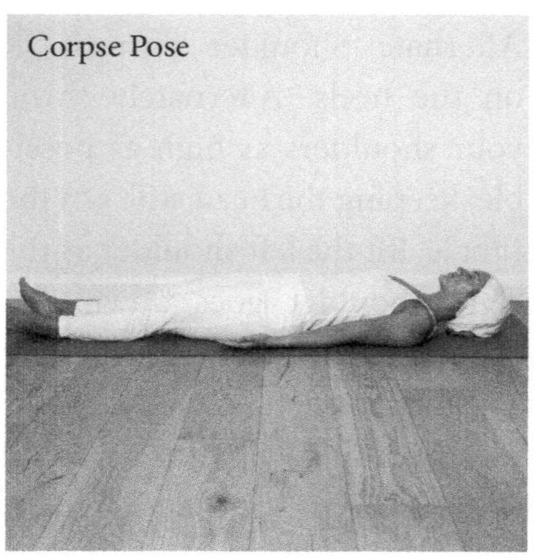
Corpse Pose

Triangle Pose: place the palms of the hands and the soles of the feet flat on the ground. Feet are approximately hip-width apart. Create a straight line between the wrists and the hips, and from the hips to the heels. The chin is pulled in. Roll the armpits towards each other. Hold this position for 5 minutes, breathing normally. Then inhale. Exhale and slowly come of the position and relax.

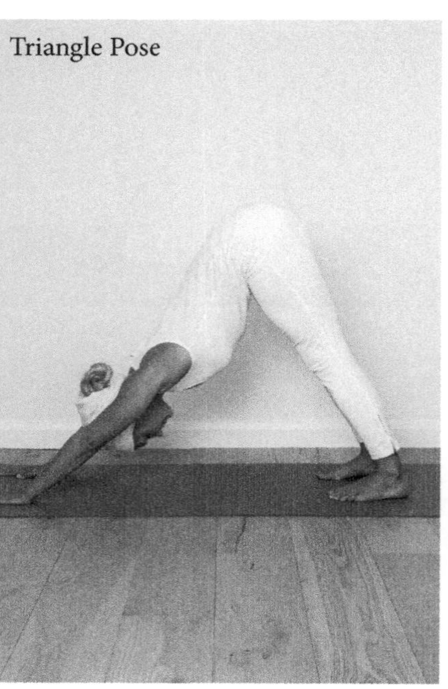
Triangle Pose

Author's suggestion: Start on all fours and lift the knees and the hips to come into the position. Come back onto all fours at the end of the exercise and sit back on the heels to come out of the position.

Elephant Walk: from a standing position, reach down and hold onto the ankles. Keeping the knees straight, begin walking around the room. Continue for 2 minutes, then return to your place. Sit down and relax.

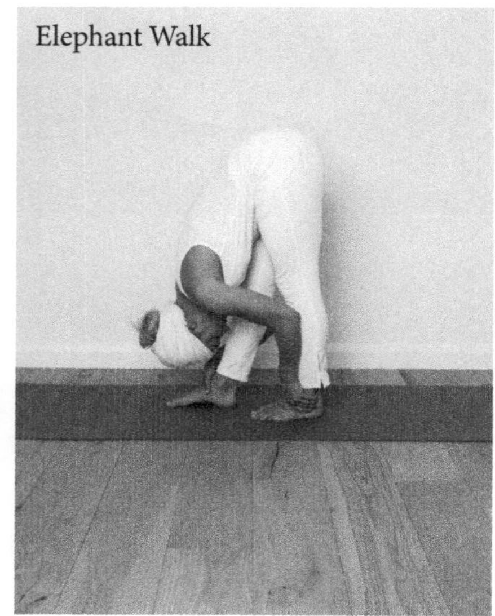
Elephant Walk

Meditation

Meditation for Projection and Protection from the Heart[137]

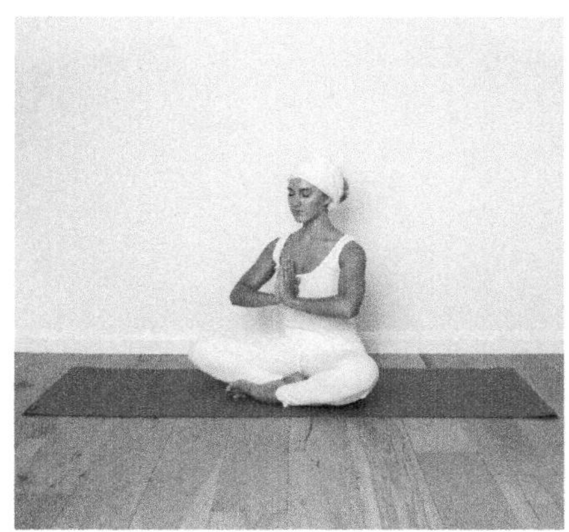

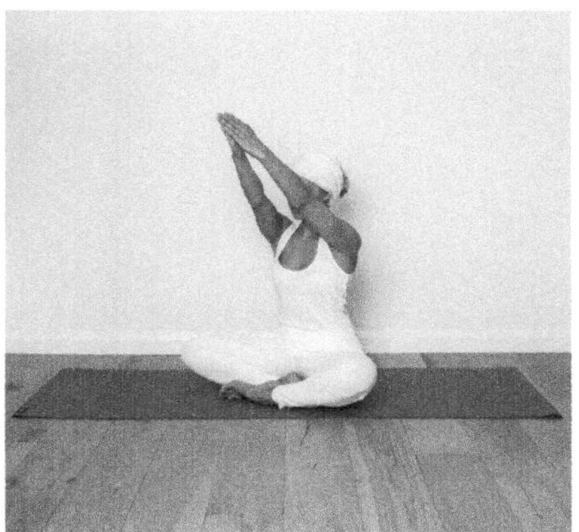

Sit in Easy Pose with your chin tucked in and your chest lifted. Place the hands together in Prayer Pose, level with the Heart Centre. The thumbs are crossed. Chant the Mangala Charn Mantra: *Aad Guray Nameh, Jugaad Guray Nameh, Sat Guray Nameh, Siree Guroo Dayvay Nameh.* As you chant each phrase, extend the arms as shown in the picture. Between each phrase, inhale the arms back into Prayer Pose at the Heart Centre.

Continue for 11 minutes.

The Mangala Charn Mantra is a protective mantra. It is said to surround the magnetic field with protective light.

[137] From the Library of Teachings. Originally taught by Yogi Bhajan in February 1975

Chapter 12
Light at the End of the Tunnel:
Breaking Free from Addictions

"First you make habits, then habits make you."
~ Yogi Bhajan[138]

Modern humans struggle with all kinds of addictions: substances (including nicotine, alcohol, caffeine, refined sugar, illegal drugs such as cannabis and cocaine and legal drugs such as sleeping pills), patterns of behaviour (sex and love addiction, internet addiction, shopping addiction, gambling, compulsive eating and bulimia) and patterns of emotional response (a compulsion towards financial or social advancement, addiction to being needed or accepted or to unhealthy relationships).

Whether patterns of behaviour and emotional response should be classed as addictions in the same way as substance addictions is a matter for debate but for our purposes, we are talking about any potentially damaging habits over which we cannot exercise control. For instance, is the person who smokes a couple of cigarettes a day, or has one glass of wine every evening with dinner, in more trouble than the person who ignores her children all day while gambling compulsively online, racking up thousands of pounds of debt she cannot repay?

The result of habits we cannot control is always the same: neurotic, compulsive behaviour and insecurity. They may also cause us other problems like debt, unhealthy weight and intoxication with dangerous chemicals. Dangerous habits damage relationships, including those we have with our children. We are their role models and they are learning from our behaviour. Any addiction can eventually be fatal because of toxic overload, illness or suicide.

[138] Quoted in *The 8 Human Talents* by Gurmukh Kaur Khalsa with Cathryn Michon (HarperCollins Publishers Inc, 2000), p.1

Exhausted parents – like anyone on the road towards burnout – are particularly vulnerable to losing themselves in addictions. This may be due to a wish to escape from the grinding relentlessness of caring for young children, or from feeling constantly tired, or from problems with significant relationships. As we have seen earlier they are also susceptible to depression, which is often linked with addictive behaviour.

All addictions share certain characteristics including denial, high tolerance, preoccupation, withdrawal symptoms, risk of damage to significant relationships and a wish for escape. Matters are complicated by the false information and advertising with which we are surrounded (there is a lot of money being made out of your habits!) and the (often well-meant but ignorant) input of friends and family. Many health professionals have little understanding about addictions unless they have personal experience.

Appendix II contains details of the main addictions which tend to relate to parents of young children (although this should not be regarded as an exhaustive list) along with contact details of the main organisations available to help or provide further information. Most organisations can be contacted by email if you don't want to speak to someone over the telephone.

"Stimulants kill you. It doesn't matter what they are."
~ Yogi Bhajan[139]

Is this You?

- Do you feel guilty about the extent to which you indulge your particular habit?
- Do you indulge your habit in order to change your mood? For example, do you have a cigarette when you feel stressed, a glass of wine when you feel bored, or go shopping when you feel lonely?
- Do you tend to "reward" yourself at the end of the day with your particular habit?
- Do you intend to have a small amount of a particular substance then feel compelled to consume more? Or intend to spend only a certain amount of time or money on your habit, but find yourself indulging more than you had planned?
- Do you hide evidence of your habit from your partner or anyone else?

[139] *Kundalini Yoga: The Flow of Eternal Power*, p.278

Reflection Points

- How would you react if you were told you could never indulge your habit again?

- Would you consider giving up your habit for a fixed period, such as a month? Could you do it if you had the additional incentive of being sponsored and raising money for a charitable cause close to your heart?

- How do you feel about people who have already given up the same habit?

- How has your relationship with your habit changed over the years? Is it as much fun as it used to be? Do you feel more guilty about it now than you used to? Have people commented on it?

- Do you fully understand the impact your habit has on your health? The consequences of sugar addiction, for example, include hyperglycemia, weight gain, tooth decay, pancreatic problems and type 2 diabetes. Bowel diseases, including cancers, constipation and excessive wind, are all commonly found in those addicted to sugar, along with poor dental hygiene, arthritis and obesity. Sugar is particularly unhelpful for anyone suffering from exhaustion because it disturbs sleep, increases any hormonal imbalance and feeds cortisol, the hormone that generates stress.

- What might your children be learning about how to manage the pressures of life if you turn to the drinks cabinet, a packet of cigarettes or the biscuit tin every time you feel stressed? What did you learn from your own parents?

- Spend some time thinking about how you have developed your particular habit. For example, do you regularly drink alcohol in the evenings as a form of escapism, because it relaxes you quickly, to spend time with your partner or because you miss the social life you enjoyed before having children? If you drink caffeine, is it because you feel you can't get going in the morning without it, or because you experience a dip of energy mid-afternoon? Does a sugary snack make you feel comforted or give you a boost of energy?

- How much money would you save if you gave up your habit?

- Can you identify any times when you particularly crave a substance you want to give up? For example, are you more likely to smoke when you feel stressed? Are you more likely to crave alcohol around 5pm, before eating, and drink less after you have eaten?

- Is there something you could substitute for a substance you want to give up? For example, if you can't imagine life without chocolate, try some raw chocolate from your local health food shop instead.

Yogic Viewpoint: Positive Habits

Physical addiction is only part of the picture; habits become associated with various aspects of our lives to such an extent that suddenly giving them up can feel like we have cut off a limb. Smokers often smoke at specific points in the day: during a morning tea-break or after lunch, for example. Caffeine drinkers associate sitting down with a cup of tea or coffee as a short break from work or housework. Alcohol can be the focus point around which people socialise; giving it up can mean completely rethinking how we spend our leisure time and maybe even who our friends are.

The fact that humans are prone to habitual behaviour is something we can use to our advantage; the yogic approach is to replace demoting habits with promoting habits. Yogi Bhajan taught it takes 40 days to master a new habit because "it takes time for a conscious action or habit to permeate the subconscious and finally command the unconscious." So we can establish a positive habit such as a daily Yoga practice and over time, "the subconscious begins to support you and *sadhana* begins to feel effortless. The subconscious, which directs about 85% of our activities and responses, has now acquired a habit – a habit to support your growth in consciousness and awareness through the practice of *sadhana*."[140]

Habits and the Lower Triangle

The lower chakras, or the "lower triangle", are also relevant to a discussion regarding addictions and how we overcome them through Kundalini Yoga. The Root Chakra, the most basic of the major chakras, is the realm of habits and automatic behaviour. It is also the chakra in which we are most alone. Feeling alone and disconnected is something with which addicts often identify.

[140] *Sadhana Guidelines*, p.30

Addictions relating to food reside in the Sacral Chakra, and the ability to make and break habits is associated with the Navel Chakra. This is the chakra where our will power resides so we need it to be strong and balanced if we are to have the courage and determination to save ourselves from addiction.

SELF-AWARENESS AND ACCEPTANCE

Having the self-awareness to recognise we suffer from an addiction is the first step to healing ourselves of it. Acknowledging an addiction is nothing to be ashamed of; it takes a lot of courage and anyone who genuinely cares about you will support you.

The *yamas* and *niyamas* of the yogic lifestyle (see chapter 6) can assist us here. Being truthful about the extent of a problem with addiction, letting go of the mask we have been hiding behind and forgiving ourselves for our actions is an application of *satya*. Detoxifying the body is an example of *shaucha*. Accepting that we are what we are is *santosha*. We need to employ determination, the principle of *tapas*, to be successful in giving up a habit. Practising *ahimsa* means giving up a habit that is causing harm to ourselves and possibly those around us, without judging ourselves or beating ourselves up about it.

THE PINEAL GLAND

Western scientific knowledge is only just beginning to understand the various functions of the pineal gland, located in the brain. We do know that it reaches maturity when a person is around 7 years old, when the gland is about the size of a chickpea, after which it shrinks and its secretions decrease until it reaches the size of a grain of wheat by adulthood[141]. Many Kundalini Yoga kriyas stimulate the pineal gland and reverse this shrinking process. In the Kundalini Yoga tradition, it is said that imbalance in the pineal gland makes mental and physical addictions seem unbreakable.

Top Tips for Breaking a Habit

- Yogi Bhajan taught it takes 40 days to change a habit and 90 days to confirm the new habit. In 120 days the new habit is who you are and in 1,000 days, you have mastered the new habit;[142]

- When giving up an addictive substance, Yogi Bhajan

[141] *Kundalini Yoga: The Flow of Eternal Power* by Shakti Parwha Kaur Khalsa, p.51

[142] *The Aquarian Teacher*, p.136

advised substituting oxygen instead. For example, a smoker should take a maximum inhale followed by a maximum exhale whenever they feel a craving and within a week or two, they will have given up smoking;[143]

- Use the "Gatga" practice referred to earlier: repeat the mantra *Ek Ong Kar Sat Gur Prasaad, Sat Gur Prasaad Ek Ong Kar* five times, every time you feel a craving for your habit.[144]

Yoga Routine for Breaking Addictions

Breathing Exercise

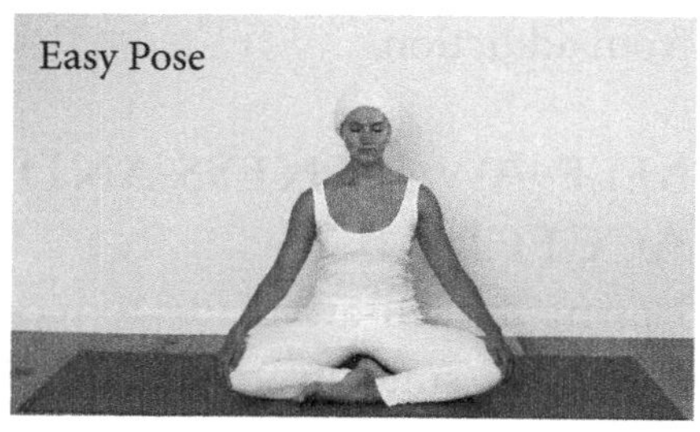

BREATH OF FIRE

Amongst other things, Breath of Fire breaks the subconscious habit patterns that fuel addictions. Sit in Easy Pose and follow the instructions for Breath of Fire from Chapter 1 for up to 3 minutes.

Kriya

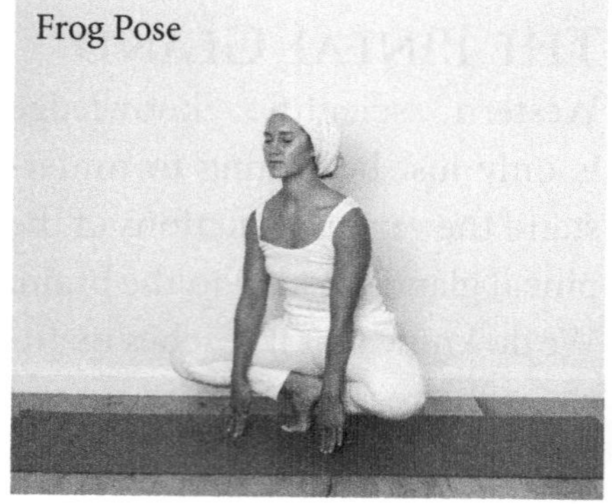

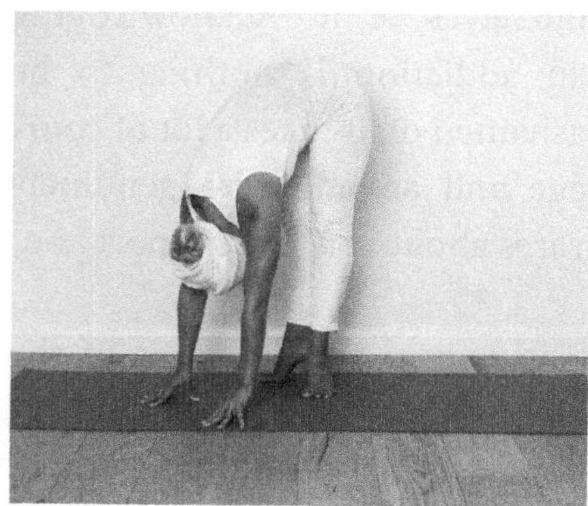

NABHI KRIYA[145]

Author's Note: Go easy with this kriya, especially the leg lifts, during the heaviest part of your Moon Cycle.

---

143 From a lecture given on 18th October 1999 in Albuquerque, New Mexico

144 *Kundalini Yoga: The Flow of Eternal Power*, p.221

145 *The Aquarian Teacher*, p.345

Prepare for this kriya by doing up to 26 "Frogs" which strengthen and balance the lower chakras, the region of habits: squat on the toes with the heels raised and touching each other, fingertips on the ground and the face forward. Inhale as you lift the hips up, lock the knees so the legs are straight, and draw the Navel Point in. The head moves last. Exhale as you bend the knees to return to the starting position.

Caution: Frogs can be done slowly but the breathing is the other way around, exhaling as you straighten the legs and inhaling as you bend the knees, and the heels may drop to the ground.

Alternate Leg Lifts: on the back, inhale and lift the right leg up to 90 degrees. Exhale and lower it. Repeat with the left leg. Continue alternate leg lifts with deep, powerful breathing for 5 minutes.

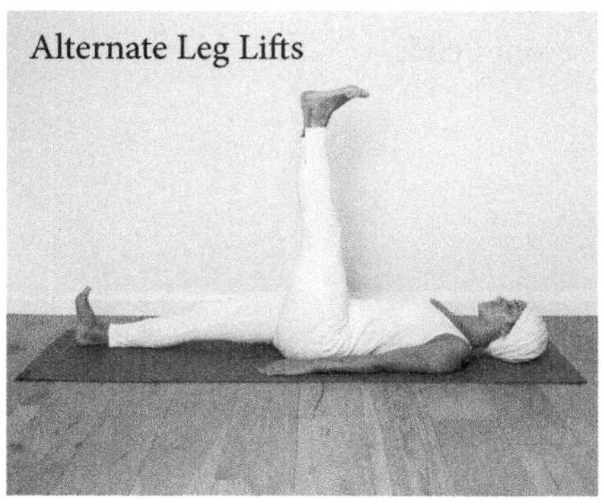
Alternate Leg Lifts

Leg Lifts: without pause, lift both legs up to 90 degrees on the inhale, and lower them on the exhale. For balance and energy, have the arms stretched straight up, palms facing each other. Continue for 2 ½ minutes.

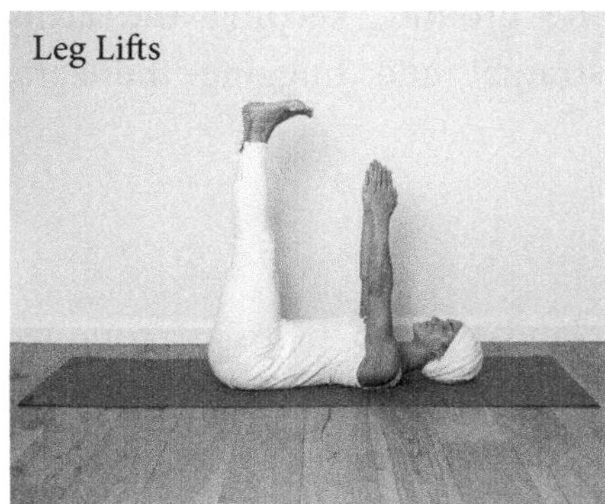
Leg Lifts

Knees to Chest: bend knees and clasp them to the chest with the arms, allowing the head to relax back. Rest in this position for 2 ½ minutes.

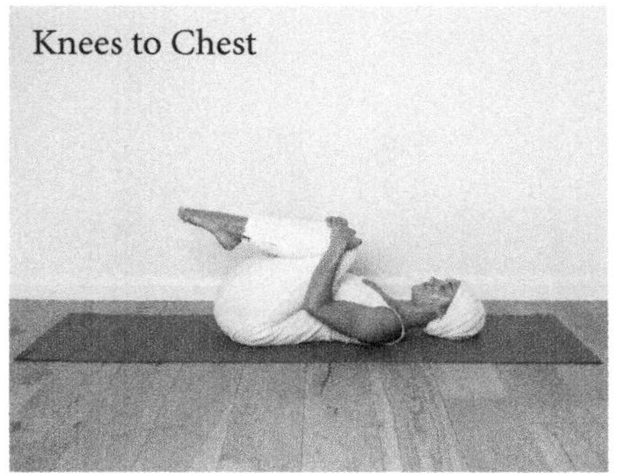
Knees to Chest

Beginning in the Knees to Chest position above, inhale, open the arms out to the sides on the ground and extend the legs straight out to 60 degrees. Exhale and return to the original position. Repeat and continue for 7 ½ minutes.

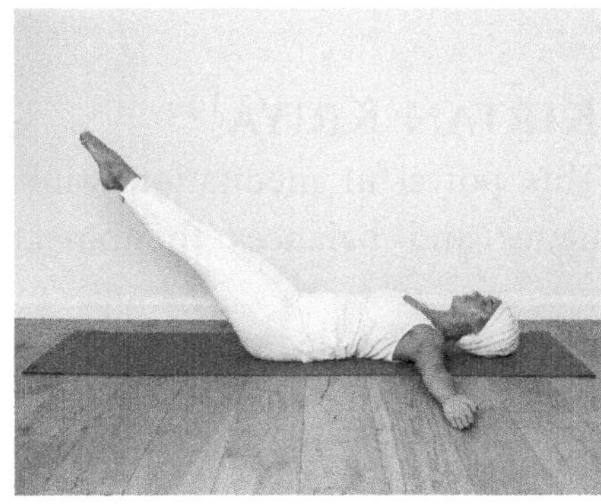

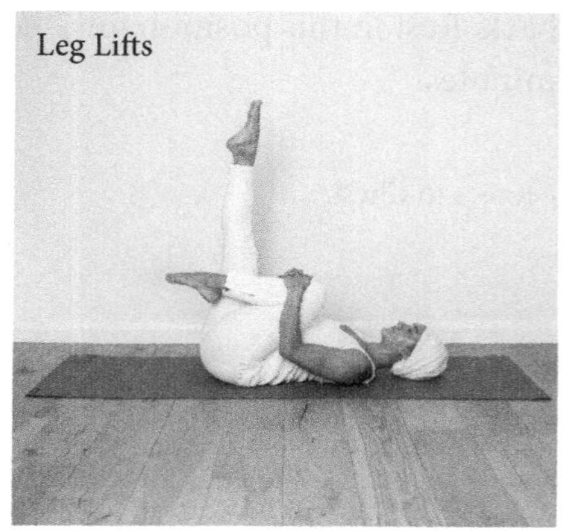
Leg Lifts

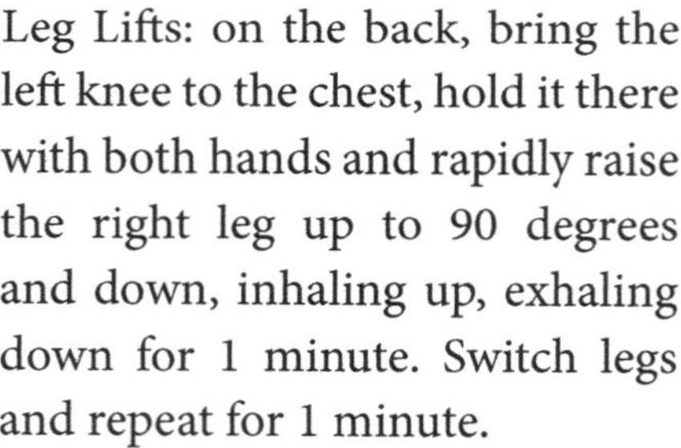

Leg Lifts: on the back, bring the left knee to the chest, hold it there with both hands and rapidly raise the right leg up to 90 degrees and down, inhaling up, exhaling down for 1 minute. Switch legs and repeat for 1 minute.

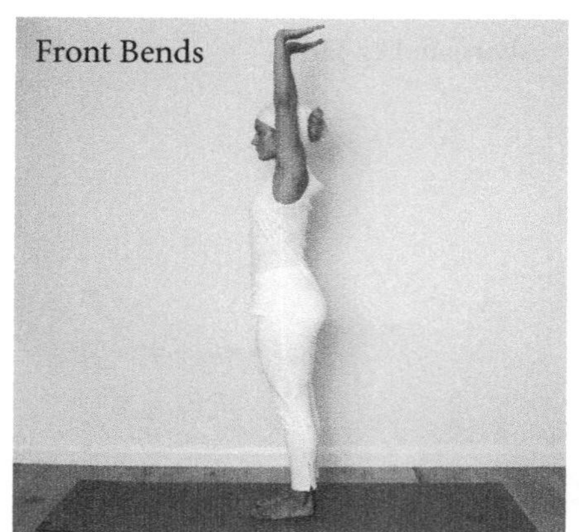
Front Bends

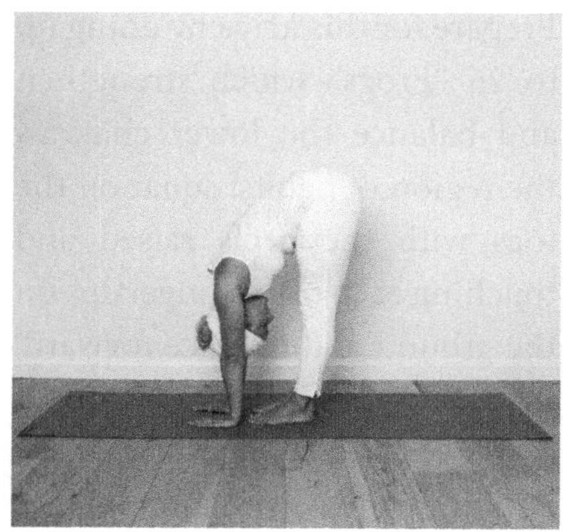

Front Bends: stand up straight, raising the arms overhead, hugging the ears and pressing the fingers back so that the palms face the sky or ceiling. Exhale as you bend forward to touch the ground, keeping the arms straight and hugging the ears, and inhaling up, very slowly with deep breathing. On the exhale, apply the Root Lock. Continue at a slow pace for 1 minute then more rapidly for 1 more minute.

Totally relax or meditate for 10-15 minutes.

Meditation

Kirtan Kriya[146]

This powerful meditation stimulates and balances the pineal gland. It also helps to conquer the fear that can make giving up addictions seem impossible.

Sit in Easy Pose. The eyes are closed, focused at the point between the eyebrows.

---

[146] *The Aquarian Teacher*, p.425

Chant: *Sa Ta Na Ma*

Each repetition of this mantra takes 3 to 4 seconds.

Begin with the hands in Gyan Mudra with the thumb and index finger touching each other. The elbows are straight while chanting, and the hand position changes as each fingertip touches the tip of the thumb in turn with firm pressure:

On *Sa* touch the index finger

On *Ta* touch the middle finger

On *Na* touch the ring finger

On *Ma* touch the little finger

Begin by chanting the mantra in a normal voice for 2 minutes, then whisper for 2 minutes, then go deep into the sound, vibrating it silently for 4 minutes. Then come back to a whisper for 2 minutes, then aloud for 2 minutes. To end, follow with 1 minute of silent prayer. Then inhale and exhale. Stretch the spine, with the hands up as far as possible, spread the fingers wide and take several deep breaths. Relax.

This sequence will take 13 minutes. The duration of the meditation may be increased up to a total of 62 minutes, as long as the proportion of loud, whisper, silent, whisper, loud is maintained.

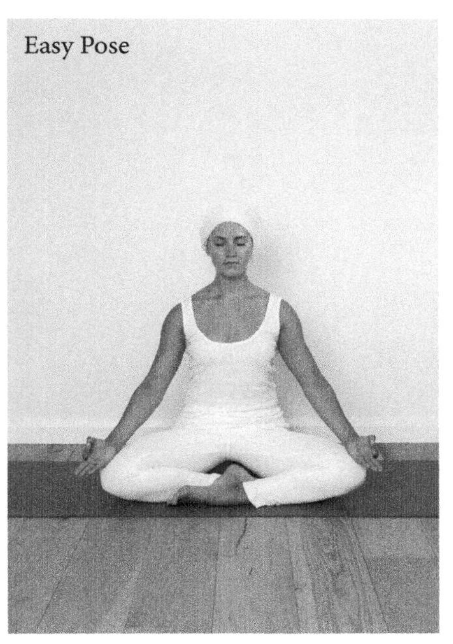

Easy Pose

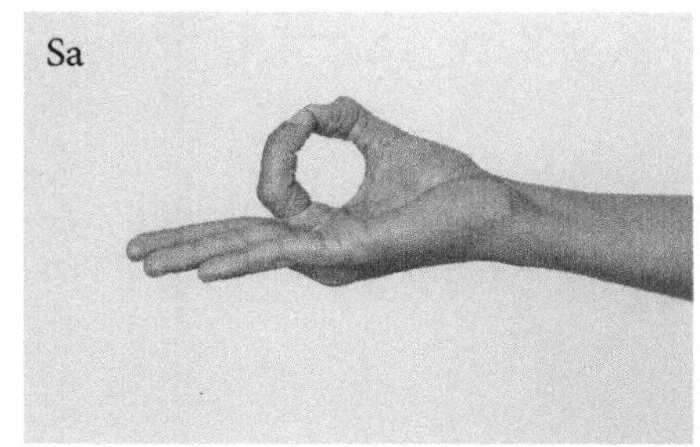

Sa

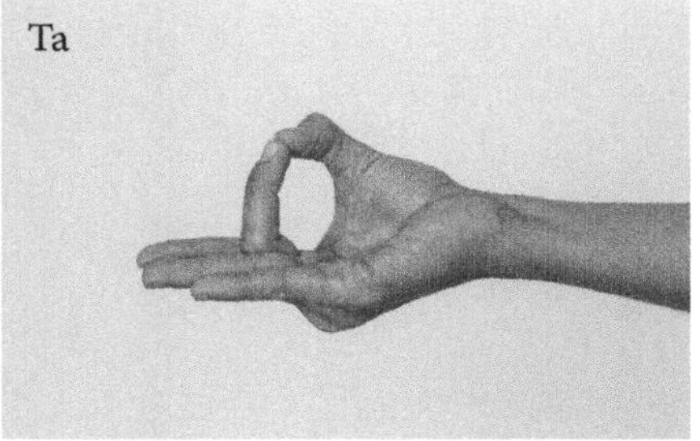

Ta

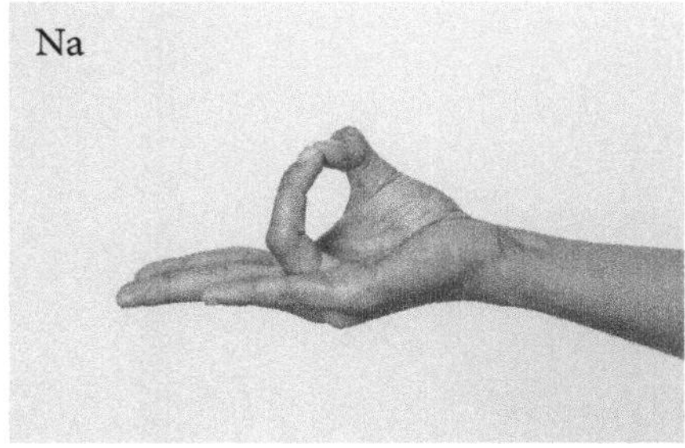

Na

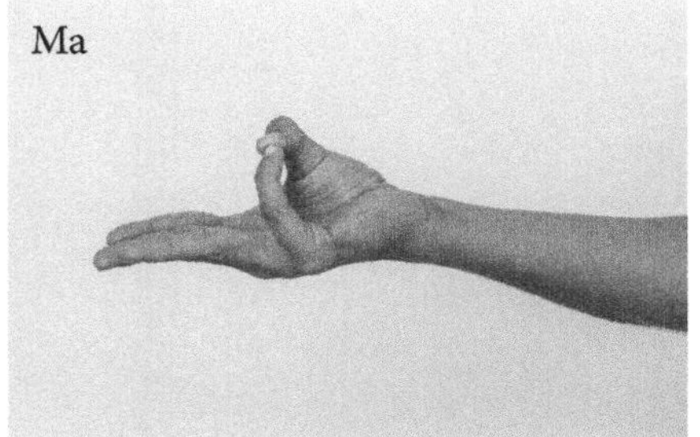

Ma

Chapter 13
Inner Radiance:
Increasing Body Confidence

"The beauty in you is in your spirit."
~ Yogi Bhajan[147]

Having children can affect the female body in many ways: it is normal to put on weight during pregnancy and it can be difficult to shift it again afterwards, especially when the restrictions of having a baby – and the associated tiredness – mean we do not fall back into exercising as we did previously. Changes to the breasts during pregnancy and breastfeeding may be irreversible. We may be left with stretch-marks or a saggy tummy that never quite recovers from being stretched to its limits! If we have had a caesarean section we will have a large abdominal scar.

At home with children, within easy reach of the kitchen all day, we may develop unhealthy habits around food: snacking at all times and finishing the kids' leftover fish fingers. If we are sleep-deprived we may reach for sugary snacks to keep ourselves going during the day.

In the western world, we are bombarded with images of how the female body "should" look. We are constantly subjected to messages about dieting and exercise that tell us we are not trying hard enough and we have failed if we do not fit a certain body type. Why can't we get back into shape as quickly as the "celebrity" mums do?! Sadly, many women often have low self-esteem about the way their post-partum bodies look.

Poor body image affects our health and self-esteem. It can also impact on our attitude towards sexual relations, which may in turn affect our relationship with our partner.

Poor body image affects children as well. However much time you

[147] *I Am a Woman*, p.47

spend lovingly preparing healthy meals for them, if they see you don't feed yourself properly, that you reach for a packet of biscuits every time you feel stressed or tired, or you belittle yourself and your dieting efforts, then you are teaching them an unhealthy way of thinking about food. Modelling healthy and consistent eating patterns and a positive body image will help your children when they become responsible for feeding themselves in the future.

Is this You?

- Has the way your body has been affected by having children had an impact on your self-esteem? Do you wish you could lose some excess weight or change your body in some way?
- Has your post-baby body affected your feelings about having sex with your partner?
- Have you developed any unhealthy eating habits since having children that have had an impact on your weight or well-being?
- Do you "diet" on and off? Do you use "fad" diets?

Reflection Points

- Are you looking after yourself enough?
- Are you eating three balanced meals a day?
- Are you getting enough sleep? Insufficient sleep is a major cause of obesity. When we are sleep-deprived we tend to over-produce an appetite-stimulating hormone called ghrelin and under-produce an appetite-suppressing hormone called leptin. Can you improve the quality of your sleep (see Chapter 3)?
- Think about how your own mother, or other people close to you, talked about food when you were growing up. What impact might that have had on how you feed yourself now?

Yogic Viewpoint: Food

The Yogic view is that the food you choose to eat is critical to your health and well-being. Yogi Bhajan described the body as the vehicle in which we travel through life;[148] it won't function

[148] *The Aquarian Teacher*, p.15

properly without adequate, high-quality fuel. Yogis prefer to eat to live, rather than live to eat. The following are recommended guidelines for a healthy way of eating:[149]

- Eat more alkaline foods than acidic foods. Acidity in the blood creates the ideal environment for the development of cancer. The optimum balance is 75% alkaline and 25% acidic. Alkaline foods are calming and build and tone organs, nerves and glands. These include green vegetables, pulses, legumes, sweet and sour fruit, yoghurt, milk and lemons (which are acidic to the taste but are alkaline-forming in the body). Acidic foods give a burst of energy but too much makes us prone to illness. These include meat, eggs, starches, sweets and butter products. Meat is among the most acid-producing foods and leaves a residue of uric acid in the bloodstream;

- To help the digestive system to function optimally, chew your food really well and only eat food you can digest within 18 hours (24 hours for men). If you can't digest it and eliminate it, don't eat it! Incorporate at least some raw food in your diet to provide enough roughage;

- Don't eat too much protein as it is very difficult to digest. The World Health Organisation recommends 35-40 grams a day;

- Avoid white sugar, salt, white bread, alcohol and caffeine, all of which are poisonous to the body and put it under pressure to de-toxify;

- Only eat when you are actually hungry and don't snack between meals. Stop eating when you are three-quarters full;

- Don't eat too late in the day. Yogi Bhajan recommends not eating after sunset.

Yogi Bhajan also recommends we eat in a pleasant, relaxing environment, take the time to eat consciously and rest after every meal. Living with young children can make these aspirations challenging, but we are all just doing our best!

Ahimsa

Ahimsa, the principle of "non-harming" or "non-violence", is one of the reasons often cited for why many Yogis are vegetarian. But it is important to remember we must also direct compassion towards ourselves.

[149] *The Aquarian Teacher*, pp.252-254

This includes loving and being kind to ourselves and not harming the body through starvation dieting or cutting out major food groups. *Ahmisa* means not judging yourself and loving the person you actually are – not the person you think you would be if only you could lose some weight.

Yoga sometimes seems to be portrayed in the media as a practice exclusively for those who are fit and flexible. This is unhelpful because Yoga is for everyone and anyone who engages with it under the guidance of a reputable teacher will benefit from the practice. When following the exercises set out in this book (or when taking part in any Yoga classes) I encourage you to always regard your mat as a cease-fire zone. Whatever issues you may have about how your body looks, or what it can or cannot do, please leave them aside when you do your practice. This is a time to nurture yourself and to feel proud of yourself for finding the time and the inclination to invest in your mental and physical health.

The Aura

The phenomenon of electrical coronal discharges said to be captured by Kirlian photography is referred to in the Yoga tradition as the Aura or electro-magnetic field. As the Earth is surrounded by a field that protects it, mainly from the charged particles of solar wind that would otherwise strip away the ozone layer, humans also have a protective shield. In the teachings of the Kundalini Yoga tradition the Aura is recognised as a chakra and also one of our **Ten Bodies**.

According to the teachings the Aura has two functions: it protects us from negative outside influences and projects us to the outside world. So when our Aura is strong we feel confident and secure in ourselves, with healthy self-esteem, and we attract positivity from others. When our Aura is weak we feel the opposite: paranoid and lacking in self-confidence. We attract negativity from others and we are vulnerable to illness. So if we are suffering from poor body image since (or despite!) having children, strengthening our personal Aura can help to rebuild our self-esteem.

Radiant Body

The tenth of the Ten Bodies gives you spiritual royalty and radiance. When it is strong you exert a magnetic presence and command the respect of all who know you. When it is weak you may dislike attention, being afraid of the energy and responsibility that come with the recognition of your inner nobility. To strengthen the Radiant Body it is recommended you do not cut your hair. Commitment (for example, to your practice and your spiritual development) also helps to strengthen this Body.[150]

Top Tips for Body Confidence

- Eat foods that help keep the digestive system functioning well: apples (eaten in the afternoon), black pepper, ginger and garlic;[151]
- Avoid caffeine, which impedes the digestive process;[152]
- Don't eat within three hours of going to bed so the body has plenty of time to finish digesting before sleep;
- Eat three proper meals so you don't need to snack in-between, allowing the digestive system to function optimally;
- Wear light-coloured clothing made of natural fibres to enhance the Aura;
- Chant the mangala charn mantra (*Aad Guray Nameh, Jugad Guray Nameh, Sat Guray Nameh, Siri Guru Dev-ay Nameh),* which surrounds the magnetic field with protective light;[153]
- Create a positive mantra and say it to yourself as often as possible. For example: *This incredible body has brought a child into the world.*

Yoga Set for Body Confidence

Breathing Exercise

RESTRAINING COMPULSIVE EATING[154]

At the time the urge to eat compulsively affects you, sit in Easy Pose with a straight spine. Block the right nostril with the thumb of the right hand. Deeply inhale through the left nostril and hold the breath in to

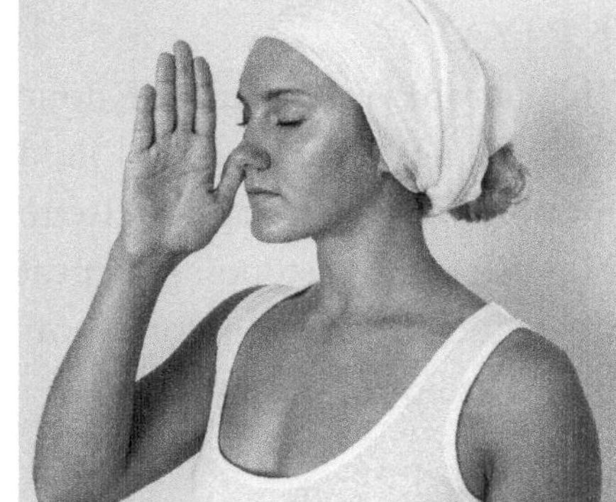

[150] *The Aquarian Teacher*, p.203

[151] *The Aquarian Teacher*, p.255

[152] *The Aquarian Teacher*, p.254

[153] *The Aquarian Teacher*, p.82

[154] *Praana Praane Praanayam*, p.109. First taught by Yogi Bhajan in 1979

your capacity. Then exhale through the left nostril and hold the breath out for the same amount of time as you held it in. Start with 3 minutes and build up to 31 minutes.

Author's suggestion: If you have high blood pressure be particularly careful about holding the breath and don't do it for too long. Hold the breath in for as long as feels comfortable to you.

"Ninety days of practising this breath technique for 31 minutes per day can take care of most chronic cases. But don't exaggerate. It should be long, deep breathing through the left nostril without pressure on the diaphragm. It makes the initial hemisphere of the left side of the brain take command and project itself against the impulse that 'I must go and eat'."

~ Yogi Bhajan

Kriya

Complete Workout for the Elementary Being (Har Aerobic Kriya)[155]

This aerobic set should be done fairly quickly and in a fluid motion, moving from exercise to exercise without stopping. Repeat the sequence five times for a thorough cardiovascular workout.

1. Standing with feet comfortably apart, clap your hands over your head 8 times. Each time you clap, chant *Har* with the tip of your tongue.

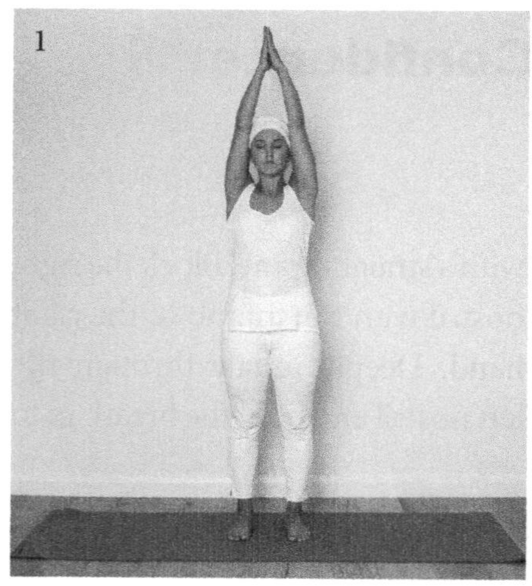

2. Bend over from the hips. Slap the ground hard with the hands 8 times. With each pat, chant *Har* with the tip of your tongue.

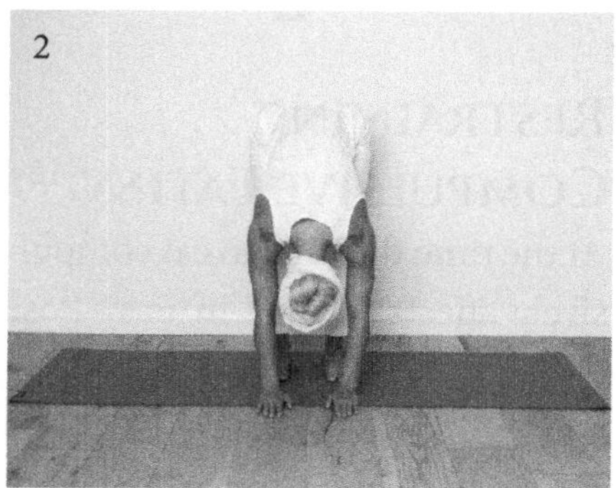

[155] The Library of Teachings: *www.libraryofteachings.com*. First taught by Yogi Bhajan on 14 and 16 July 1985

3. Stand up straight with arms out to the sides parallel to the ground. Raise and lower the arms, patting the air, one foot up and one foot below the shoulder height, as you chant *Har* with the tip of your tongue. Do this 8 times.

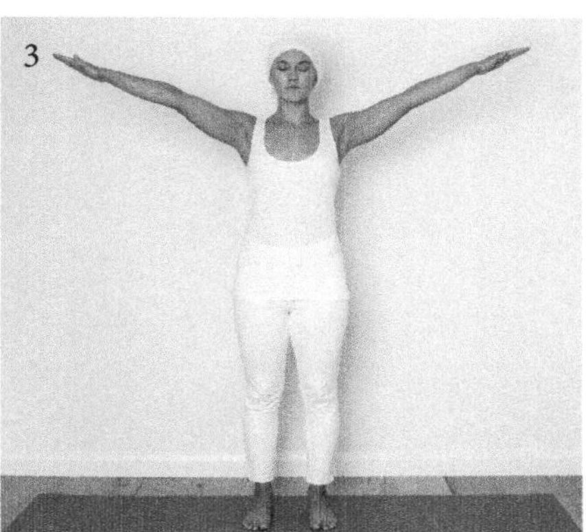

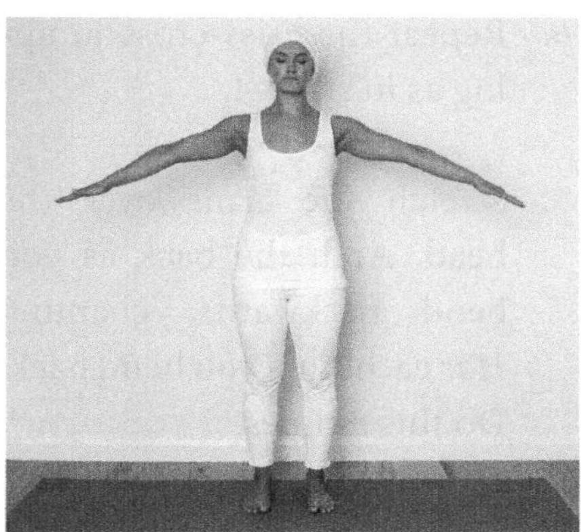

4. Still standing, jump and criss-cross the arms and legs chanting *Har*, both as the arms and legs cross and when they are out at the sides for a total of 8 chants of *Har*.

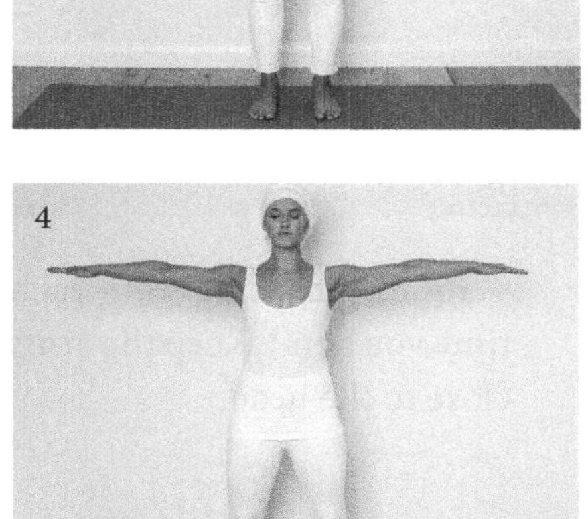

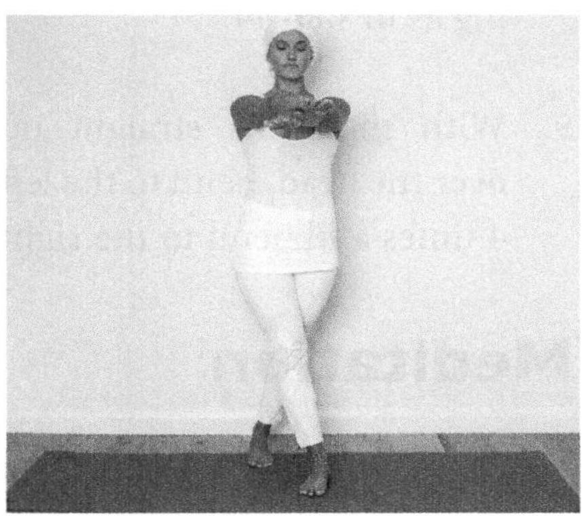

5. Come into Archer Pose with the right leg forward, left leg back. Bend the right knee, extending in and out of the full stretch of the position, chanting *Har* each time you bend forward. Do this 8 times. Switch sides, with the left leg extended forward chanting *Har* each time you bend forward. Do this 8 times.

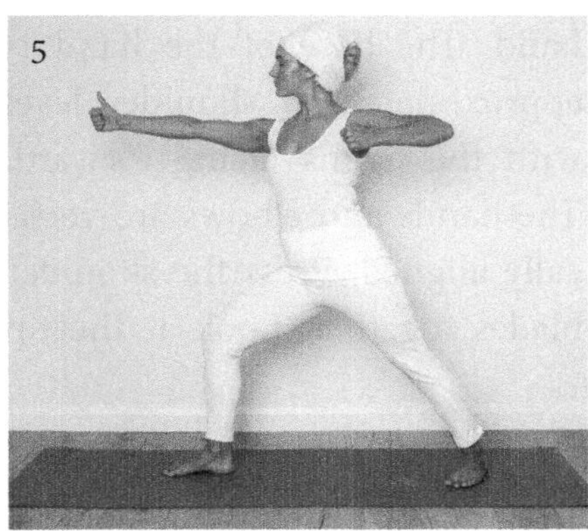

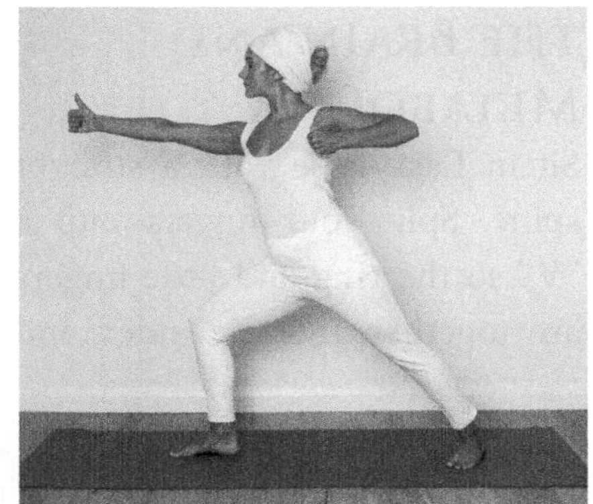

6. Repeat the criss-cross jumping as in step #4.

7. Stretch the arms over the head. Arch the back as you bend backwards, chanting *Har* each time you bend back. Do this 8 times.

8. Repeat the criss-cross jumping as in step #4.

9. With the arms straight up over the head, bend to the left 4 times and bend to the right

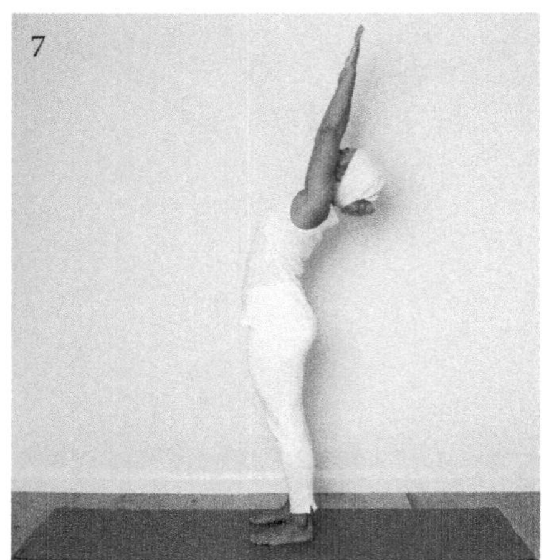

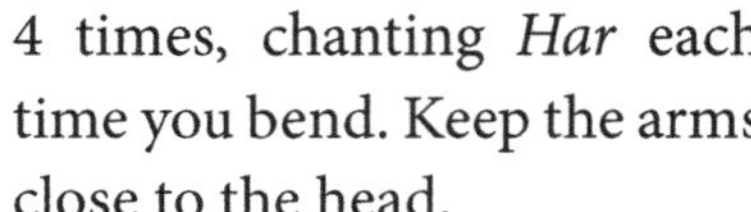

4 times, chanting *Har* each time you bend. Keep the arms close to the head.

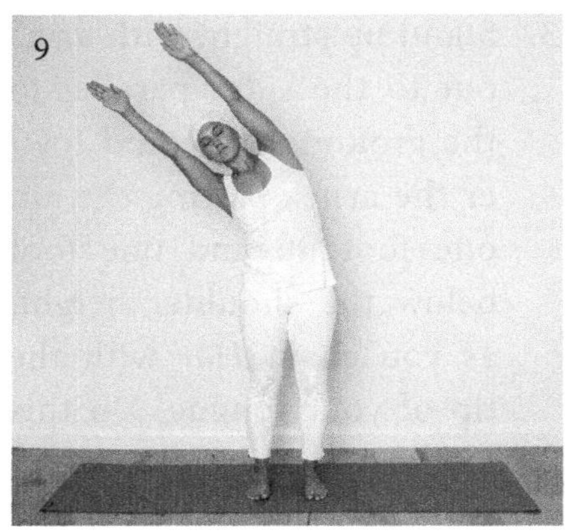

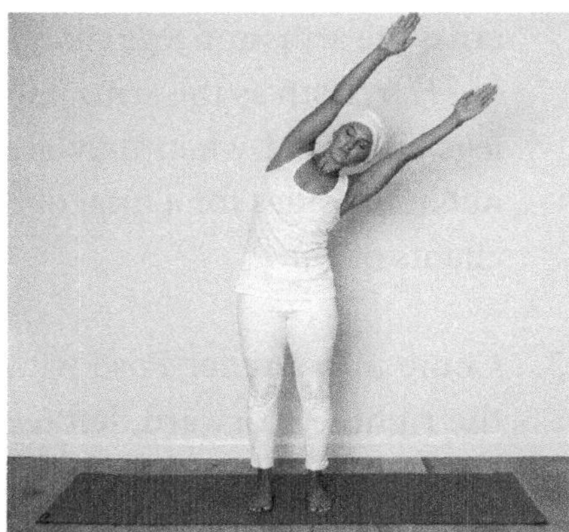

Meditation

Ten-Stroke Breath to Balance the Brain and Metabolism[156]

Sit in Easy Pose with a straight spine. Split your fingers into a "V" so the ring and little fingers are together and the index and middle fingers are together. The thumbs spread away from the hand. The base of the hand is approximately at shoulder level with the palms facing forward. The hands and elbows are vertically aligned. Press the shoulder blades together. Look at the tip of your nose. Inhale through the nose in ten quick strokes or parts (about 2 strokes per second). Hold the breath in and mentally chant: *Aad Such, Jugaad Such,*

[156] *Praana Praanee Praanayam*, p.170. First taught by Yogi Bhajan on 13th February 1979

Haibhay Such, Nanak Hosee Bhay Such.

The total time the breath is held in is 5-6 seconds. Exhale through the nose in ten quick strokes (about 2 strokes per second). Hold the breath out and mentally chant: *Aad Such, Jugaad Such, Haibhay Such, Nanak Hosee Bhay Such* .

The total time breath is held in is 5-6 seconds.

Continue in this pattern for 11 minutes.

Caution: do not attempt to drive immediately after doing this practice.

See my website for a demonstration of the mantra: www.karmaparent.com/about-me.

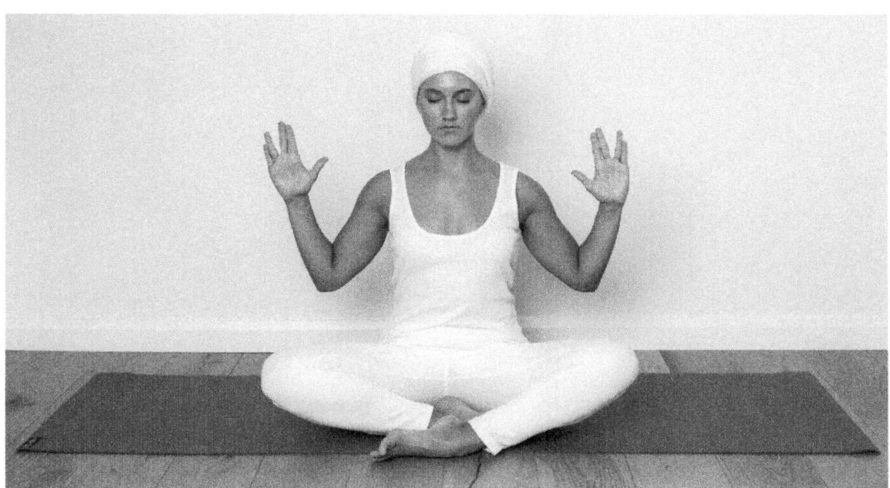

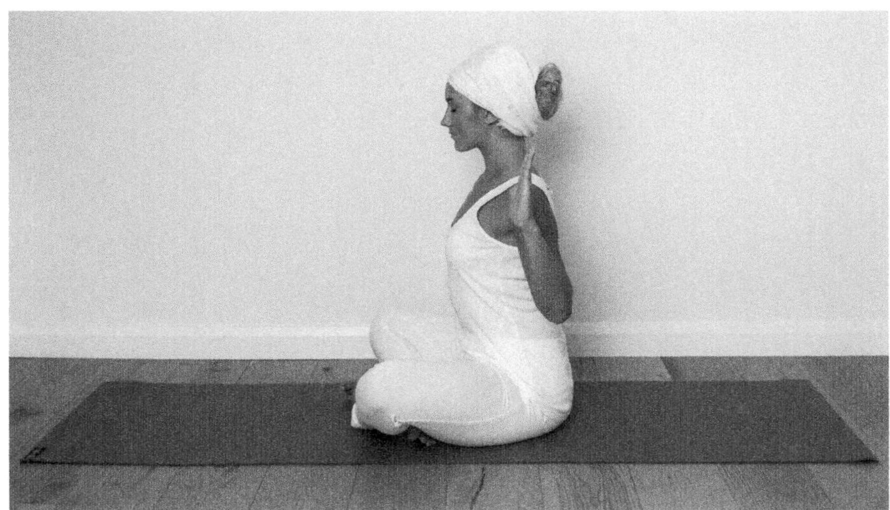

Chapter 14
A New Dawn:
Strengthening Relationships

"Women are exactly the opposite from men – they have nothing in common. It is only this mysterious thing called love which brings them together. We cannot know what is going on inside the other's head. Admit that you do not know what the other's world is like – just agree that you have the right to be you and he/she has the right to be him/her."

~ Yogi Bhajan[157]

Becoming a parent is a massive life change and everything we have learned before that point is thrown into a new light. We are no longer able to regard ourselves as just ourselves; we now have a unique relationship with our child that affects us in a very deep way and may even change the way we decide to lead the rest of our lives. We may find ourselves reviewing our priorities and our core values. We may realise we don't have as much control as we thought we had. There may be things we had planned to do but now can't. We may find issues from our own childhoods surfacing and affecting how we feel about parenting. Perhaps our life partner does not take to parenting in the way we had anticipated. Perhaps relatives and friends express views about our child or our parenting that surprise and even irritate us. We can't hide any more: we have to decide who we are, what is important to us and what we believe in.

Although many parents feel their relationship is strengthened in the long run by having children, it is hardly surprising such a huge and exhausting life change often creates tension between couples. Many marriages are dissolved when the parties are aged between 36 and 45.[158] Some relationships are just not strong enough to withstand the pressure

[157] Winter 1974

[158] *The Aquarian Teacher*, p.238

of parenting together; according to the Office for National Statistics[159] it is now expected that 42 per cent of British marriages will end in divorce. Of the 118,140 couples who divorced in 2012, 48 per cent had a child under the age of 16 living with them.

Is this You?

- Has your relationship with your partner been more strained since you had children?
- Has sex become more of an issue between you than it was before you had children?
- Do you feel sufficiently supported, emotionally and physically, by your partner?
- Do you feel your partner understands how your needs have changed since you had children?
- Do you find yourself complaining about your partner to others?
- Have your relationships with your friends and relatives felt more strained or distant since you had children? Have any relationships improved with the common bond of a child?

Reflection Points

- Spend some time thinking about the people in your life. Which are the relationships that are really important to you? Are there any you feel are important to maintain for the sake of your children? How might your own childhood impact on your feelings about that? Are there any you could describe as dysfunctional or even toxic? What might your children be learning from them?
- Focus on a difficult relationship, such as with a partner or close relative. Can you identify any major issues you come back to time and again with them? Are there underlying issues you know you will need to resolve if the relationship is to be healed? Are there issues that seem to have become worse since you had children but were still there in the past?
- Think back to previous relationships. Can you identify any patterns that might be repeating in your current relationships?

---

159 Divorces in England and Wales, 2012, published by the Office for National Statistics on 6th February 2014 and downloadable from the ONS website: www.ons.gov.uk

Yogic Viewpoint: The Chakra System

Understanding a little about the Chakra system helps us in our relationships with others. A journey through the main chakras takes us from our most selfish position – at our root, where we keep ourselves as safe and secure as we can, through our Heart Centre, where we move from "me" to "we", to our crown, where we move beyond our individual consciousness to the Universal Consciousness. The strength or otherwise of our Aura, which combines all of our chakras, determines how we project ourselves to others.

Several of the chakras are particularly important to our relationships with others: the second, which relates to our sexual functioning, the fourth, which relates to the heart, and the fifth, which is the centre for communication.

If the second chakra is blocked, sluggish or overactive this can manifest in problems with our sexual functioning, which can in turn put pressure on intimate relationships. A blocked second chakra can manifest as frigidity. An overactive second chakra can lead to sex addiction and seeing everything in terms of sex, as well as irresponsible relationships: promiscuity and infidelity that damage a more meaningful relationship. A second chakra that is balanced and clear enables us to have a healthy attitude towards sexual functioning.

A strong, balanced heart chakra enables us to be kind, to forgive people and to give and receive love. It enables us to speak kindly but honestly. If our heart chakra is weak or blocked, we may be dependent on love and affection from others, easily hurt, or afraid of rejection. We may be heartless towards others. Or we may experience "helper syndrome", in which we display a strong drive to make other people feel better, in order to ease or divert from our own pain. Helper syndrome can lead to burnout and depression. It can also contribute to abusive relationships and is often typified by imbalanced relationships (one partner being the other's teacher or manager, for example) with the helper deliberately keeping the other person dependent.

"Don't become so bitter that somebody will throw you away or so sweet that someone can eat you up."

~ Yogi Bhajan[160]

[160] *The Aquarian Teacher*, p.227

Communication is the foundation of any successful relationship. The fifth, or throat, chakra is our centre for truth, language and communication; strength in this chakra enables us to be authentic. A strong navel chakra allows us to know who we are and a strong, balanced fifth chakra gives us the ability to express this effectively to others. If the fifth chakra is not functioning well, we are likely to have difficulties with intimate and other relationships: we feel shy and insecure and don't speak up when we should; we say what we think the other person wants to hear rather than what we know to be the truth; or we talk too much and don't listen to the other person's point of view.

THE CYCLES OF LIFE

According to Yogi Bhajan, we are all subject to three cycles of development throughout our lives which can be regarded as opportunities to review our progress. Even if we are not aware these cycles are happening, we may have experienced times in our lives that feel "transitional": perhaps we feel unsure of ourselves, or that there are important decisions to be made about our purpose and our relationships.

Every 18 years we review our physical health, vitality and overall life quality. Every 11 years we review our applied intelligence and how it affects our actions. Every 7 years we review our level and style of consciousness. How do we understand things? What are our priorities? I noticed some profound changes in my eldest son when he was 7 years old, and I remember my own consciousness changing significantly when I was the same age.

The following visual depiction of these Cycles of Life indicates there are some major transition points at which the cycles converge ("clusters"):

Linear time

0__________25__________50__________75__________100

Cycle of Consciousness

0___7___14___21___28___35___42__49___56___63___70___77___84___91___98

Cycle of Intelligence

0____11____22____33____44____55____66____77____88____99

Cycle of Life Energy

0______18______36______54______72______90______108

The main clusters are: 11-14, 18-21-22, 33-35-36, 42-44, 54-55-56, 63-66 and 72-77. During these periods we experience changes to our energy levels, relationships, awareness, values, intelligence and means of action. The '7-year itch' has long been established as a phenomenon of intimate relationships; these clusters are times when extra effort is required to maintain a relationship, or to decide whether to move on from it. The mid-thirties is a time which often coincides with having young children, just when you are likely to be reviewing your relationships and life path,[161] and as we have already seen, it is a very common time for people to divorce.

The Soul Body

The first of the Ten Bodies, the Soul Body connects you to your inner infinity. When it is weak, you may act from your head rather than from your heart. Opening the heart (see the recommended set below) and raising the Kundalini[162] strengthen the Soul Body. In a successful relationship the parties are able to express themselves openly and with authenticity; they speak and act from the heart rather than the head.

Ahimsa

The Yogic principle of non-harming is relevant here as well, because having young children is a time when we have to make extra efforts to take care of ourselves. Most parents do their best to look after their children, but many do not look after themselves anywhere near enough. Remember how on an aeroplane you are always instructed to fix your own oxygen mask first before helping your children? If you aren't able to breathe, you aren't going to be much good to anyone else. It's the same with all our relationships: we can't give our best to nurturing them if we are in a bad way ourselves. In Yoga, the work is always with ourselves.

"Your heart has not to open to others. Your heart has to open to yourself."

~ Yogi Bhajan[163]

Top Tips for Improving Relationships: Yogi Bhajan's 5 rules for harmonious communication[164]

1. You are communicating for a better tomorrow, not to spoil today;

[161] *The Aquarian Teacher*, p.228

[162] *The Aquarian Teacher*, p.201

[163] *The 8 Human Talents*, p.93

[164] *The Aquarian Teacher*, p.142

2. Whatever you are going to say is going to live forever. And you have to live through it. Therefore, take care you don't have to live through the mud of your communication;
3. One wrong word said can do much more wrong than you can even imagine or estimate;
4. Words spoken are a chance for communication. Don't turn them into a war;
5. When you communicate, you have to communicate again. Don't make the road rough.

Yoga Set for Improving Relationships

Breathing Exercise

Developing Your Human Kindness[165]

Sit in Easy Pose with the spine straight, chin in and chest lifted. The elbows rest alongside the rib-cage. The hands are in front of the chest, palms facing upwards, with the little fingers touching and the outside part of the base of the palms touching. Keep the ring and index fingers straight and the thumbs pulled back. Touch the tips of the middle fingers so they form a triangle. The

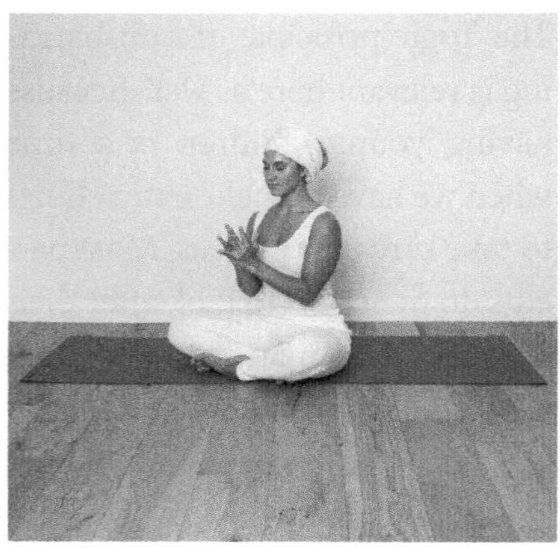

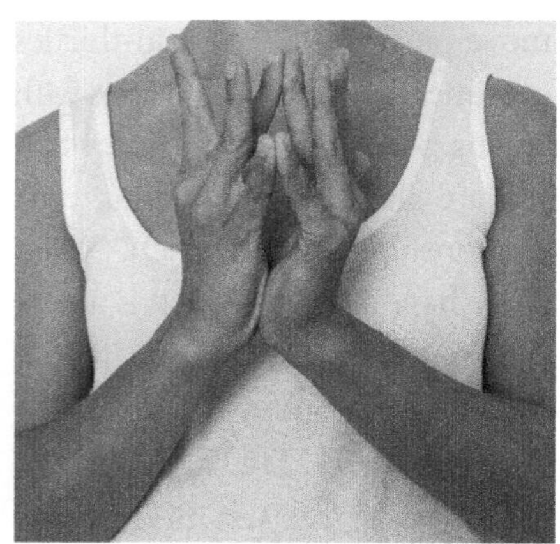

mudra is held before the heart centre in a comfortable, prayerful position, but does not touch the chest. Inhale through the nose in eight strokes (break the inhalation into eight equal segments like "sniffs"). Each stroke is about one "nose length": i.e. you can

[165] *Praana Praanee Praanayam*, p.200. First taught by Yogi Bhajan on 27th October 1975

feel the breath travel the length of the nose from the nostrils to the eyebrows. Each count of a stroke is about one second. Exhale completely and totally with a whistle through puckered lips. Continue for 11 minutes.

Kriya

Kriya to Open the Heart Centre[166]

This set creates open, loving feelings. It opens the heart, increases compassion and sensitivity to others, and helps you to drop emotional defensiveness. Its calming effect allows you to eliminate unnecessary thoughts and feelings, so you can be more in the present and experience your feelings more clearly.

Stand with palms together in Prayer Pose at the centre of the chest and do a steady Breath of Fire for 3 minutes. Inhale and hold briefly at the end.

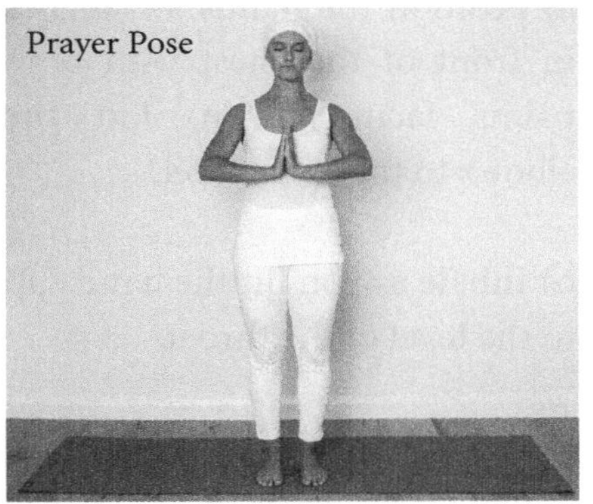
Prayer Pose

Stand or sit with an erect spine. Keep the eyes open and look to the horizon. Make fists of both hands. Begin alternately punching with one fist then the other. Together the hands create a piston-like motion with one arm pulling back to balance the other arm punching forward. The hands do not turn or twist. Exhale with each punch forward and punch rapidly so the breath becomes like a Breath of Fire. Continue for 3 minutes.

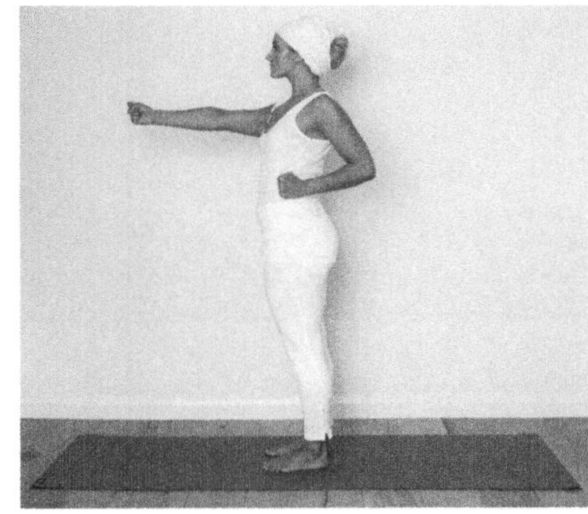

To end: inhale, draw both elbows back, tighten the fists, apply root lock and suspend the breath for 5 seconds. Exhale and relax.

[166] *Transformation Volume Two*, Sat Purkh Kaur Khalsa, editor (Kundalini Research Institute, 2010), pp.46-47.

Stand straight, extend the arms out to the sides and begin to make big circles with both arms at the same time. Inhale as they come forward and up, and exhale as they go back and down. Continue for 2 minutes.

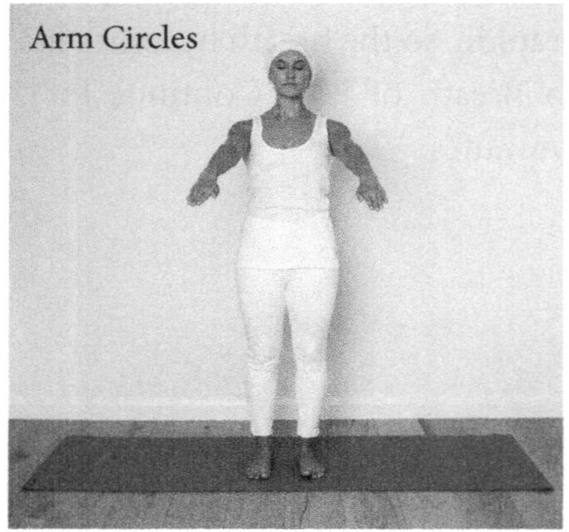
Arm Circles

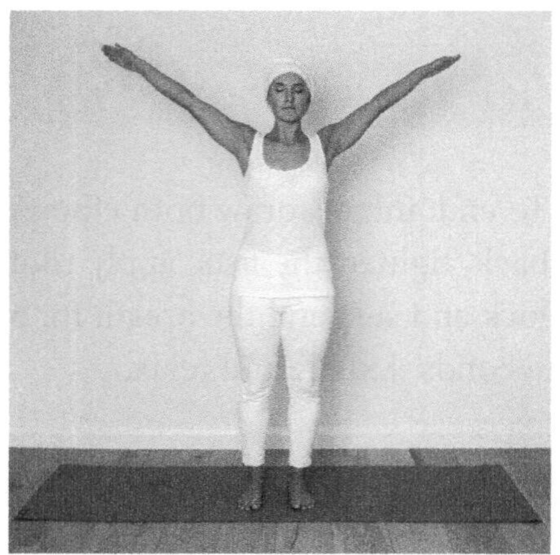

To end: Inhale and stretch both arms straight up over the head. Exhale and relax.

Sit straight. Interlace the fingers with the thumbtips touching:

a) Position the hands 4-6 inches in front of the chest with both palms facing down. Lift the elbows to the same level.

b) Inhale as you lift the hands up to the level of the throat.

c) Exhale as you sweep them down to the level of the Navel. Create a steady pumping motion with a powerful breath, and continue for 3 minutes.

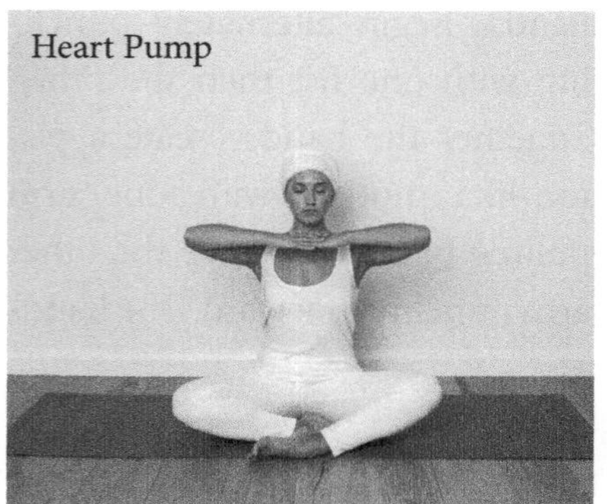
Heart Pump

To end: inhale, bring the hands to the level of the heart, and suspend the breath for 10 seconds. Exhale and relax.

Stand or sit with a straight spine. Place the hands beside the shoulders with elbows by your sides and palms facing forward. Close your eyelids halfway and fix your gaze downward. Begin to slowly inhale and exhale. Your breath should be equal on the inhale and the exhale. Mentally repeat the following primal sound scale on both the inhale and exhale:

Sa Ta Na Ma

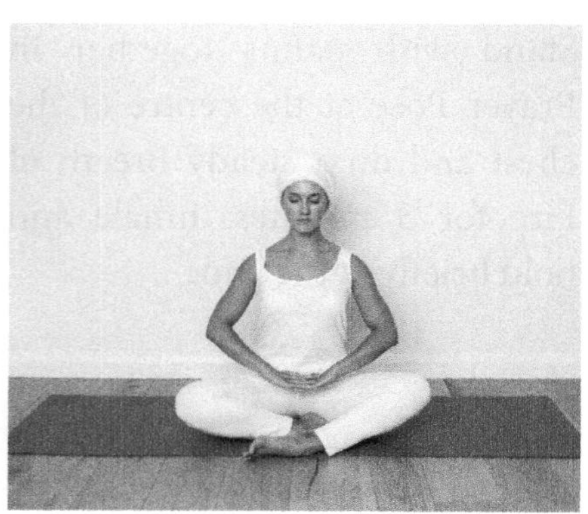

Press the thumb tips to the finger tips sequentially from the first finger tip to the little finger tip with *Sa Ta Na Ma*, while you vibrate the mental sounds as you would with Kirtan Kriya (see Chapter 12). Continue for 3-5 minutes

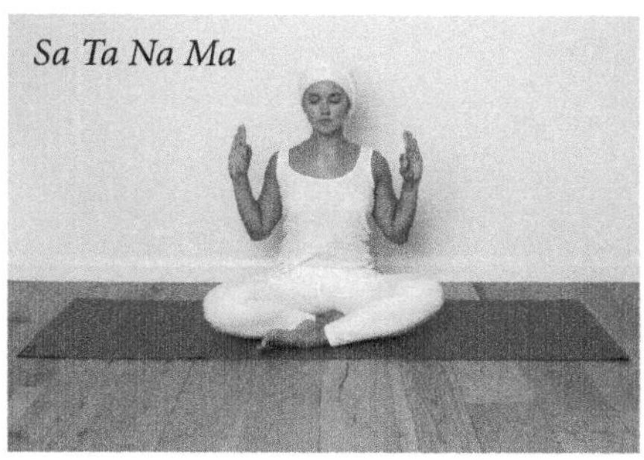
Sa Ta Na Ma

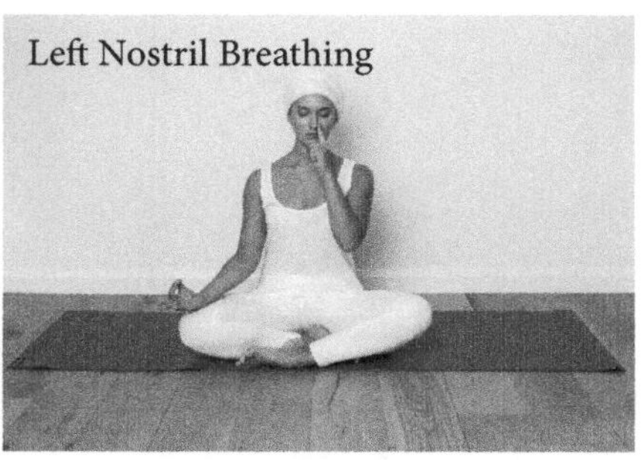
Left Nostril Breathing

Sit with a straight spine. Block the right nostril gently with the index finger of the right hand. Inhale slowly through your left nostril, exhale slowly through rounded lips. Match the duration of the inhale and exhale, with each one lasting about 10 seconds. Continue with this slow breathing pattern for 3 minutes. Then relax and follow the natural flow of your breath for another 2 minutes.

Meditation

Meditation to Open the Heart[167]

(See next page for illustrations.) This meditation is for when you feel your heart is closed and there is no flow of love. Sit in Easy Pose, with a light Neck Lock. The eyes are closed, looking up, focusing at the Brow Point. Chant the mantra *Sat Kartaar*:

As you say *Sat*, the hands are pressed together in Prayer Pose at the centre of the chest.

As you say *Kar*, the hands are extended out from the shoulders, halfway towards the final position. Fingers are pointing straight up.

As you say *Taar*, the arms are fully extended out to the sides and parallel to the floor, fingers pointing up.

Make the transition from step to step a flowing movement. Continue for 3 minutes.

---

167 *The Aquarian Teacher*, p.436. First taught by Yogi Bhajan in 1971

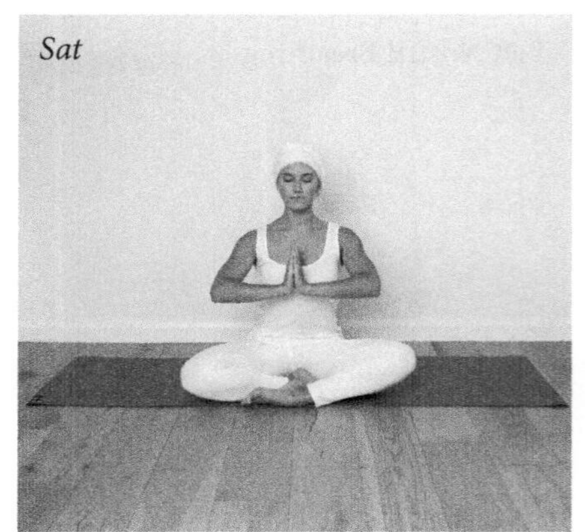
Sat

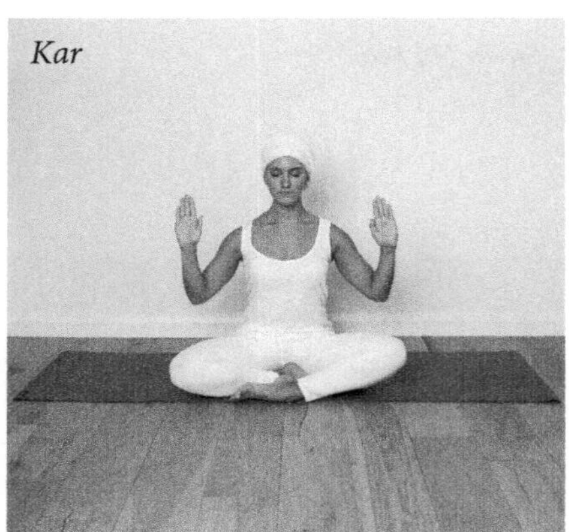
Kar

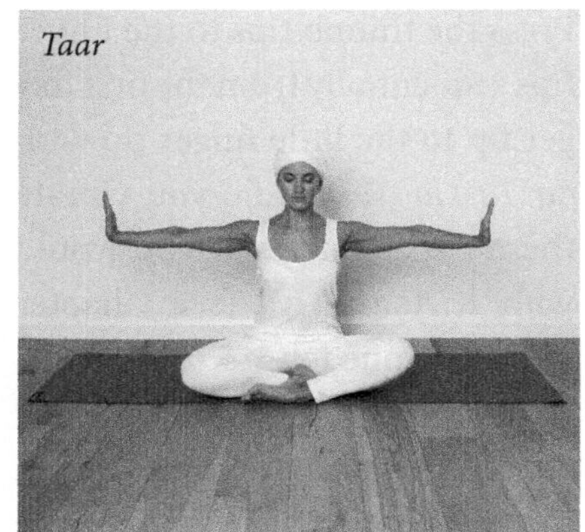
Taar

Conclusion

"The purest thing is the world is the heart of the mother… It can move the universe… The heart of the mother is the greatest power of Infinity ever given to any finite being."

~ Yogi Bhajan[168]

When Yogi Bhajan first arrived in the West in the late 1960s he was shocked by the exploitation of women and the breakdown of family life he witnessed. Female empowerment was central to his teachings and he established women's summer camps that taught skills such as self-defence as well as Kundalini Yoga. He emphasised the importance of the mother and the respect which motherhood should receive.

The practice of Kundalini Yoga has the potential to empower mothers by giving them the tools to improve and maintain their physical and mental health, to determine their life's purpose – whatever that may be – and to give them the strength to pursue it.

In particular, unblocking and balancing our chakras helps us in our role as mums in many ways:

Balancing the Root Chakra enables us to feel secure in ourselves and in our various roles, including that of mother. We can start to feel we belong, and are stable and grounded.

Balancing the Sacral Chakra enables us to have a positive, relaxed attitude to our sexual functions which may have been thrown into disarray after childbirth and the transition from partner to mother (and partner). It can help us to develop the huge reserves of patience we need with children. It can help minimise the problems caused by unnecessary guilt.

Balancing the Navel Chakra enables us to strengthen our self-esteem and sense of personal power, and to stop always putting the needs of others before our own.

Opening the Heart Centre develops our compassion and our empathy for others (including children who don't behave the way we think they should) and allows us to speak truthfully

168 Women's Camp 1977 www.3ho.org

but with compassion. This is an important skill for parents; we often have to tell our children things they don't want to hear ("no, you can't eat a whole packet of chocolate biscuits"). A balanced Heart Chakra enables us to give them good parental guidance with kindness.

Opening the Throat Chakra gives us the ability to express ourselves in a positive way. With an effective voice, we can communicate our concerns to our partner if we feel the childcare and household responsibilities are not being shared fairly, or to relatives who may be teaching our children values that are incompatible with our own. On a wider scale, we can express the inadequacies of a parenting system in which it seems to be quite common for mothers of young children to struggle but to feel unable to talk openly about it, and for mental health issues such as Postnatal Depression to be so common. We can contribute to a discussion about how to change the role of the mother to create a more supportive and healthy framework for families, and start to initiate change.

Balancing our Third Eye strengthens our ability to rely on our intuition. It can set us free from depression and confusion about our lives. It enables us to understand our purpose, which is fundamental to our psychological health and emotional well-being.

Balancing the Crown Chakra elevates us and connects us with our soul or our highest Self. A strong and balanced Crown Chakra frees us from the fear of being separated from our children by death, allowing us to enjoy the time we do have with them.

When we radiate a strong, balanced Aura people, including our children, respond positively to us. We are also protected from the pressure our society puts on us because we are mothers, and the negativity other parents can emit as a way of affirming their own parenting choices.

Kundalini Yoga allows us to re-establish our personal identity and to accept that this may bear little resemblance to who we thought we were before we had children. It gives us the energy we need to approach our new life, and to regain a sense of choice over where that life is going.

Armed with a technology that gives us a clear mind, a body that functions well and the ability to connect to our spirituality, we have the opportunity to enjoy a much happier experience of parenting.

May the long-time sun shine upon you,

All love surround you,

And the pure light within you,

Guide your way on.

Appendix I
Mantras and Meanings

Key to Pronunciation[169]

A	like the "a" in about
AA	like the "a" in want
AY	like the "ay" in say
AI	like the "a" in hand
I	like the "i" in bit
U	like the "u" in put
OO	like the "oo" in food
O	like the "o" in go
E	like the "ay" in say
EE	like the "e" in meet
AAU	like the "ow" in now

Aad Guray Nameh, Jugad Guray Nameh, Sat Guray Nameh, Siri Guru Dev Nameh
~ I bow to the primal wisdom, I bow to wisdom through the ages, I bow to True Wisdom, I bow to the great, unseen wisdom

Ek Ong Kar Sat Gur Prasaad, Sat Gur Prasaad Ek Ong Kar
~ God and We are One, I know this by the Grace of the True **Guru**. I know this by the Grace of the True Guru. That God and We are One

Ong Namo Guru Dev Namo
~ I bow to the subtle divine wisdom, the divine Teacher within

Sat Kartaar
~ God is the One doing this action

Sat Naam
~ Truth is my identity

Sat Narayan Wahe Guru, Haree Narayan Sat Nam
~ Sat Narayan is the True Sustainer, Wahe Guru is Indescribable Wisdom, Haree Narayan is Creative Sustainer, and *Sat Nam* (pronounced *Naam*) means True Identity

Sa Ta Na Ma
~ This mantra describes the continuous cycle of life and creation: Sa means infinity or the totality of the Cosmos, Ta means life, Na means death or transformation, Ma means rebirth

Wahe Guru
~ I am in ecstasy when I experience the Indescribable Wisdom

[169] *Kundalini Yoga: The Flow of Eternal Power*, p.201

Appendix II
Sources of Help for Addictions

Alcohol

Have you ever decided to stop drinking for a week or so but only lasted for a couple of days? Do you wish people would mind their own business about your drinking and stop telling you what to do? Has your drinking caused trouble at home? Do you have "blackouts": periods when you were drunk that you later cannot remember at all?

If you suspect you have a problem with alcohol there is a questionnaire on the Alcoholics Anonymous website: www.alcoholics-anonymous.org.uk. They can also be contacted in confidence on 0845 769 7555.

Sugar or Food Addiction

Beating Addictions offers help and support in relation to all addictions, including sugar and food: www.beatingaddictions.co.uk.

Drugs

Frank is a confidential 24-hour helpline for unbiased information about drugs. Call free on 0800 776600 or visit www.talktofrank.com.

Sex Addiction and Love Addiction

It is estimated that at least 6 per cent of the population experience sex addiction, of whom around one in five are women. Sex addiction is any sexual behaviour that feels out of control, and may include frequent casual sex, multiple affairs when you're in a relationship, wanting to stop or change your sexual behaviour but feeling unable to, using sex as a way to cope with other problems, spending large amounts of time planning or engaging in sex, or feeling very low or guilty afterwards. The consequences of sex addiction include the breakdown of meaningful relationships, sexually transmitted infections and unwanted pregnancy. For help, visit Sex and Love Addicts Anonymous www.slaauk.org or call 07984 977884.

Internet Addiction Disorder (IAD)

If you are worried about your Internet use – you stay online longer than you originally intended, you use the Internet as a way of escaping from problems or of relieving feelings of helplessness, guilt, anxiety or depression, or you have repeatedly made unsuccessful efforts to control, cut back or stop Internet use – you may well be an Internet addict. Visit Beating Addictions (see above) or www.helpguide.org (a non-profit guide to mental health and well-being which features help and advice on IAD as well as other addiction disorders).

Gambling

Gambling is fast becoming a much bigger problem for women than it used to be now people can gamble online in the safe anonymity of the Internet. For help, visit www.gamcare.org.uk or call (Freephone) 0808 8020 133.

Compulsive shopping or Compulsive buying disorder

If you regularly buy things even though you don't need or can't afford them, hide purchases from family or friends, feel anxious, guilty or ashamed after a buying binge or avoid opening your mail or answering your phone because you don't want to face the consequences of your buying, visit www.beatingaddictions.co.uk. If you are in debt contact Debtors Anonymous on 020 7644 5070 or visit www.debtorsanonymous.org.uk.

Yogic Approaches to Recovery from Addiction

SuperHealth® is a yogic therapeutic technology that addresses alcohol, drugs, smoking, food issues, co-dependency, gambling, work and computers and includes stress, depression, fatigue and anxiety. Developed by Yogi Bhajan, the approach combines the ancient wisdom of yogic science with the innovations of western sciences.

Personal consultations are available with Mukta Kaur Khalsa, PhD. These incorporate yogic counselling, diet, nutrition, clinical knowledge and Kundalini Yoga and meditation. Email SuperHealth12@gmail.com to arrange a consultation by telephone or Skype. See the SuperHealth® website for more information: www.super-health.net.

Glossary

Adi Mantra	the mantra to begin Kundalini Yoga practice
Adrenal glands	sitting on top of the kidneys, these produce essential hormones and adrenaline
Affirmations	positive statements
Ahimsa	one of the *yamas* from Patanjali's Eight Limbs of Yoga, which is usually translated as "non-harming"
Aquarian Age	the period that started in 2011, based on experience, commitment and universality, ushering in a new level of consciousness and civilization
Apana	the eliminating force in the body
Arcline	the sixth of the Ten Bodies, the Arcline is the balance point between the physical realm and the cosmic realm
Asana	posture
Aura	the electro-magnetic field surrounding the body, referred to by Yogi Bhajan as the eighth major chakra and also the seventh of the Ten Bodies
Breath of Fire	one of the foundational breath techniques used in Kundalini Yoga, it accompanies many postures and has numerous beneficial effects
Brow Point	the location of the Third Eye, between or just above the eyebrows
Chakra	energy centres which spiral through, and emanate from, the body
Crown Chakra	the seventh of the major chakras, located at the crown of the head
Easy Pose	a common posture for meditation and many Kundalini Yoga exercises

Functional Minds	the three minds (Negative, Positive and Neutral) that act as guides for the personal sense of self
Golden Chain	the chain of Teachers who have come before and passed on the Teachings through the technology of transference. When we tune in with Adi Mantra, we are connecting with the Golden Chain and becoming part of it.
Guru	Infinite Teacher or wisdom; what takes you or the person who shows you how to go from darkness to light or a person who helps you. The Guru is not a living, human teacher, but a catalyst for transformation that exists in each of us.
Guru Nanak	a great yogi, healer, and founder of the Sikh lifestyle who lived from 1469-1539
Guru Ram Das	the 4th Sikh Guru, who lived from 1534-1581, Yogi Bhajan's spiritual teacher
Gyan Mudra	a commonly-used hand posture in which the thumb and index finger touch each other and the remaining fingers are extended
Heart Centre	the middle of the chest
Heart Chakra	the fourth of the major chakras, located in the middle of the chest on the breast bone level with the nipples
Hydrotherapy	the technology and science of hydrotherapeutic massage
Hypothalamus	an area no bigger than a walnut in the midline of the brain, just below the thalamus and connected to the pituitary gland by blood vessels. It receives information from all parts of the body and sends information in the form of chemical messengers to the body and mind.
Ida	the *nadi* which ends at the left nostril and brings in the cooling, soothing, mind-expanding energy of the moon
Inversions	postures in which the head is lower than the heart

Japji Sahib	the first section of the Siri Guru Granth Sahib, comprised of forty *paurees* (or steps) including many mantras as captured by Guru Nanak. One of the core sources for mantra in Kundalini Yoga.
Kriya	completed action; a set of Kundalini Yoga practices which cumulatively have a particular effect
Kundalini energy	the energy which lies dormant at the base of every human spine, the creative potential of the human being
Kundalini Yoga	the unitive discipline of the power of awareness and the potential in each individual. Once called the science of the serpent power (kundalini-shakti).
Long Deep Breathing	a breathing technique that uses all three chambers of the lungs with many beneficial effects
Mantra	the creative projection of the mind through sound. The science of mantra is based on the knowledge that sound is a form of energy having structure, power and a definite predictable effect on the chakras and the human psyche.
Mantras	formulae that alter the patterns of the mind and the chemistry of the brain, according to physical and metaphysical laws
Meditation	the practice of controlling and transcending the waves of the mind, the flow of radiance from the soul
Meridian points	reflex points in the body
Moon Cycle	the menstrual cycle
Mounds of Mercury	the mounds at the base of the little fingers
Mudra	a hand position that locks or seals and guides energy flow and reflexes to the brain. Each area of the hand corresponds to a certain part of the body or brain, representing different emotions and behaviours.

Mul Mantra	the first words of *Japji Sahib*, known as the Ballad of Enlightenment. The Mul Mantra was given by *Guru Nanak* and is considered to be the highest of all mantras.
Naad	the essence of all sound, the vibrational harmony through which the Infinite can be expressed
Naad Yoga	a science, thousands of years old, that focuses on vibrating the creativity in the universe and in your inner being, through the use of sound
Nadis	channels of flow for *prana*. The three *nadis* which are most crucial to the flow of Kundalini energy are *ida, pingala* and *sushmuna.*
Navel Chakra	manipura, the third of the major chakras, located at the *Navel Point*
Navel Point	a centre of energy transformation in the body, located below the navel and in front of the lower spine. It encloses within itself the starting point of the 72,000 *nadis.*
Neck Lock	keeping the chin tucked slightly in so the neck is long and energy can flow through it freely
Negative Mind	the second of the *Ten Bodies.* Warns whether there is danger in a situation.
Nerve plexes	branching networks of intersecting nerves
Neutral Mind	the fourth of the *Ten Bodies.* Observes the actions of both the *Negative* and *Positive Minds* and judges and assesses without attachment in relation to the higher Self.
Niyama	a discipline which the Yogi aspires to observe
Patanjali	creator of the Yoga Sutras of Patanjali, a masterpiece of yogic philosophy written between 200 and 600 CE

Physical Body	the fifth of the Ten Bodies, and the temple where the other nine play out their parts. The balance of the Physical Body affects the rest of our capacity and experience.
Pineal gland	produces hormones that regulate levels of sex and thyroid hormones and affect brain activity
Pingala	the *nadi* which ends at the right nostril, bringing in the stimulating, energising, heating energy of the sun
Pituitary gland	regulates the secretion of the thyroid, adrenal and reproductive glands
Positive Mind	the third of the *Ten Bodies.* Sees the positive essence of all situations and beings.
Prana	the subtle life force in the body, the first unit of energy
Pranayam	the science of breath, controlling the movement of *prana* through the use of breathing techniques
Pranayama	energy management using the science of the breath
Pranic Body	the eighth of the *Ten Bodies.* Continuously brings the life force and energy into the system.
Radiant Body	the tenth of the *Ten Bodies.* Gives spiritual royalty and radiance.
Rock Pose	sitting on the heels with the hands resting on the knees, the chin tucked slightly in and the spine straight
Root Chakra	the first of the major chakras, located at the base of the spine between the anus and the sex organs
Root Lock	a gentle squeeze of the muscles at the base of the spine, including the perineum, anus, sex organs and navel
Sacral Chakra	the second of the major chakras, located in the sex organs
Sadhana	a daily spiritual practice

Sevadar	someone who performs a service without any expectation of result or reward
Shabd	the sound current or vibration that cuts away the ego which obstructs truth and prevents us from perceiving and acting from our True Self
Shabd Guru	sound current as Teacher, a quantum technology of sound which directly alters our consciousness through the power of the Naad
Siri Guru Granth Sahib	1,430 pages of the words of seven of the ten Sikh Gurus plus enlightened people of other faiths
Solar Plexus	a complex network of nerves located in the abdomen, behind the stomach and in front of the diaphragm
Soul Body	the first of the *Ten Bodies*. Connects you to your inner infinity.
Sushmuna	the central *nadi* through which Kundalini rises
Subtle Body	the ninth of the *Ten Bodies*. Carries the Soul at the time of death.
Sutra	a thought-laden aphorism; literally translated as “thread”
Ten Bodies	powerful capacities of the psyche comprising the physical body, three mental bodies and six energy bodies
Third Eye	ajna, the sixth of the major chakras, located between or just above the eyebrows
Throat Chakra	vishuddha, the fifth of the major chakras, located at the throat
Thymus gland	involved in maturing white blood cells that help support the immune system
Thyroid gland	controls body metabolism and growth along with the development of the nervous system
True Self	our authentic or higher Self, our true identity
Tuning in	starting any Kundalini Yoga class or personal practice by chanting *Adi Mantra*

Upanishads, the	the earliest Yogic writings, over 2,500 years old. Upanishad means to sit near and be attentive and relates to the way knowledge was passed on from teacher to student.
Venus Lock	a mudra in which the fingers are interlaced with the right little finger at the bottom and the right thumbtip just above the base of the left thumb on the webbing between the thumb and index finger. The right thumbtip presses the fleshy mound at the base of the left thumb. For men the sequence of alternating the fingers is reversed and the left thumbtip is on the webbing between the right thumb and index finger.
Yama	qualities to which the Yogi should aspire in his or her external interactions
Yoga	a technology of awareness, a manual for human consciousness that explores your dimensions, depth, nature and potential as a human being. *Yoga* connects the individual consciousness to the Universal Consciousness.
Yogi Bhajan	born Harbhajan Singh Puri, Yogi Bhajan brought the technology of Kundalini Yoga, which had previously been kept secret, to the West in the late 1960s

Further Reading and Music Sources

Kundalini Yoga

Yogi Bhajan: www.yogibhajan.org

The 3HO Foundation: www.3ho.org

The Kundalini Research Institute: http://kundaliniresearchinstitute.org

Kundalini Yoga Classes Near You

The Kundalini Yoga Teachers Association offers a search facility: www.kundaliniyoga.org.uk

Kundalini Yoga and lifestyle

The Aquarian Teacher by Yogi Bhajan, PhD, (Level One Instructor textbook published by Kundalini Research Institute, 2003)

Kundalini Yoga: The Flow of Eternal Power by Shakti Parwha Kaur Khalsa (First Time Capsule Books, 1996)

The Chakra System

The Eight Human Talents by Gurmukh Kaur Khalsa with Cathryn Michon (HarperCollins Publishers Inc, 2000)

Teaching Kundalini Yoga

The Kundalini Yoga Teachers Association in the UK: www.kundaliniyoga.org.uk

The International School of Kundalini Yoga: www.i-sky.net

The Mind

The Mind: Its Projections and Multiple Facets by Yogi Bhajan, PhD (Kundalini Research Institute, 1998)

More kriyas and meditations

The Library of Teachings on Yogi Bhajan's website: www.libraryofteachings.com

The 3HO Foundation: www.3ho.org/kundalini-yoga

I am a Woman: Essential Kriyas for Women in the Aquarian Age (Kundalini Research Institute, 2009)

Sadhana Guidelines: Create Your Daily Spiritual Practice (Kundalini Research Institute, 2007)

Music

www.spiritvoyage.com

Pranayam

Praana Praanee Praanayam (Kundalini Research Institute; 2006)

Puran Prem Kaur

www.karmaparent.com

www.facebook.com/karmaparent

@KarmaParent

Index

Acknowledgements

The Teachers who have come before me, especially Yogi Bhajan, who made it his life's mission to preserve and share these teachings for the benefit of future generations, and my own Teachers.

All the people who have helped me create this book: Emily Johnston of Photographic Blonde who took the photos, Danni Everdell who modelled the postures, Siri Neel Kaur Khalsa of the Kundalini Research Institute for all her guidance, Alison Jones of Practical Inspiration Publishing and The Expert Author programme, my sister Sally Bland and my friends Rachael Moulder Phillips and Helen Lewis for providing valuable feedback, Guru Dharam for writing the Foreword, and last but not least, my family and my children for inspiring me to write it in the first place.

Lightning Source UK Ltd.
Milton Keynes UK
UKOW07f1623210216

268793UK00004B/24/P

9 781910 056363

Bath

History and Guide

Trevor Fawcett and Stephen Bird

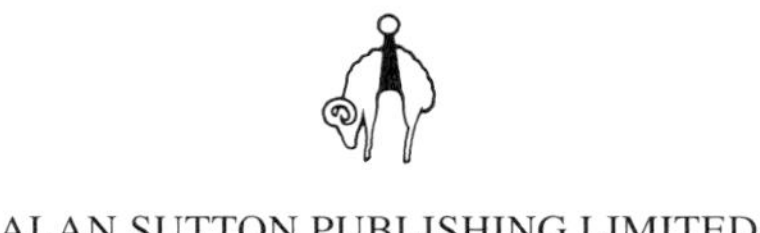

ALAN SUTTON PUBLISHING LIMITED

First published in the United Kingdom in 1994
Alan Sutton Publishing Ltd
Phoenix Mill · Far Thrupp · Stroud · Gloucestershire

First published in the United States of America in 1994
Alan Sutton Publishing Inc.
83 Washington Street · Dover · NH 03820

British Library Cataloguing in Publication Data

A catalogue record for this book is available from the British Library

ISBN 0–7509–0425–9

Library of Congress Cataloging-in-Publication Data applied for

Jacket illustration: The Roman Baths, with their late Victorian additions, and Bath Abbey (photograph by Stephen Bird).

Typeset in 10/13 Times.
Typesetting and origination by
Alan Sutton Publishing Limited.
Printed in Great Britain by
Redwood Books,
Trowbridge, Wiltshire.

Contents

One of the saddest moments in Bath's history occurred in 1978 when an amoeba was discovered in the spa water, which cost the life of a child. This was a tragedy in itself. It also put an end to at least two millennia of therapeutic bathing. This book is dedicated to the hope that the spa water, the life-blood of the city, will once again be restored to use for the benefit of the people of Bath and its visitors.

Introduction

Renowned for its Roman and Georgian past and characterized by images, often trivial and misleading, of life in those periods, Bath is in reality a city whose appearance is moulded by the deep valley of the River Avon and its tributaries scored into the plateaux of the southern Cotswolds, and textured by its man-made landscape of pale oolitic limestone hewn from the downs to the south and east. But the beating heart of the city is surely the geothermal springs that rise within a loop of the river in the valley bottom. Originating as rain or snow on the Mendip Hills to the south-west, the water reaches Bath through cave systems in the Carboniferous limestone, is heated at a depth of between 2,700 and 4,300 m (8,800–14,000 ft), expands and is forced up through fissures to break the surface in three locations. Other fissures in the valley bed are known to be choked by alluvium and river gravel, which prevent the thermal water from breaking through.

The three hot springs are all located within the ancient walled area of the city centre. The Hetling Spring, rising in an eighteenth-century stone tank beneath Hot Bath Street, no longer reaches the surface and is only betrayed in the coldest winters by the damp patch where the hidden warmth below prevents snow from settling. A few metres to the north the Cross Bath Spring, open to the sky, can only be glimpsed from the street, while 100 m (325 ft) to the east the visitor must penetrate the Pump Room complex to gaze down on the principal spring in the King's Bath. Here the flow is by far the greatest, yielding about 90 per cent of the total – over one million litres (*c*. 250,000 gallons) each day at a temperature of 46 °C (115 °F). Trapped beneath the hard man-made environment of the city centre, the springs convey little of the mystery and drama they must have given the empty valley in its natural state. There can be little doubt that early man was fascinated by, perhaps fearful of, this powerful natural phenomenon that welled up ceaselessly from the mud, stained a bright ochre by iron oxide deposited as the steaming water soaked away to the river.

As befits a city of Bath's historic pedigree, there is a legend to explain its origins. In the ninth century BC, it is said, Prince Bladud, son of Ludhudibras, King of Britain, contracted leprosy, was banished from the court and became a country swineherd. In time he noticed that when his pigs went to wallow in a steaming swamp in the valley bottom they emerged cleansed of their warts and sores. Convinced that his own condition could be cured in this way he plunged into the mire and, true to all good legends, scrambled out without a blemish. He was accepted back into his father's court and, in grateful thanks to the hot springs, founded the city of Bath on the site.

CHAPTER ONE

Bath Before Bath

The earliest evidence for human activity at Bath comes, appropriately, from the hot springs and their immediate environs. Small flint blades or 'microliths' dating to around 5000 BC attest the presence of small bands of hunters at the springs, and the many waste flakes found with them indicate that they paused here long enough to fashion their tools and weapons from flint nodules brought from sources several miles away. The deciduous forests that had populated much of lowland Britain since the final recession of the ice sheets several thousand years earlier were home to animals such as deer, ox and wild pig which, attracted to the springs to lick at the mineral deposits, would make easy prey. These early inhabitants were wholly dependent on their environment for survival and followed an annual cycle of winters spent in the river valley and summers on higher, more open ground. Similar flint tools and chisel-ended arrowheads from the downs around Bath are evidence for this migratory cycle.

During the fourth millennium BC agriculture and stock-raising were introduced into southern Britain and the semi-nomadic existence of the indigenous population gradually gave way to a more settled lifestyle. Heavy polished flint and stone axeheads from around Bath show that land was cleared of trees for farms, fields and pastures. Cattle, goats, sheep and pigs were domesticated, although flint arrowheads show that diet was still supplemented by hunting. Fragments of pottery and extensive scatters of flint implements and waste material on the downs overlooking the Avon valley suggest a dense population, bringing flint nodules from the chalk some distance to the east and south to domestic sites and fashioning them into tools and weapons there.

The chambered tomb at Stony Littleton, south of Bath, is the best surviving of numerous such structures known in the vicinity. These funerary monuments represent the upper echelons of an increasingly complex society in which dynastic tombs may have served as a focus for the surrounding population. All recorded examples are several kilometres from the city centre, suggesting that the hot springs may have been on the boundaries between tribal groupings. They belonged to a megalithic building tradition that extended from the

Mediterranean along the Atlantic seaboard to the northern isles, indicating that the passage of ideas and customs, if not of people, took place over great distances. The Jurassic Way, extending from the Wash to the Dorset coast and one of Britain's great prehistoric routeways, crossed the River Avon at Bath, doubtless interlinking with other more local tracks. The river valley itself was a natural corridor of communication from the Bristol Channel towards the Ridgeway and the Salisbury Plain. These and other routeways enabled the widespread transmission of materials, people and ideas over great distances; the inhabitants of the Bath vicinity would have been accustomed to, and would have benefited from, the passage of trade through and across the Avon valley.

Around 2000 BC the search for metals brought fresh newcomers to southern England and with them new burial practices, single inhumations under round barrows. Flints continued to be used extensively but, as the secrets of metalworking were mastered, isolated copper objects started to appear among the grave goods. Early Bronze Age occupation of the Bath area is represented almost exclusively by barrow cemeteries on the downs, occupying the same areas as the neolithic flint scatters and indicating continuity of a predominantly stone- and flint-using population. The paucity of bronze and copper finds from these areas may be due to the fact that broken tools would be exchanged for new ones by travelling bronzesmiths who, on occasion, seem to have hidden their stock-in-trade, perhaps because of danger and with the intention of collecting

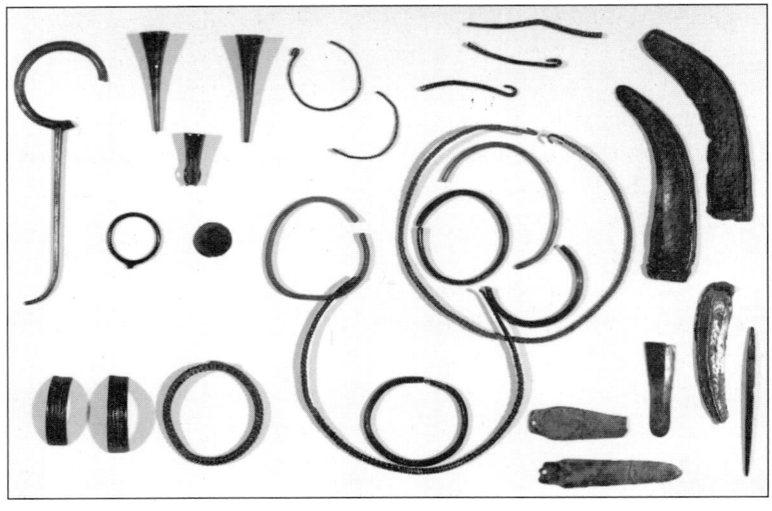

The Monkswood Hoard (*c.* 1250–1050 BC), found during the construction of Monkswood Reservoir north-east of Bath in 1894

it later. The hoard found at Monkswood Reservoir, Batheaston, contains sickles and items of personal adornment, demonstrating the range of equipment that could now be made in bronze. Perhaps the most enigmatic metal item from this period is a gold 'sun-disc', possibly of Irish origin, found under a barrow on Lansdown. Such finds are rare and it must have belonged to a person of considerable wealth or influence. The proximity of this find to the hot springs has prompted the suggestion that it may allude to the natural heat of the springs, although no Bronze Age material has been found in them. One might expect the springs to have been particularly significant to the later Bronze Age population at a time when the climate was deteriorating and religious practices appear to have been shifting from sky-oriented sites such as stone circles to more watery sites like springs, rivers and bogs.

This climatic deterioration in the first millennium BC led to exposed moorland sites being abandoned in favour of lower-lying areas. Competition for the use of available land may be reflected in the development of more aggressive weapons like the leaf-shaped slashing sword and the emergence of a new, perhaps equestrian, warrior élite. At the same time Celtic people started migrating into southern England from France and the Low Countries, creating yet more tensions but bringing with them new forms of art and material culture. Two votive bronze spoons found in 1866 in a stream in Weston village, close to one of the routes of the Jurassic Way through Bath, are decorated with typical flowing curvilinear ornament and are an indication that watery sites continued to be revered into the Celtic period.

The Iron Age is characterized by the appearance of hillforts in the landscape, several of which are known around Bath. Little Solsbury above Batheaston was occupied by circular wooden huts erected on clear land away from the escarpment. Later a defensive rampart and drystone wall were built, although these did not protect the settlement from a violent destruction by fire. New huts were erected over the rubble, associated with new forms of pottery that also appear on domestic sites at Rush Hill and Sion Hill, and which may represent the conquest of the Bath area by a neighbouring community. At Rush Hill the pottery was found on a settlement outside a possible hillfort which, together with the new undefended settlement on Little Solsbury, suggests that a particular period of danger had passed. These are rare domestic sites, however, and the extensive 'Celtic' fields and tracks on Charmy Down and Bathampton Down represent a fairly dense population whose settlements have, as yet, escaped discovery.

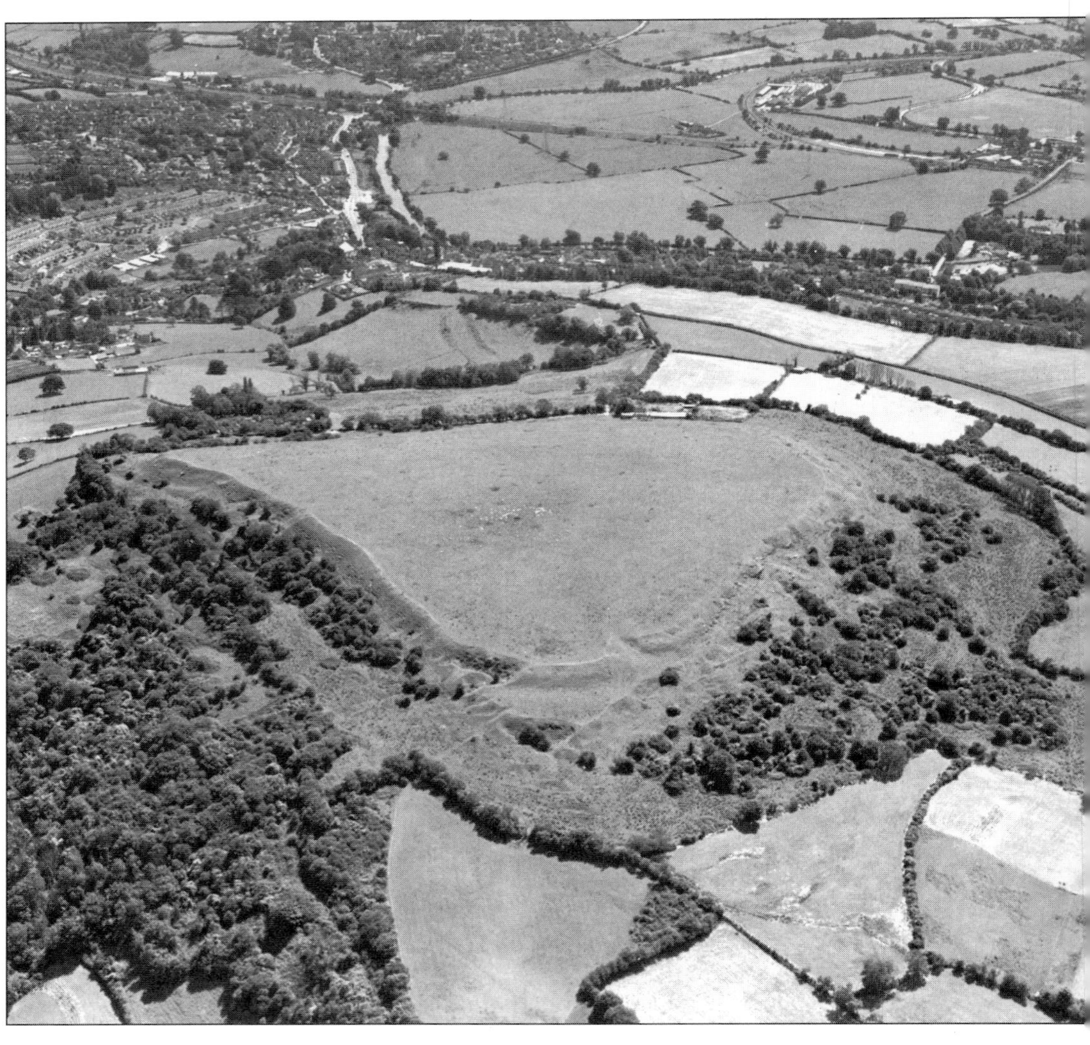

Little Solsbury Iron Age hillfort: the site may have been occupied during the later Bronze Age but had been abandoned by the first century BC

The invasions of south-eastern England by Julius Caesar in 55 and 54 BC had little discernible effect on the Bath area. Little Solsbury hillfort was finally abandoned between 100 and 50 BC, its occupants moving elsewhere, perhaps to the large undefendable enclosure on Bathampton Down. Caesar's campaigns were followed by ever closer contacts between the British Isles and occupied Gaul. Roman influence was already prompting the issuing of gold coins by the kings of British tribal areas, not as a means of market exchange but more probably as symbols of power or favour, although similar coins in baser metals may have served as an early form of currency. Numerous coins of the Dobunni, the

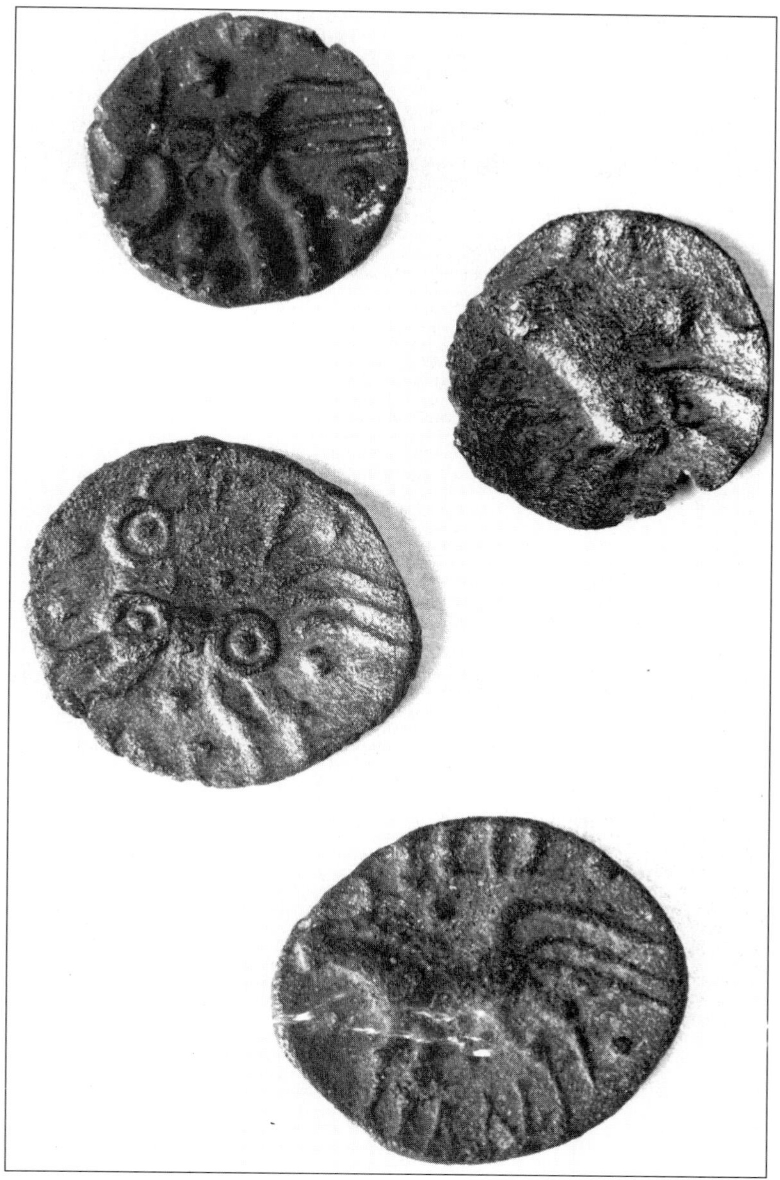

Celtic coins from the Sacred Spring, probably deposited during the early first century AD prior to the Roman invasion

kingdom whose territory included Gloucestershire and north Somerset, have been found in Bath and, in particular, in the hot springs, suggesting that these held some significance for the local population. Others have been found close to likely tracks, such as the small group near the foot of Bathwick Hill and one from a native farmstead near Marlborough Lane.

CHAPTER TWO

The Rise and Fall of *Aquae Sulis*

The Roman invasion of Britain under the Emperor Claudius in AD 43 quickly established control of England as far as the rivers Severn and Trent. Roman rule over the new territory was exerted by a network of timber forts and military roads, in particular the Fosse Way from Dorset to Lincolnshire, which was laid out to enable rapid communication along the new frontier zone.

The Bath valley encountered by the Roman army seems to have been a peaceful landscape of fields, woods and hutted settlements. Several prehistoric routeways traversed the valley, linking major native centres of influence at Bury Hill to the north and Camerton to the south. Doubtless these tracks were used by the army, with some being metalled and cleared of scrub to form part of the Fosse Way. Very soon a fort would have been built to guard the principal river crossing and house troops to police the native population. This fort has yet to be discovered. Antiquarians in the early nineteenth century recorded substantial rectangular camps on opposite sides of the river at Walcot and Bathwick, and more recently early Samian pottery has been found in the Forester Avenue area of Bathwick.

Despite the apparent absence of resistance, the Romans were determined to stamp their authority on the area and, as an act of suppression and humiliation, drove a substantial military road through the native sanctuary around the hot springs. A possible reason for this was a serious breach of the new frontier in the winter of AD 48–9, probably by the Silurian tribes of South Wales, which led to punitive measures being taken behind the frontier once the incursion had been repelled. But despite this brutal act the springs excited the curiosity of the Roman garrison, and word about them must have spread quickly within the army; some veterans may even have retired here to be close to them.

Dialogue between Celts and Romans quickly established the qualities of the presiding deity Sulis – perhaps healing and wisdom –

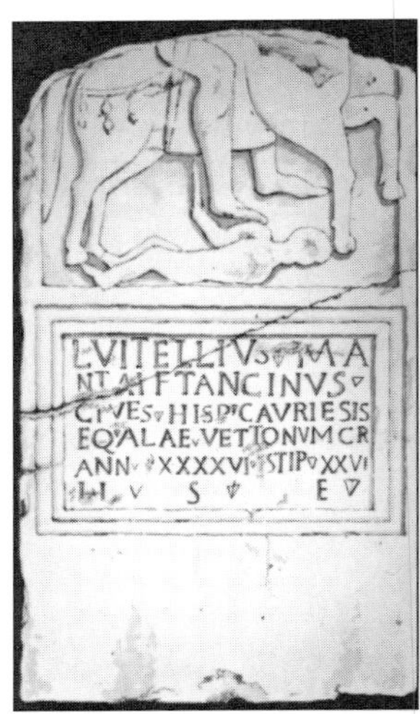

Roman military tombstones from the early cemetery beside the London Road, recording an auxiliary cavalryman (top) and an armourer of the Twentieth Legion (above) (Samuel Lysons *Reliquiae Britannico-Romanae*, 1813)

and a classical equivalent was promptly found in Minerva. In the 60s, when major Roman investment was being poured into civilian building projects in southern England, work began to construct a religious spa, dedicated to the combined deity Sulis Minerva, around the springs. In deference to the site's Celtic origins the settlement was named *Aquae Sulis* – the waters of Sulis. The geographer Ptolemy later referred to it as *Aquae Calidae* – hot waters; evidently he was more interested in the site's physical properties than in its religious significance.

Using the engineering, surveying and architectural skills of the army, and doubtless carefully directed by priests, a range of classical buildings was laid out around the principal spring, which was itself enclosed within a substantial lead-lined stone reservoir. This performed two functions: it created a head of water to supply three rectangular pools to the south while at the same time providing a focus for worship of Sulis Minerva on the north side where the temple stood. Doubtless there was much approval when the open-air temple yard enclosed within a colonnaded walk was laid out over the military road that had earlier desecrated the native sanctuary. The hatchet was buried; repression was replaced by harmony.

Nowhere was this harmony better demonstrated than on the highly decorated pediment of the temple, which stood on a podium in the centre of its precinct. A Gaulish sculptor was engaged to create a

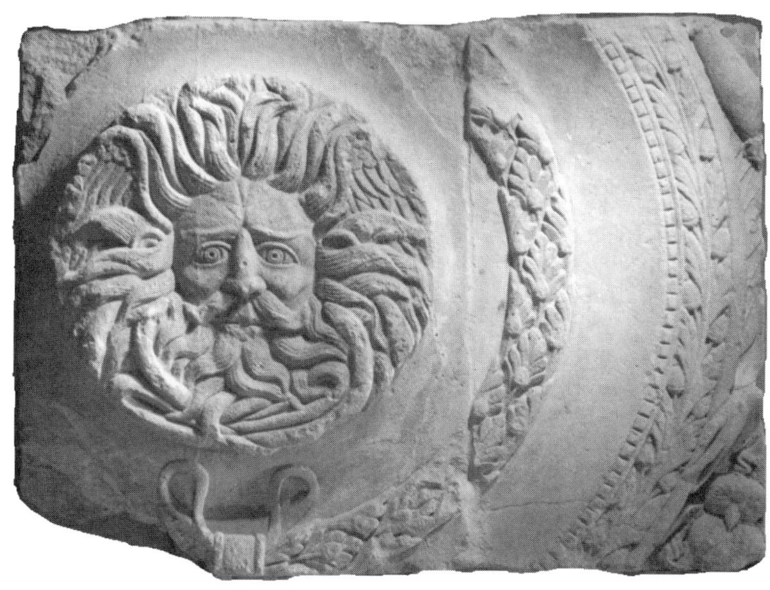

The 'Gorgon's Head' relief carving in the *tympanum* of the Temple of Sulis Minerva, which dominated proceedings in the busy inner precinct

blend of Celtic and classical imagery to satisfy both traditions. In this he succeeded brilliantly. The central face is unmistakably Celtic in its inspiration but hints at the Gorgon, a symbol of Minerva; it is reminiscent of other water deities but at the same time resembles the sun, giver of heat to the springs, while around it other devices explain and enhance the presiding goddess. Other aspects of the site were purely classical. The arrangement of the temple complex, with its large altar centrally sited in part of the temple, had its origins in the Mediterranean world where the convention was for public worship to take place in the open air. The bathing range of three pools fed from the spring and two heated rooms was austere and monumental, as would be expected from its military designers.

As the complex took shape during the 60s and 70s, the area around the springs must have appeared chaotic. Building materials – locally felled timber, stone from the surrounding downs and ingots of Mendip lead – were assembled in vast quantities to be fashioned and finished on site. By around AD 75 the painting of the temple was completed, the plumbing of the baths in place and functioning. Bath's valley now sported a gleaming range of buildings the like of which the local population had never seen before. These may have included a theatre adjacent to the temple, while clustered around may have been lodgings for priests and visitors and outbuildings for service and maintenance purposes. The massive stone structures must have appeared all the more imposing for, unlike public buildings being erected in new towns elsewhere, they were not at the centre of an extensive urban development of regular streets and *insulae*. Travellers approaching along one of several new roads converging on the valley cannot fail to have been impressed by the grandeur of their destination in an otherwise largely rural environment. A suburb of dwellings and workshops along the main road in the Walcot area may represent the beginnings of the community that serviced and maintained the temple and baths throughout the Roman period.

Although baths were the social focus of towns, those of *Aquae Sulis*, with their emphasis on immersion in water, were built to function in harmony with the temple of Sulis Minerva. Visitors seeking cure for illness or injury, or simply relaxation and therapy, might first pay their respects to the goddess at the temple and petition her for healing before turning to the baths to seek and receive that healing in the curative water provided by the goddess.

Acts of public worship took place on the large altar in the temple forecourt, where the organs of sacrificed animals were scrutinized by a *haruspex* or augur, watched by onlookers waiting to hear the

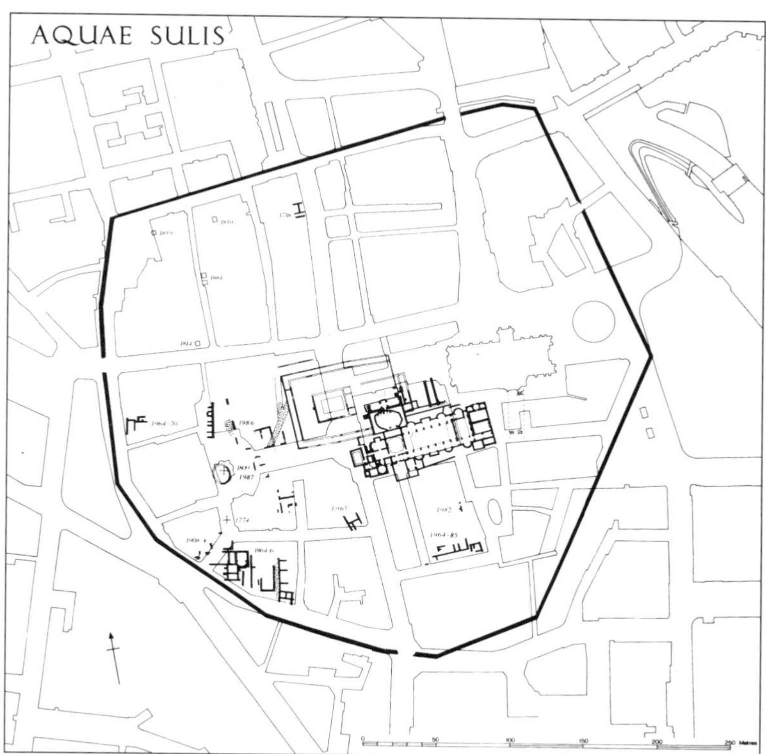

The walled area of *Aquae Sulis* with the baths and temple at its centre. The extra-mural settlement stood a few hundred metres to the north

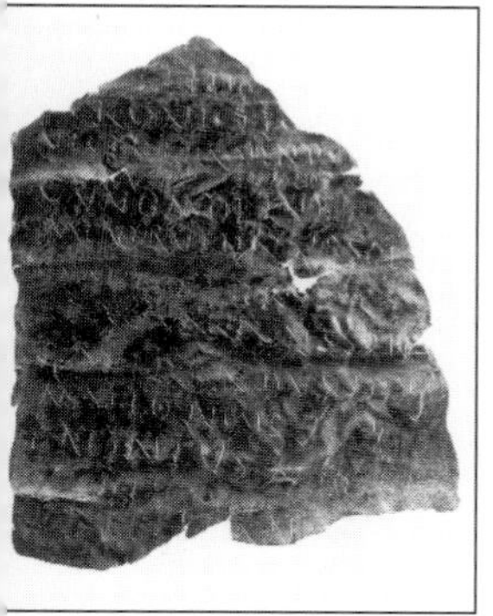

Pewter curse tablet with gabled top, from the Sacred Spring; among the people mentioned in the incised text is one *Minervina*, possibly named after the patron goddess

portents for the future. One such priest, Lucius Marcius Memor, is known from a dedication stone he erected close to the altar. Other ceremonies may have taken place on the steps of the temple, which gave those officiating, such as Gaius Calpurnius Receptus, 'priest of the goddess Sulis', a commanding view over the precinct, altar and sacred spring. Serious pilgrims here to perform a particular act of duty or devotion conducted private ceremonies at inscribed stone altars positioned in the outer precinct around the base of the temple. The steaming reservoir in the corner of the precinct would be approached with some respect, and a personal petition, in the form of a coin, item of jewellery or other symbolic offering, might be cast into the spring to curry the favour of Sulis Minerva. Those seeking vengeance for grievances done to them would, perhaps using a scribe, scratch their request on a small pewter sheet. These messages, though carefully formulated, could be unbridled in their quest for revenge. The secrets were then sealed as the curse tablets were folded up and dropped into the spring for the goddess to act upon. It was never imagined that, centuries later, archaeologists would have the audacity to retrieve them from the grasp of the goddess and expose the petty irritations that, in an impassioned moment, had once seemed so important.

From the other side of the sacred spring the bath-house cast a shadow over this corner of the temple yard. Its interior could be glimpsed through three arches and, conversely, bathers could look out across the spring towards the temple. On both sides these views reminded people that the roles of temple and baths intertwined, the sacred spring being the common central feature. After paying their respects to Sulis Minerva, visitors would then enter the baths to cleanse themselves, relax with friends or await restoration to health.

In the early years the choice of bathing facilities was limited to three pools through which water from the spring passed, gradually cooling as it went. Two steam rooms, heated from beneath by hypocausts, formed a simple suite of Turkish baths – providing the basic cleansing facilities a Roman would expect to find anywhere. But nowhere else in the province of *Britannia* offered the same endless supply of hot water, and the bath-house erected to use it must have been one of the wonders of Roman Britain, the creation of Mediterranean people who could hardly believe the beneficence of the gods in providing such liquid bounty in this cold northern land. The opportunity was not wasted. The largest and warmest pool was constructed to standing depth, and its level bottom and steps were lined with lead sheets to keep out cold ground water. Along each side, steps to the surrounding ambulatory gave bathers unrestricted movement in and out of the water, while recesses in the walls enabled them to sit, dry off and chat. Above them a pitched timber-framed roof, supported by square stone columns, covered the high echoing chamber whose steamy gloom was relieved only by daylight from high-level windows. Unlike the picture of bustle and commotion normally painted for town bath-houses, the atmosphere here is likely to have been more solemn and contemplative, without the population of an ordinary town to provide for and with its role as an adjunct to the temple. Doubtless the arrival of squads of soldiers, either on leave or in transit, enlivened proceedings somewhat.

Those who planned the baths may not have anticipated the effects of a constantly humid environment on timber-framed roofs and may have underestimated the popularity that *Aquae Sulis* was to achieve. Within a hundred years the roof structure, weakened by the constant exposure to steam, was replaced by an impressive brick and tile vault spanning the chamber on strengthened stone piers. At the east end the smallest

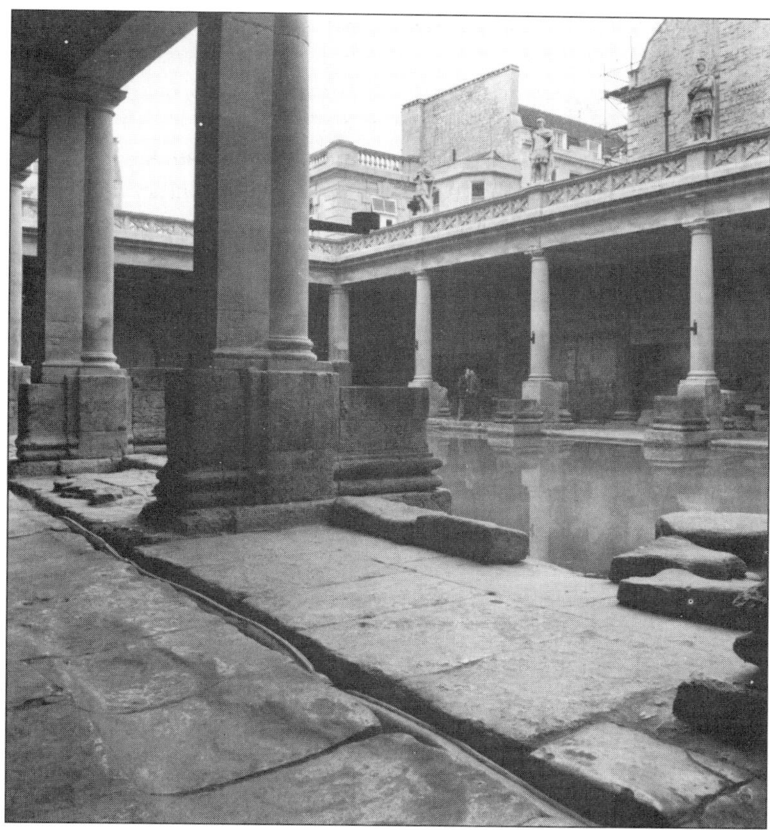

The massive Bathstone pillar-bases of the Great Bath and a lead water-pipe set into the blue lias ambulatory

and coolest of the baths was sacrificed to make way for an additional suite of hypocaust rooms, perhaps in response to Hadrian's instruction that public baths should take steps to prevent mixed bathing. The original hypocaust rooms at the west end were extended and furnished with a small sauna and a circular cold plunge rinsing pool. Hereafter both suites were intermittently extended and improved so that in its final form the bath-house was an eclectic and complicated range of adjoining rooms, still dominated by its central vaulted pool.

Changes to the temple complex were slower in coming, but when they did their effect was dramatic. In the late second or early third century changes in ritual practice occurred and the open reservoir tank was enclosed within a vaulted rectangular building, separating the sacred spring from the outside world. The three arches still overlooked the spring from the baths, but access from the temple precinct was possible only through a small doorway, whose well-worn step still testifies to the traffic of priests and pilgrims visiting the spring. At the same time the purely classical temple took on a more hybrid or Romano-Celtic flavour with the addition around it of an ambulatory, possibly with a lean-to roof, and two lesser temples or treasuries at its front beside the steps. Still later the building over the spring was strengthened with buttresses and a central portico, which faced the altar and enhanced the doorway giving access to the spring. On the other side of the altar stood a lesser-known building, possibly a dormitory for the sick awaiting their cure. The effect of these changes was to create a more intimate inner precinct around the altar in front of the temple. All around, painted relief carvings displayed a pantheon of Roman and Celtic deities; symbols of the seasons and the elements made reference to the natural phenomenon at the heart of the site, while inscriptions recorded renovation and repainting of the temple buildings. The visitor, approaching through the arched entrance, was greeted by a brightly coloured array of reliefs and inscriptions on buildings whose arrangement restricted sightlines and stimulated the spirit of enquiry about what lay around corners and beyond doorways – the spring inside its mysterious steamy chamber, the cult statue inside the temple, attended only by the priests who kept perpetual flames alight. It must have been an emotionally satisfying experience; some of the symbolism was obvious while the significance of other icons was more obscure, but gradually the pattern would take shape and the nature and qualities of the spring and its presiding deity would become clear.

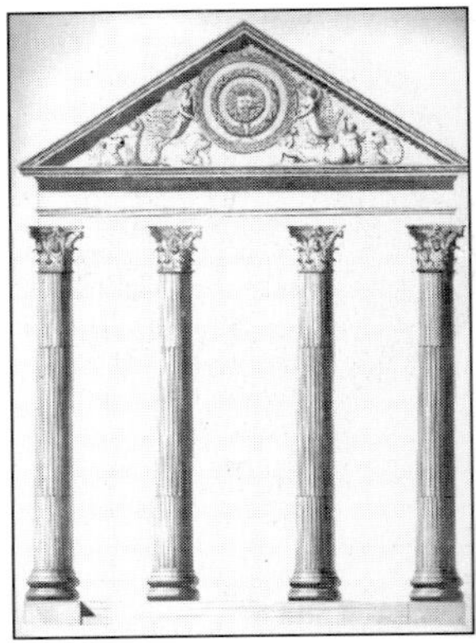

The Temple of Sulis Minerva as reconstructed a few years after fragments of the columns and pediment were discovered (Samuel Lysons *Reliquiae Britannico-Romanae*, 1813)

Who, then, were the people of *Aquae Sulis*? Most of those known from inscriptions were probably visitors; many locals, perhaps without cause to erect an altar and lacking the wealth for an elaborate memorial, will have gone unrecorded – baths personnel, tradesmen, retired residents and the artisan community of Walcot among them. The healing waters, presided over by Minerva whose martial prowess was well known to the army, quickly attracted the attention of soldiers serving in the garrison, and *Aquae Sulis* became a resort for legionaries and auxiliaries seeking rest and recuperation. In its very early years the spa must have resembled a military transit camp, although the cemetery of tombstones lining the main road from London served as a reminder that for some at least the cure did not work. It was not long, however, before civilians were visiting. The colossal funerary memorial of a woman's head, whose hairstyle dates the deceased to the later first century, shows that already the spa was attracting pilgrims of considerable wealth. Some were evidently a long way from home. A Spanish cavalryman and

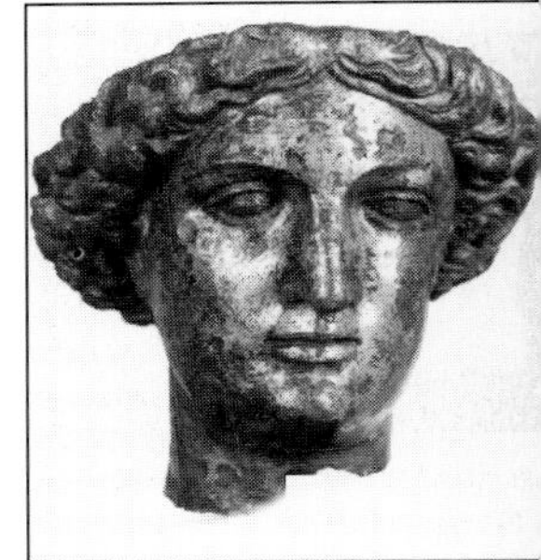

Head of the cult statue of Sulis Minerva; the jagged neck suggests that it met a violent end. The body has never been found

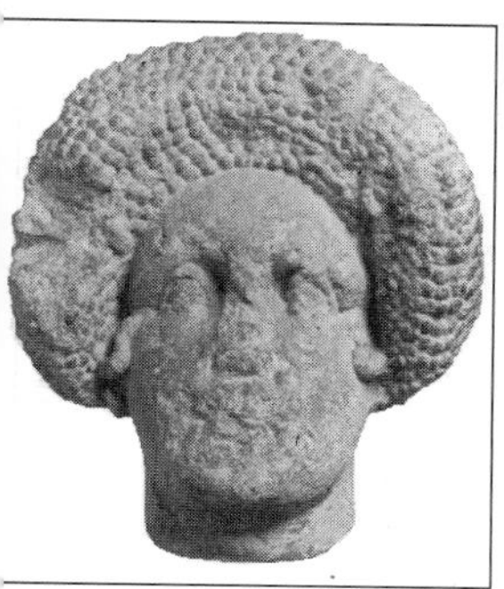

First-century AD tomb sculpture commemorating a wealthy woman. Found during roadworks in Walcot in 1714 or 1715

legionaries from Germany and southern France were already serving in Britain when they came to *Aquae Sulis*, while others, like Peregrinus of Trier and fifty-eight-year-old Rusonia Aventina from Metz, probably made the journey especially. Priscus, a stonemason from Chartres, probably saw an opportunity to ply his trade in stone-rich Bath. Very young to very old are recorded on inscriptions, from eighteen-month-old Mercatilla to the eighty-six-year-old town councillor from Gloucester who retired to *Aquae Sulis* for the cure.

Although *Aquae Sulis* was never intended to perform the economic and administrative roles of a provincial town, it gradually acquired other buildings that gave it the appearance of a small, albeit well-endowed, town. Shrines stood over the other two hot springs, one of which supplied another bathing complex. One would expect a theatre close to the principal temple for the enactment of ceremonies and religious plays, and a massive decorated cornice block from immediately north of the temple precinct may indicate its location. A circular Greek-style temple, or *tholos*, may have stood in its own precinct to the east of the temple of Sulis Minerva, perhaps a legacy of the visit by Hadrian, a Graecophile, to the province in the AD 120s. Early domestic timber-framed buildings with painted wall plaster were replaced in the second century by masonry houses, but areas were left undeveloped as work areas or maintenance yards. Late in the second century a defensive rampart and ditch was thrown around the settlement, being consolidated with a masonry wall in the third century, which effectively inhibited any further organized growth of the town. Thereafter, with the exception of the well-established extra-mural settlement in Walcot, new developments took place within the wall by infilling unused areas or by demolition and rebuilding. Close to the wall at least three substantial town houses, variously sporting hypocaust rooms, elaborate geometric mosaics and window glass, were built in the third and fourth centuries; whether these related to the operation of the spa in any way, or belonged to the owners of estates in the surrounding countryside, is unknown.

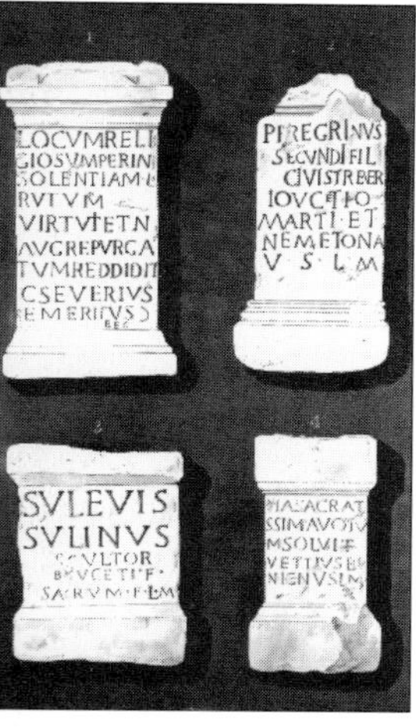

nscribed altars erected by) G. Severius Emeritus, enturion of the region',) Peregrinus from Trier,) Sulinus a sculptor, and) Vettius Benignus (Samuel ysons *Reliquiae Britannico-omanae*, 1813)

It is difficult to compare *Aquae Sulis* with normal Romano-British towns, as its hot springs and religious spa set it apart from other settlements. Although the population of Britain remained overwhelmingly rural throughout the Roman period, towns were central to the administration of the province. Regional capitals, ranging in size from 45 to 240 acres, governed cantons somewhat larger than present counties. *Aquae Sulis* lay within that of the *Belgae*, which stretched from the Severn to the Solent with its capital at *Venta Belgarum* (Winchester) at its eastern end. It is possible that in the

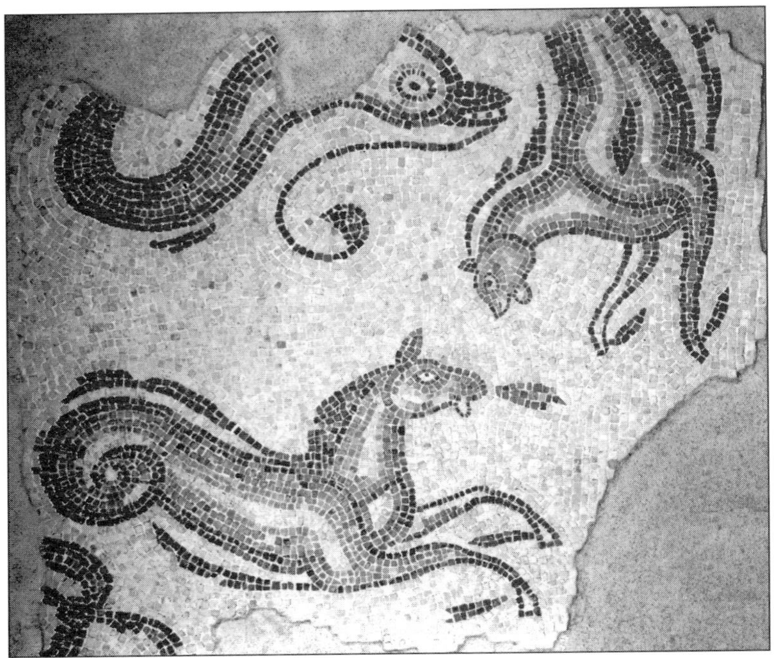

Fragment of a mosaic, probably fourth century, depicting a dolphin and sea horses; found in the north-west corner of the walled settlement in 1859

fourth century an administrative role was thrust upon *Aquae Sulis* after the surrounding countryside had become populated by influential villa owners demanding a market centre for their agricultural and industrial products. But neither the walled area, which occupied just 23 acres, nor the undefended artisan suburb in Walcot, demonstrate any of the characteristics of towns planned as regional capitals.

The occupation of a new province put considerable strain on the ability of the Roman administration to maintain a regular supply of food for the army and the vast quantities of building materials needed for the many construction projects being undertaken in southern England. To meet these demands imperial estates were established in key areas, and around Bath these were maintained for many years. Lead and silver production on Mendip was under way as early as AD 49, grain production in the fertile Chew Valley intensified, and at Combe Down stone quarrying was almost certainly put under military administration. Gaius Severius Emeritus, recorded as 'centurion of the region' on an altar he erected in the temple precinct, may have worked there. This estate was still functioning in the early third century when Naevius, an imperial freedman, supervised the reconstruction of its headquarters. A lead seal of the procurator's office suggests official business here, also in the third century. With so much land apparently under military control, no villas were built in the countryside around Bath until the later third century, and the absence of these highly civilized farmsteads in the vicinity must have highlighted the sense of isolation of the religious spa of *Aquae Sulis*. When land was finally released from official hands, however, there was clearly a demand for it that quickly led to a landscape dotted with stone-built farm dwellings, many equipped with hypocaust rooms and mosaics, and some, like that at Keynsham, of almost palatial proportions.

Mosaics at Bathwick and Norfolk Crescent attest two of the villas within the present city, while others at Marlborough Lane and Sion Hill were built on the sites of earlier native farmsteads. Although many villa estates were agricultural or livestock farms, some undertook industrial activities such as pewter manufacturing (which took place on Lansdown and was probably managed by a nearby villa), while others may simply have been residential retreats with little or no economic activity. The villa dwellers, Latin-speaking and familiar with the art and literature of the classical world, surrounded themselves with Roman trappings and luxuries and looked towards the sanctuary of *Aquae Sulis* as their principal social focus and contact with the civilized world. Sculptors like Sulinus, son of Brucetus, must have found a ready market for statuary and ornamention in the wealthy surrounding villas, and it was evidently worth his while having a workshop at Cirencester in the Cotswolds, where another concentration was to be found. Yet for every villa there must have been numerous more humble Romano-British farms in the landscape that, due to their insubstantial nature, escape detection.

During the fourth century Britain was increasingly beleaguered by barbarian attacks from northern Europe and Ireland. Between 350 and 370 villas around Bath were attacked and burned; many were not reoccupied, the survivors preferring to seek refuge within the walls of *Aquae Sulis*. The very late presence of hypocaust rooms with mosaics in the outer temple precinct suggests extreme pressure on available building land.

As travel became unsafe the number of visitors declined, although small numbers of coins continued to be deposited in the spring to the end of the century. Flooding from the River Avon up the drains made maintenance of the baths and temple increasingly difficult, while the rising popularity of Christianity must have undermined the appeal of a major pagan cult. It may have been around this time that the statue of Minerva was toppled and desecrated. Mud and rubbish started to accumulate in the inner precinct and exposed fragments of decorated stonework fell or were knocked off the temple buildings, although attempts were made through cobbled paving to maintain some kind of activity here. This was clearly a community fighting to preserve its existence, and Bath may have been one of the British cities that petitioned the Emperor Honorius in AD 410 for protection, only to be told to see to their own defence. Within the walled area of *Aquae Sulis* some domestic buildings remained in use well into the fifth century. While the regular supply of visitors to the religious spa had long since dried up, the resident Romano-British population survived. They dropped out of the archaeological record but they did not go away.

CHAPTER THREE

The Growing Borough: Anglo-Saxon to Tudor Bath

During the period between the Roman abandonment of Britain and the Saxon conquest of the west country in the sixth century, the surviving population maintained a communal life of sorts, throwing their rubbish into the swamp that now engulfed the temple and baths. Yet it was a period of great uncertainty. In the 440s Saxon raiders overran the south and east of England; in the west the population either cowered behind the walls of Roman towns or fled to the hills and reoccupied Iron Age strongholds and Romano-Celtic temples. From these Dark Age communities new leaders emerged, semi-legendary warrior-kings like Arthur and Ambrosius, who led the defence against the West Saxon advance from the Solent area, culminating in Arthur's renowned victory around 517 at the Battle of *Mount Badon*. Many sites have been claimed for this battle but it is likely to have been fought somewhere on the heights overlooking Bath; certainly Badon is one of numerous Saxon names later given to the city. Arthur's victory only temporarily halted the West Saxon expansion, and in 577, at the Battle of Dyrham, Cuthwine and Ceawlin captured the cities of Gloucester, Cirencester and Bath, killing three kings in the process. The reference to cities and kings may have been to magnify the importance of the victory, which put paid to British resistance east of the Severn, but it does suggest that Bath was a town ruled by a local king, perhaps controlling a considerable tract of surrounding land.

The victory at Dyrham established West Saxon rule as far as the Cotswolds to the north and the River Severn to the west, but it also brought them into contact with the Saxon kingdom of Mercia. In

628, at Cirencester, Mercia defeated the West Saxons who withdrew to south of the Avon. It may have been at this time that the West Wansdyke earthwork was thrown up, from Odd Down to Maes Knoll south of Bristol, as a political frontier between Mercia and the new Kingdom of the West Saxons, or Wessex. Bath, now just inside Mercia, became the gateway between the two.

In 676 King Osric of the Hwicce in Mercia granted 100 hides of land around the city of *Hat Bathu* to the Abbess Berta on which to build a nunnery, possibly a double house of nuns and monks. Although its site is unknown it probably stood in the city centre, where a ready supply of building stone was available in the crumbling Roman buildings; indeed this may have been the time when the temple pediment with its blatant pagan symbols was removed from public view and laid face down as a pavement in the new religious house. Augustine, who had passed through Bath in 603, would have approved; Pope Gregory had instructed him to make use of pagan temple buildings but to destroy the images in them.

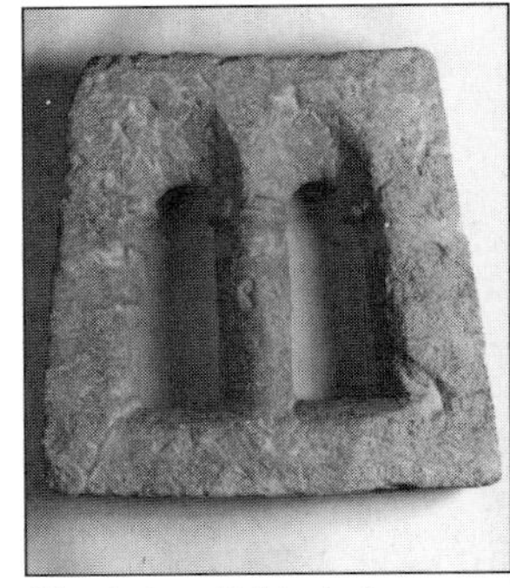

Simple two-light window carved from a single block, probably from the late Saxon monastery. Found near the present Abbey

A house of monks certainly existed by 758, and when he took possession of 'that most famous monastery at Bath' at the synod of Brentford in 781, King Offa of Mercia may well have ordered the reconstruction of the church, again using stone from the nearby Roman buildings. It may have been at this time that a monk of the priory recorded in verse the towering ruins that still cast a shadow over the monastery before they were attacked for their stone. The poem *The Ruin* is incomplete and the fragments that survive contain no name, although many phrases strike a chord with the Roman remains we know today:

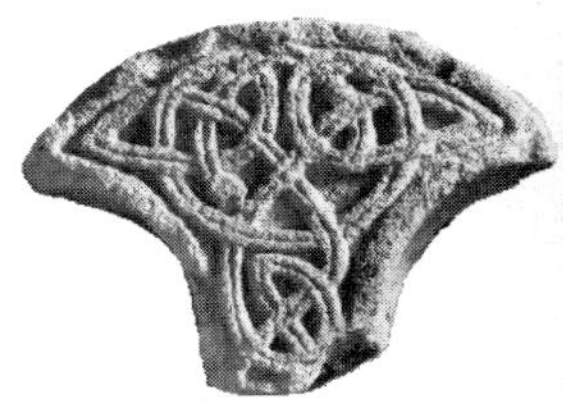

Decorated cross-head fragment found near the Cross Bath; one of several elaborate crosses that stood in the late Saxon town

> . . . Stone courts stood here:
> the stream with its great gush sprang forth hotly;
> there the baths were hot in its centre . . .

In the ninth century Nennius, in his *De Mirabilibus Brittanniae* (The Wonders of Britain), describes the hot lake 'where the baths of Badon are'; clearly the springs remained an awe-inspiring sight. Yet as the Roman buildings disintegrated so the Saxon monastery grew in fame, and around it Bath became a market centre, with well-constructed roads of locally quarried stone linking it with neighbouring villages and towns. These roads were important to the growing economic role Bath was assuming; trade and travel were vital and it was important for merchants to move freely and easily about the country. Furthermore, various royal laws forbade any

Opposite:
Coins of Edward the Elder (899–924/5), Aethelred II (978–1016) and Edward the Confessor (1042–66), struck at the Bath Mint

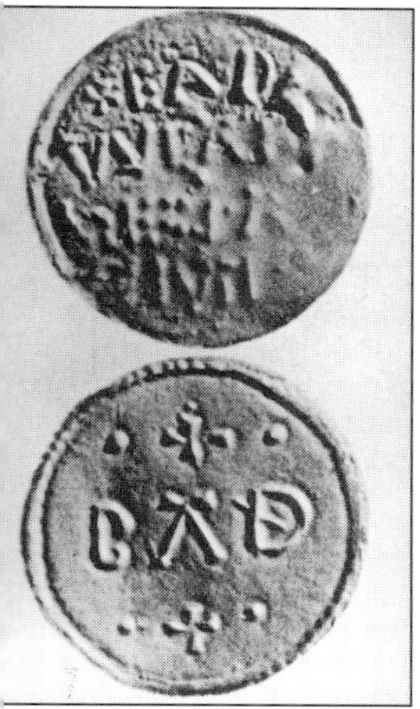

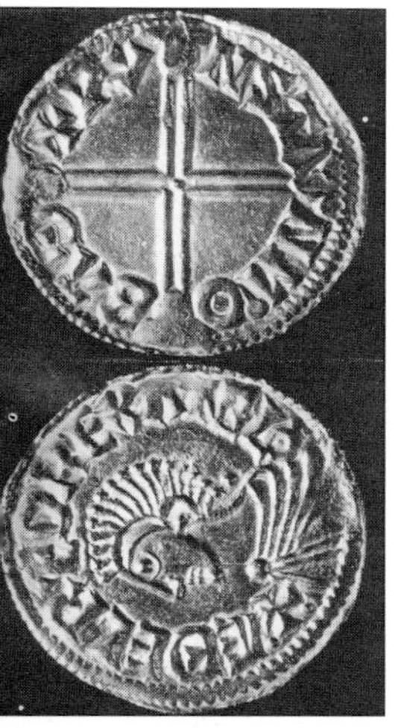

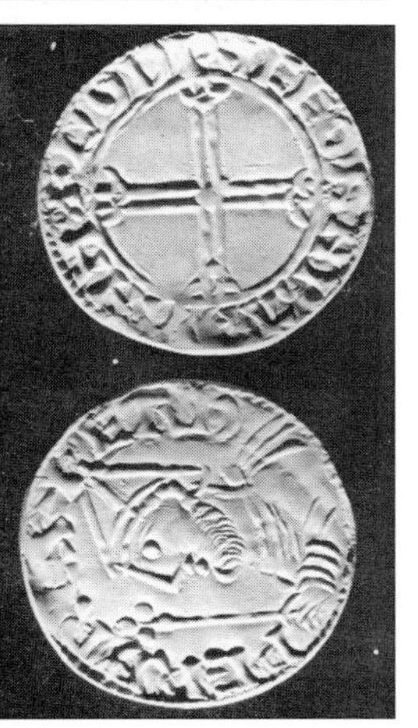

significant trading outside town walls, and this enhanced the economic development of towns in the tenth century.

By then Bath had passed from Mercia into Wessex. The date for this is unclear; in 864 Burgred, King of Mercia, held his court at Bath but Alfred the Great, King of Wessex from 871 to 899, is known to have strengthened the city's defences against possible Danish attacks. Alfred's successor Edward the Elder (899–924/5) continued to organize the defence of Wessex and ordered the compilation of the Burghal Hidage, a list of seventy-two burhs, or defended sites, in Wessex, which included Bath. He may also have been responsible for establishing a mint here, perhaps to emphasize Bath's status as a prized possession of the Kingdom of Wessex. Bath was already an impressive town. Surrounded by substantial walls and fortified gates, its mint issued fine silver coinage while the monastery was described in 957 as being 'of wondrous workmanship'. Athelstan (925–40) 'enriched the monastery with lands, relics and books' and, mindful of the needs of the poor and sick, founded a lepers' hospital near the two smaller springs. Increased prosperity in the monastery and the confidence offered by reinforced defences must have stimulated trading activities and population growth in the city, all set within the framework of a new regular street plan. It may have been during this period that the parish churches of St Michael by Westgate, St Mary intra Muros, St Mary de Stalles and St James were built.

Edgar succeeded to the throne in 959, having become King of Mercia and Northumbria two years earlier, and for the first time there was the prospect of a peaceful, united England under the rule of one monarch. But there was still work to be done. The monasteries needed revival and Edgar appointed Dunstan as Archbishop of Canterbury to perform the task. St Peter's at Bath was refounded as a Benedictine house, and charters soon followed, gathering nearby lands for the monastery. Such gains were, nevertheless, modest and the Domesday survey of a century later reveals that in Bath church-owned property amounted to no more than an eighth of that held by the king and his nobles. But though a small monastery, it possessed two important qualities. It was a splendid building, probably displaying impressive chunks of reused Roman masonry, and it was situated on the frontier of Mercia and Wessex, kingdoms united by Edgar's succession. What better stage than this for the coronation of the King of England? On Whit Sunday 973 and amid much ceremony Edgar was crowned in St Peter's church, in a service devised by Dunstan which has been used at coronations ever since. The tenth-century *Winchester Chronicle* describes the celebrations at 'the ancient town of Akemanceaster, also called Bath by the inhabitants of this island', when 'a great congregation of priests, and goodly company of monks and wise men gathered together'. The name used here is interesting; it occurs nowhere else and some have suggested that it was coined especially for the coronation. Interpretations of the word include 'sick man's town' and 'place of the oak tree'.

The optimism generated by Edgar's coronation was short-lived. Edgar died suddenly two years later without adult offspring to ensure a secure succession. Worse still, the Viking menace was looming again, and although there is no evidence of an assault on Bath, no one in the city could fail to have noticed the frantic activity at the mint, churning out tens of thousands of coins of Aethelred II (978–1016) – by far the mint's most productive period – not to service the requirements of a thriving economy, but simply to pay off the Danes. These coins of the Bath mint appear in vast quantities in hoards of Danegeld and heregeld in Scandinavia. In 1013 the thegns and ealdormen of the western shires surrendered to King Sweyn of Denmark at Bath, and in 1016 Cnut acceded unopposed as King of the English. Such political union inevitably meant personal contacts. A runestone erected at Småland in southern Sweden remembered the burial of Gunnar by his brother Helge 'in a sarcophagus in England in Bath'. A cross carved on the stone and the use of a stone coffin suggest that this funeral was conducted according to the new Viking Christian belief.

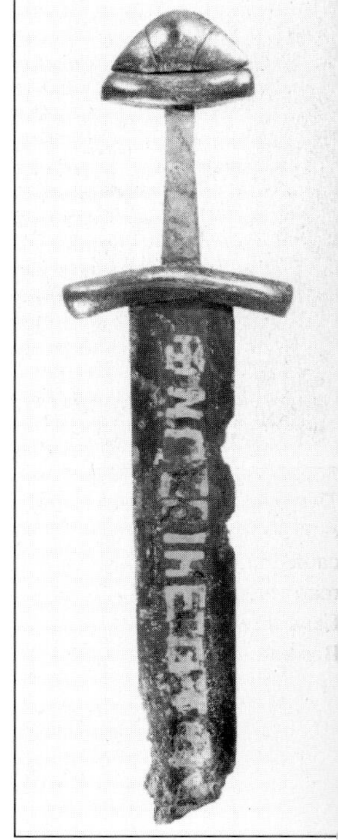

Tenth-century Viking sword inlaid with the maker's name; probably made in England. Found in the city ditch outside the North Gate

The Norman Conquest of Britain had little immediate effect on Bath. The mint continued to function, issuing coins of the early Norman kings up until the middle of the twelfth century. Bath's moment of destiny was to come twenty years after the Conquest with the destruction of the city during the Rufus Rebellion. Yet during the next 500 years the city saw the growth, decline and disappearance of the monastery, the development of baths and almshouses for the relief of the poor and sick, and the emergence of secular and civic influence in the city.

Although the Domesday Survey of 1086 was made nearly twenty years after the Norman Conquest, it is a picture of late Saxon England that emerges. The Survey reveals that while the church owned a minority of property in the city, it held many of the manors in the surrounding countryside. The livestock recorded in these communities shows an overwhelming majority of sheep over other animals, early evidence for the importance of wool to the local economy. Many villages now within or close to Bath are recorded in

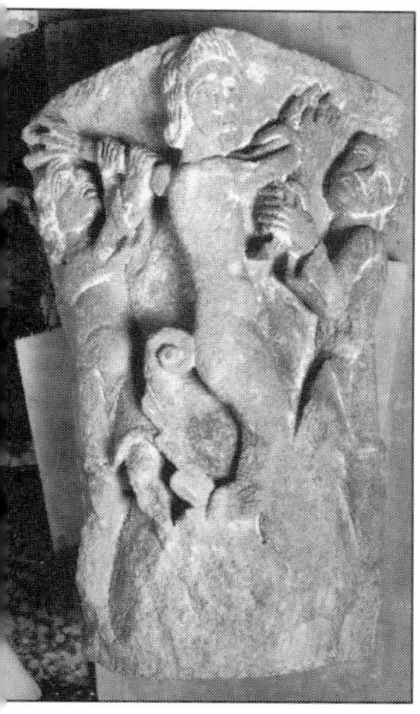

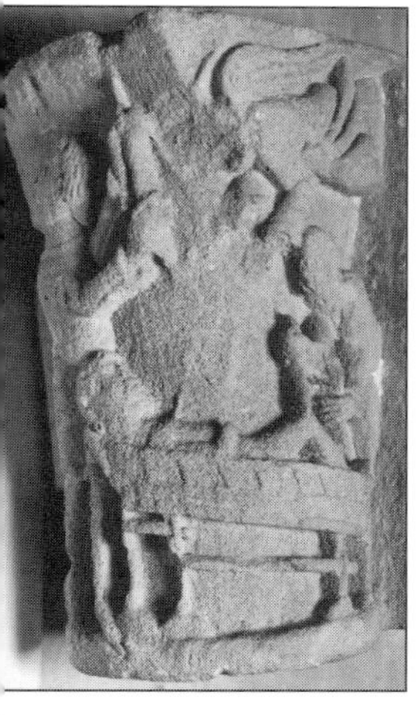

Two respond capitals of c. 1130 from the Norman cathedral, depicting two martyrdoms, possibly Saints Lawrence (top) and Bartholomew (above)

great detail, such as Bathford, Batheaston, Bathampton, Bathwick, Weston, Lyncombe, Twerton and Charlcombe.

William the Conqueror died in 1087 and his kingdom was divided between his sons Robert of Mowbray, who inherited Normandy, and William Rufus who received England. Dissatisfied with this outcome, the bishops of Bayeux, Coutances and Durham rebelled in support of Robert against his brother and, using Bristol Castle as a base, ravaged Bath and the surrounding area. The extent of the damage is unknown, but when Bishop Giso of Wells died that same year, William Rufus installed his former chaplain and physician, John de Villula from Tours, in the see and soon had granted him possession of the Abbey of St Peter and its lands. In accord with the current practice of moving sees from villages and small towns to larger communities, the new bishop transferred his seat to Bath, perhaps as a means of breathing new life into the devastated city. Before long the king had thrown in the rest of the town as well, possibly because its shattered remains were of little value to the Crown.

John de Villula turned disaster into opportunity. The rebellion may well have destroyed large areas of the town and he seized the chance to re-plan the monastery, now a cathedral priory, and at the same time explore the medical properties of the hot springs that came under his jurisdiction. John ignored the late Saxon street plan and laid out a new religious precinct of generous proportions, including within it the King's Spring and the churches of St Mary de Stalles and St James. He began a vast new cathedral, 350 ft long by 90 ft broad, on the site of the Saxon church, with cloisters on the south side and his own episcopal residence nearby. He also rebuilt the King's Bath. The rectangular Roman building that had enclosed the spring still survived, and this he lined on all four sides with stone seats in individual niches for bathers to sit in. The new bath, said to have been named the King's Bath around this time after John's patron Henry I (1100–35), evidently attracted much interest from the sick and the curious, being described in the *Gesta Stephani* of 1138 as ' . . . warm and wholesome and charming to the eye. Sick persons from all over England resort thither to bathe in these healing waters and the fit also. . . .'

Bishop John died in 1122 but his vision was caught by his successors. Bishop Robert of Lewes (1136–66) added many new buildings, including the Prior's Lodgings between the cloister and the King's Bath and an infirmary immediately beside the King's Bath. The smaller springs, both outside the monastery grounds, also came under the bishop's rule and were probably developed around this time. It is said that Bishop Robert founded a lepers' hospital in

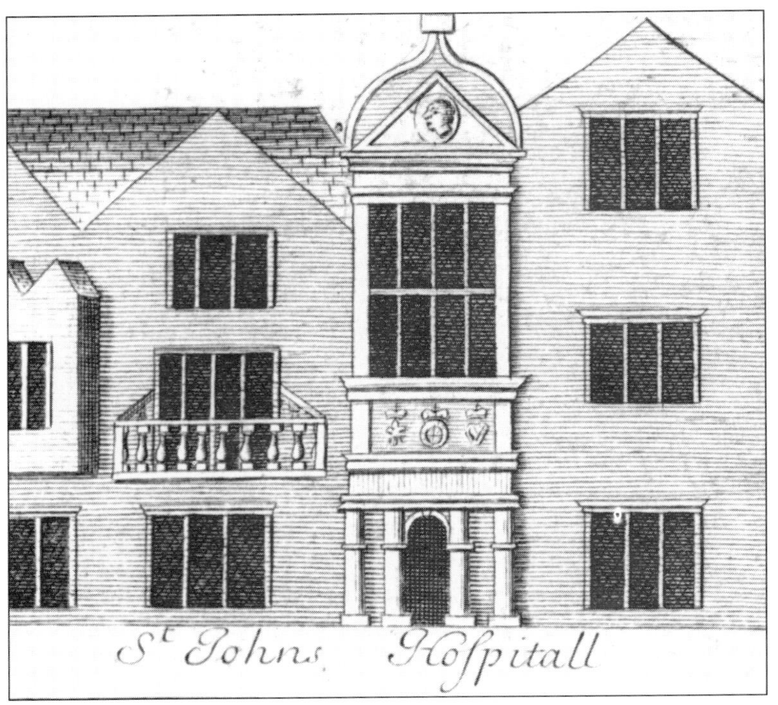

Hospital of St John the Baptist founded in 1174, as depicted on the border of Joseph Gilmore's map of 1694 (see p. 43)

1138 near the Hot Bath, tucked away against the city wall; more certain, however, is the founding in 1174 by Bishop Reginald Fitzjocelin of the Hospital of St John the Baptist beside the Cross Bath. This south-western corner of the walled city was to become home to two other almshouses – St Catherine's and Bellot's Hospitals – and additional facilities were later built in the form of the Lepers' Bath beside, and fed from, the Hot Bath.

Only one scholar of note seems to have flowered at the priory library. He was Adelard, who in the early twelfth century travelled extensively through Europe and the Middle East studying and translating Greek and Arabic literature, and who later returned to write his treatise on the astrolabe back in Bath. Around the time that Bishops John de Villula and Robert of Lewes were making therapeutic use of the springs, the legend of Bladud was first recorded by Geoffrey of Monmouth, although he acknowledged an earlier unnamed source. It may be that by now medical practice at the baths involved the use of mud, the magical element central to the legend. Certainly the mineral-rich mud that accumulated on the floors of the baths was lauded by later writers as a remedy for skin complaints.

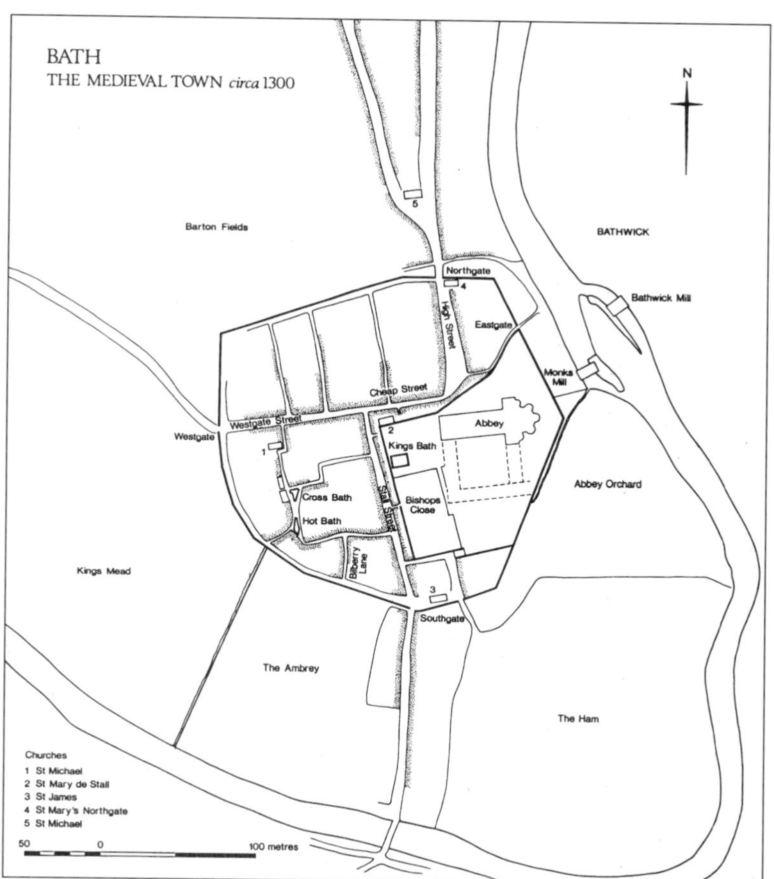

Early medieval Bath, its form still determined by the Roman defensive circuit. The late Saxon street-plan is evident in the northern and western parts

By the time he died in 1166 Robert of Lewes had completed the ambitious undertaking of his predecessor; in just seventy-five years they had between them created one of the largest churches in England with an extensive range of ancillary buildings – chapter house, cloister, refectory, infirmary and Prior's Lodging equipped with at least one bath fed from the King's Bath spring. In the precinct's south-western corner stood the Bishop's Palace in its own close with the Saxon church of St James. In 1279 St James's nave was converted into the bishop's personal chapel, and a new church of the same name was built inside the South Gate. By this time, however, the focus of the episcopacy was shifting back to Wells where a new cathedral and palace had been completed. In 1245 the Pope decreed that Wells should have equal status with Bath and that thereafter the see was to be 'Bath and Wells'. The palace in Bath seems subsequently to have been empty for long periods as bishops preferred to reside at Wells; in 1328 it was rented to the prior, confirmation that Wells was now more or less permanently the seat of the bishop. This lack of attention was reflected in poor morale, inadequate maintenance, intermittent financial troubles and occasional moral laxity among the monks. In 1349 the Black Death reduced the community from forty in number to under twenty, a setback from which it never really recovered.

If the fortunes of the monastery waxed and waned during the early medieval period, those of the secular community enjoyed a steady improvement. In most of the town outside the monastery the late-Saxon street grid survived along with the three churches of St Michael intra Muros near the Cross Bath, St Mary within Northgate and St Mary de Stalles. Timber-framed houses with thatched roofs lined the streets, only the wealthier citizens being able to afford stone-built dwellings. Outside the long north–south monastery wall flimsy stalls were pitched, paying rent to the prior for the privilege, perhaps giving the name Stall Street to the new road that led down to the South Gate and the road across the meadows to the medieval bridge. The city had in its walls two other substantial gates – the West Gate for the road to Bristol and the North Gate that greeted travellers approaching on the London road. Economic activity, encouraged by the confidence in Bath shown by John de Villula's ambitious monastic development and fuelled by a buoyant wool trade, escalated during the twelfth century. Merchant guilds emerged, keen to assert their autonomy by seeking freedom from tolls levied by the Crown on the movement of their goods. With consummate timing the guilds obtained their charter on 7 December 1189 at Dover, granted by Richard I who was desperate to raise funds for the Third Crusade. The king sailed four days later and the merchants returned to Bath with their charter.

Subsequent charters extended new freedoms to the citizens of Bath, and strengthened its growing economic role as a market centre. Permission to hold fairs on certain days of the year was granted, either by royal warrant or by papal decree. Despite competition from neighbouring towns and villages similarly empowered to hold markets and fairs, Bath's regional influence continued to grow, and out of it emerged the first Corporation, the office of mayor and the official seal of the city.

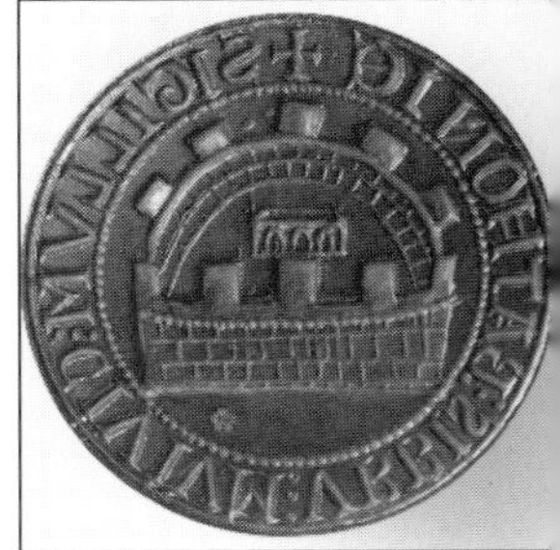

Early fourteenth-century civic seal; the simple building within the stylized city wall may be the medieval Guildhall

By the thirteenth century Bath had a guildhall, an unprepossessing single-storey structure in the lane to the East Gate. The city walls, however, were now showing signs of neglect. They had been strengthened in 1138 by Stephen who, mindful of the city's destruction only fifty years earlier, ordered the construction of outworks, which may have included the major new defence from the south-western city wall to the river, protecting the approaches to the South Gate. As the threat of siege receded during subsequent years, the walls became a quarry for the growing town. The prior, the prior's miller and the Master of St John's Hospital are all recorded as having plundered stone from the city wall, and in the later thirteenth century and again in the fourteenth, murage grants were necessary to put right the damage. As the power and identity of the Corporation grew the city walls took on new roles; they were the boundary within which the privileges granted by royal charter pertained and they created a strong identity for the community whose citizens enjoyed those rights.

The growth in economic activity also led to growth in the town. With the monastery occupying so much urban space new land was needed, and by the twelfth century suburbs were spreading along the roads outside the South and North gates. The houses outside the South Gate, mostly on the east side of the road, had long narrow gardens or plots ending at the drain that took down to the river the spa water that had passed through the Bishop's Close. This lowest and most airless suburb, flanked by marshes and prone to winter flooding from the river, must have been the least pleasant to inhabit. The one outside the North Gate, on the other hand, was well above the river with ready access to higher ground; it was close to the top end of town and the High Street inside the gate, where the markets were held. To meet the spiritual needs of this district, the church of St Michael by Northgate was built in the junction of Broad Street and Walcot Street, facing the gateway into the city.

Inevitably with a town as small as medieval Bath a strong relationship existed between the urban community and the surrounding countryside. The prior, whose establishment stood within the town walls, was nevertheless the principal rural landowner in the vicinity and citizens would cultivate arable strips and graze their animals on church lands. The Barton Farm, outside the north-west corner of the city and also owned by the Priory, consisted of meadows at Kingsmead, arable land on 'The Barton' and a pasture called Westfield, which was to become common land and which survives as High and Lower Common today. The links between town and country are best illustrated by the wool trade, the mainstay of the local medieval economy. It was sufficiently important to the economic well-being of the Priory, which owned extensive grazing lands and a mill on the river by the weir, for a shuttle to be incorporated in its coat of arms. The local cloth industry won the acclaim of Geoffrey Chaucer in the *Canterbury Tales* whose Wife of Bath outmatched the cloth-makers of Ypres and Ghent.

Strictly speaking, she was '. . . *of bisyde Bathe* . . .', recognition of the fact that cloth-making also took place in many places nearby. The city and its environs were well suited to cloth-making; the downs provided pastures for sheep and fuller's earth for removing the grease from newly-woven cloth, while the valleys provided water and power. Many tradesmen in the city were involved in the industry, such as spinners, fullers, weavers, dyers and tailors.

By the fifteenth century the medical qualities of the baths were attracting the attention of writers, from Thomas Chaundler, who in 1452 described 'the perennial flow of heated springs marvellously supplied for the benefit of man' to the more pragmatic William Caxton, who in *The Description of Britain* in 1480 observed 'hot baths which wash away pus, sores and scabs'. But despite being a comfortably prosperous community with a strong wall and three ornate gates that reflected a growing civic pride, Bath was not without its blemishes. No one could have failed to observe that while the town's streets and market-place showed all the signs of a busy wool town, over a quarter of its area was taken up by a monastery whose near-ruinous church and crumbling buildings were occupied by barely twenty monks. Small wonder that in 1495 Prior Cantlow built the Magdalen chapel on Holloway as a private chapel to which he could escape. Four years later Bishop Oliver King visited Bath to see for himself the state of the monastery. He found an undisciplined, demoralized, depleted community and a church beyond repair. Prior Cantlow died soon afterwards and was replaced by William Birde, to whom Bishop King entrusted the tasks of restoring discipline and morality to the house and rebuilding the cathedral priory.

Henry VIII's masons, William and Robert Vertue, were employed for the task. The remains of the Norman cathedral were to be pulled down and a smaller one erected over its nave. The Vertues, masters of fan vaulting, promised Bishop King the finest chancel vault in England and France. By 1535 much of the church had been built in the light restrained Perpendicular style that was to close the era of English medieval cathedral building. The south transept was still incomplete and the nave lacked a roof, but time had run out. Henry VIII assumed the role of head of the Church of England and dispatched commissioners to the monasteries to assess the moral and material condition of his new spiritual realm. The reports from Bath were not encouraging. The prior, William Holloway, perhaps sensing that the monastery's days were numbered, began to dispose surreptitiously of its properties to wealthy local landowners. In 1539 he and the other members of the fraternity signed over the house to the Crown. The

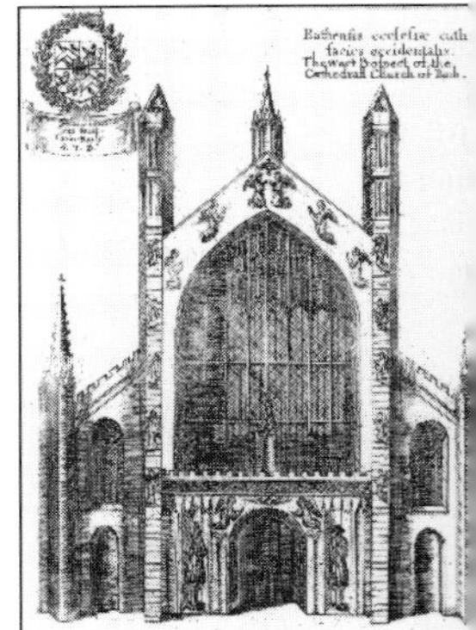

The earliest view of the west end of the Abbey Church, by Daniel King *c.* 1640, showing it prior to later alterations

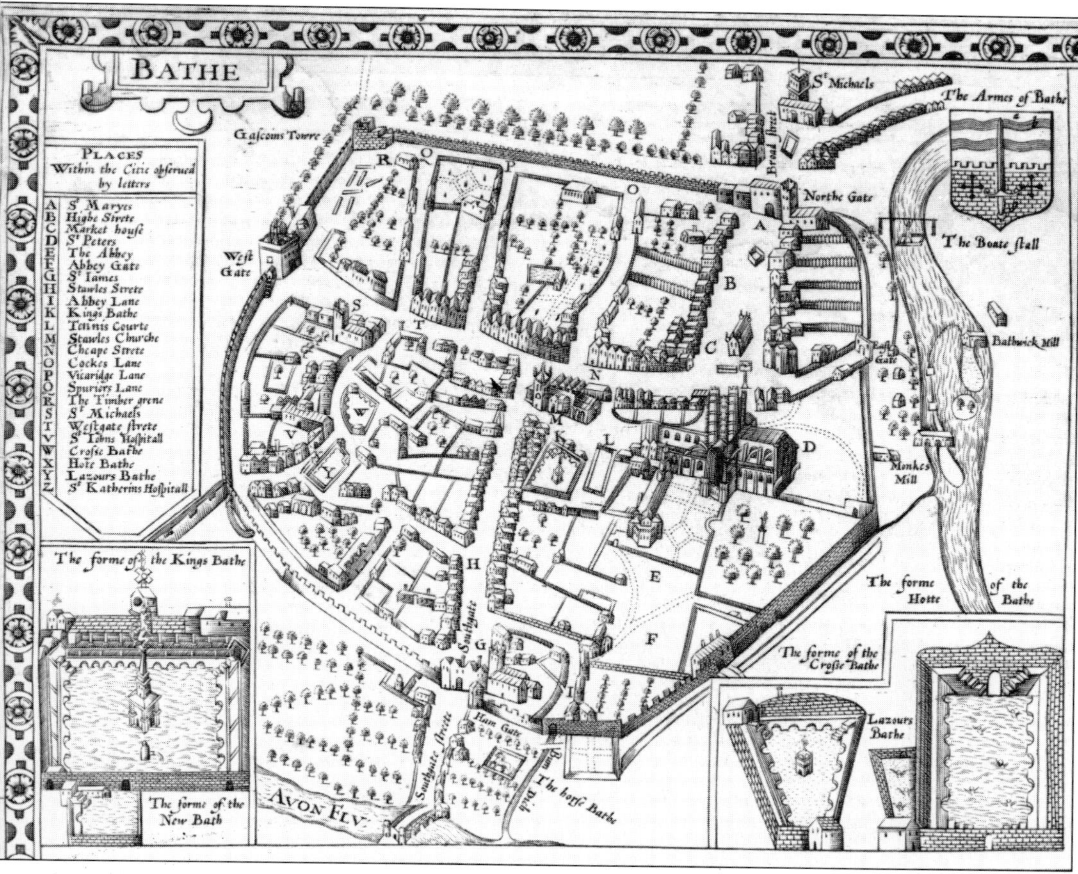

ohn Speed's map, published 610 but drawn somewhat arlier, shows the principal ndmarks of the post-issolution city, including the complete Abbey Church

monks were pensioned off and Prior Holloway retired to a house in Stall Street. For the first time in over 850 years Bath was without a monastery. The new church remained incomplete.

The state of the city during these critical years was vividly recorded by John Leland, who visited Bath around the time of the Dissolution. He was much taken with the picturesque valley, 'a fruitful and pleasant Botom', and its many cold water springs channelled to the city through lead pipes. Leland cites a catalogue of Roman inscriptions and relief carvings re-used in the city wall. The baths he describes one by one: the Cross Bath 'much frequented of people diseased with lepre, pokkes, scabbes and great aches', the Hot Bath 'that would scauld the flesch', and the King's Bath 'very faire and large. . . . to this bathe do Gentilmen resort'. Of the monastery he noted the dilapidated Bishop's Palace, of which 'one great square tour of it with other ruines yet appere', and was clearly fascinated by the new church apparently rising out of the ruins of the Norman cathedral, in whose overgrown east end he found the tombs of John de Villula and 'other divers bisshops buried there'.

Leland also commented on the decline in the fortunes of the cloth industry in Bath. Property values had collapsed since 1525, probably causing neglect, even dereliction, of houses in the city. By 1540 Bath was in such poor physical condition as to be one of thirty-six towns and cities whose rebuilding was enforced by an Act of Parliament. Despite the downturn in the fortunes of the cloth industry, the Corporation was fortunate in being able to exploit its other assets – its newly acquired properties and the medical properties of the spa waters.

Following the Dissolution the monastic buildings had been sold off, and by the end of the sixteenth century had largely disappeared. The church itself was stripped of its valuable trappings and left to disintegrate. The shell, together with the priory lands, passed rapidly through several hands before being vested in the Corporation, and in 1552 more properties, including unsold priory lands, were transferred to the Corporation by Edward VI. Some income from these endowments was intended for the refurbishment of St Catherine's Hospital and for establishing a free school, thus restoring an academic tradition that had ceased with the demise of the monastery. The Corporation now owned much of the city centre and revenues from these properties contributed much to its prosperity. With its new responsibilities and the opportunities afforded by its increased income the activities of the Corporation expanded considerably. In 1551–2 it built the market house in the High Street, perhaps more in hope than belief that it would bolster the flagging fortunes of the cloth trade. The City Chamberlain's Accounts, which survive from 1569, show the Corporation taking responsibility for repairs to the city walls, baths, almshouses and Guildhall, for clearing rubbish dumped in the city ditch and for cleaning and repairing the streets.

The Act of Uniformity of 1559, intended to bring Roman Catholics into line with the Anglican Church, was only partly observed in Bath, with some Roman Catholics dutifully attending services before going on to a secret location to celebrate Mass. More noticeable would have been the disappearance of publicly held Catholic rituals and celebrations such as Corpus Christi processions. Queen Elizabeth herself was instrumental in shaping the city's ecclesiastical life; in 1572 she licensed the creation of one Anglican parish out of all the parish churches, including St Thomas-à-Becket at Widcombe, under the Abbey Church of St Peter and St Paul. At the same time she ordered a collection to be raised throughout the kingdom for the restoration of the Abbey itself. The collection was insufficient for the task and it was not until around 1617, and a determined campaign of works by Bishop Montague, that the work was finally completed.

The baths were another potential source of income and the Corporation, some of whose members had inns or lodging-houses nearby, was keen to invest in the new health and leisure industry. Henry VIII, suspicious of the Catholic tradition of seeking miraculous cures at holy wells, had suppressed their use, but this merely resulted in Catholics resorting to continental spas. Fearful that seditious English Catholics might assist an invasion from the Spanish Netherlands, the Privy Council under Queen Elizabeth relented and began to encourage the secular promotion of certain English spas. In 1562 Dr William Turner, Dean of Wells, published his *Treatise on the Bath Waters*, a scientific assessment of the medical benefits of spa bathing in which, among other things, he criticized the inadequate facilities, poor drainage and general neglect of a precious natural asset. Other expositions followed, including Dr John Jones's *The Bathes of Bathes Ayde* (1572) while a year earlier the Italian writer Andrea Bacci had included the baths of Bath in his *De Thermis*, published in Venice. These publications, combined with the patronage of noblemen like the 2nd Earl of Pembroke and the influential Cecil family, attracted a new courtier clientèle to Bath and, in 1574, the Queen herself.

This royal endorsement of Bath as a fashionable resort prompted a new wave of improvements. Heeding Dr Turner's advice the Corporation built the Queen's Bath for women adjacent to the King's Bath, the Lepers' Bath for those with skin complaints beside the Hot Bath, and the Horse Bath outside the city wall. The Cross Bath was enlarged and improved in the 1590s. The amalgamation of all four city churches in 1583 enabled the Corporation to acquire yet more land on which fine new stone lodging-houses were built. Some physicians, keen to win the custom of the increasing numbers of aristocrats resorting to the city, took lodgers into their own homes; thus in 1591 Dr Robert Baker leased from the Corporation a new house, known today as Abbey Church House which, like many new houses in the city, boasted wide, extravagant windows made possible by cheaper glass.

Rising population and rapid inflation during the Elizabethan period, exacerbated by famines in the 1550s and 1590s, brought increasing numbers of vagabonds in search of relief of their ailments – access to the baths appears to have been without charge – and to beg from the city's affluent visitors. An Act of Parliament in 1572 restricting the numbers of poor and diseased people entering Bath

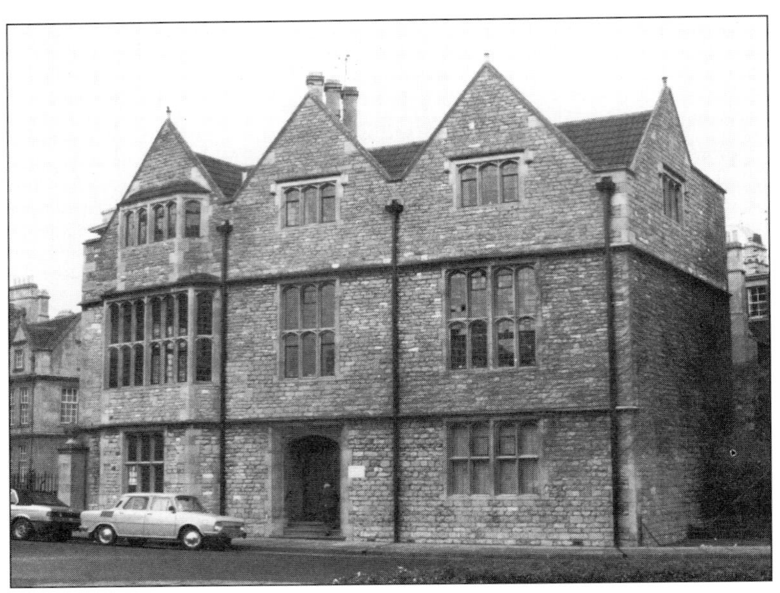

Abbey Church House, built in 1591 and much altered in the eighteenth and nineteenth centuries; it was bombed in 1942 and subsequently rebuilt

coincided with the transfer of the hospitals of St Catherine and St John to the Corporation. In 1576 Dr John Feckenham built a poorhouse for lepers beside the Hot Bath to complement the new Lepers' Bath, and around 1590 St John's Hospital was substantially enlarged. Further provision for almsfolk was made in 1609 when Thomas Bellot, one-time steward of Lord Burghley, contributed a hospital bearing his own name in Bell Tree Lane, now Beau Street.

Despite the spa's fast-growing reputation, its patronage by visiting nobility and those closer to home like Sir John Harington, godson of the queen and owner of local property that included the tennis court beside the Abbey and Kelweston (Kelston) outside Bath, the city remained essentially a small, walled, West Country town. The Corporation had benefited hugely from the acquisition of former priory lands, of non-church property granted by Edward VI and of yet more endowments received from Queen Elizabeth in 1585, all of which left it owning far more land than came under its jurisdiction. In 1590 it neatly secured from the queen a charter that not only greatly extended its boundaries to include properties it held outside the city walls, but confirmed the rights and privileges of previous charters and accorded full powers of government to the mayor, aldermen and citizens of Bath.

CHAPTER FOUR

A 'Little Pretty City' Under Strain

A stray comment in 1606 from a German wholesaler at Stade (on the Elbe estuary) about the slow turnover of fabrics from Bath is rare evidence for the marketing of undyed broadcloth, the city's staple product. Despite the strong development of the health spa over the past thirty years, Bath still displayed the characteristics of a West Country woollen town. Its textile industry was organized and financed by a handful of independent clothiers, men of some substance such as William Sherstone, William Clift, Edward and John Parker, three of whom served as mayor between 1600 and 1620. These were the entrepreneurs who oversaw each stage of production: carding and spinning (mostly by women), plain weaving (the domestic looms being concentrated most heavily in St Michael's parish outside the North Gate), scouring and fulling (at the river-powered Monks Mill), and finally tentering to re-stretch the cloth. Once the lengths of material had been transported to Blackwell Hall in London, middlemen took over – for the clothiers depended on metropolitan dealers, Merchant Adventurer shippers and foreign merchants to see the goods safely to the Low Countries or Germany for dyeing, finishing and onward distribution. The process was lengthy, financially risky and always at the mercy of events. Ever since its heyday the broadcloth trade had fluctuated, sometimes buoyant, sometimes depressed. In 1596, for example, when Sir John Harington thought the Bath industry in definite decline, it was in fact on the eve of another recovery that lasted until the serious crisis stemming from the misguided national Cockayne project of 1614–17, which banned the sending of undyed cloth abroad. The damage this caused the West Country broadcloth trade was further exacerbated by the outbreak of the Thirty Years' War in 1618 and subsequent disruption of the crucial German market. By 1622 distress was widespread among the cloth producers. Many of Bath's clothworkers were on poor relief, and the mayor, finding the government unremitting in its tax demands, felt obliged to point out that the manufacturers of this 'very little poor city' had much decayed. Yet once again textiles proved resilient. The revival, when it came, seems to have relied on a switch from exporting to the home market – so much can be guessed from the emergence of a weekly cloth mart in the manufacturing suburb just beyond the North Gate. But documentation is scanty. It remains unclear to what extent the volume of production had been sustained, or whether the success of lighter, coloured fabrics woven in the vicinity (especially at Freshford) persuaded Bath clothiers to innovate – though the eventual presence of dyeworks beside the Avon suggests they did. For some decades yet cloth-making continued to count in the local economy. In 1660 over a hundred looms were reportedly still at work. Tenter racks stood in the surrounding fields as late as the 1690s, though by then production had largely migrated to the external parishes of Bathwick, Lyncombe-Widcombe and Twerton, free from interference by the Merchant Taylors of Bath.

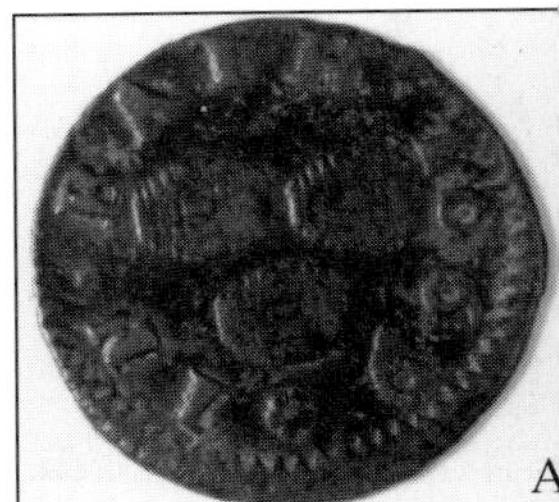

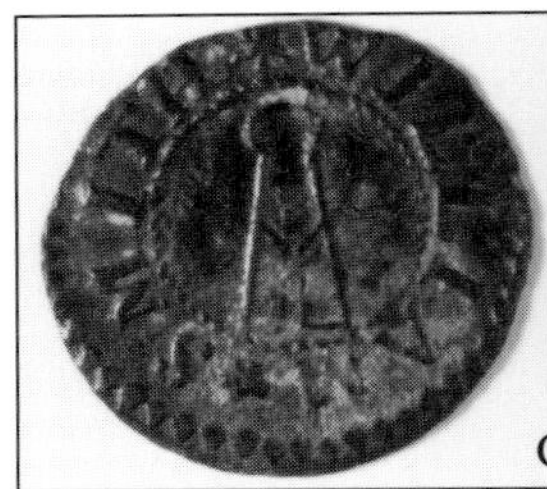

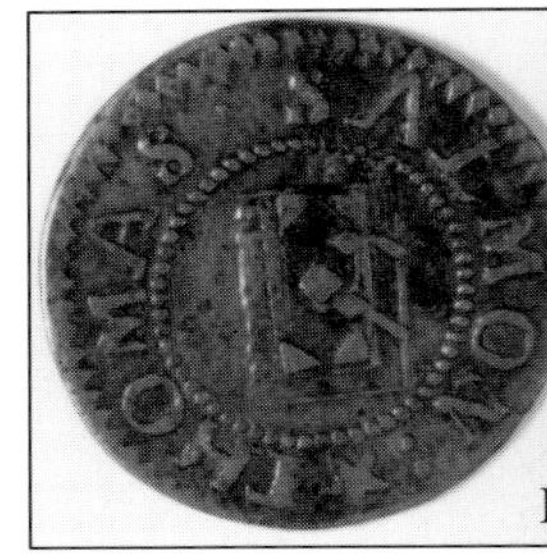

Farthing tokens issued by Bat[h] tradesmen. A William Landicke, innkeeper, 1669, B John Pearce, mercer, 1652, C William Smith, clothier, 1666, D Thomas Salmon, bookseller, 1667

Organized in 1629, the Merchant Taylors company was one of the guilds that helped to regulate the various trades, keep out competitors and supplement Corporation income through the purchase of freedoms. A typical mix of urban occupations turns up in contemporary records, including drapers, shoemakers, bakers, butchers, grocers, chandlers, smiths and farriers. Bath's growing functions as county town for east Somerset and as a nationally signficant health resort enabled it to support a wider range of specialists than its size might otherwise have warranted: before 1640 it boasted several mercers, a hatmaker, bookbinder, scrivener, vintner, confectioner, cutler and goldsmith. Building work and the frequent repair of municipal property gave employment to stonemasons, carpenters, plumbers and glaziers, plasterers and tilers (thatch being finally prohibited in 1633). These years saw the Abbey Church at last completed thanks to private benefactions (1617), the erection of a prominent new Guildhall-cum-Markethouse (1625–7), and the conversion of existing buildings into a workhouse or bridewell (1632–5). Accommodation for visitors also continued to grow.

The hot springs brought business not only to inns, lodging-houses and tradespeople but to medical practitioners and personnel at the five baths. Three or four resident physicians attended patients both in town and within riding distance around. Others arrived during the spring-to-autumn season from London and Oxford, sometimes accompanying

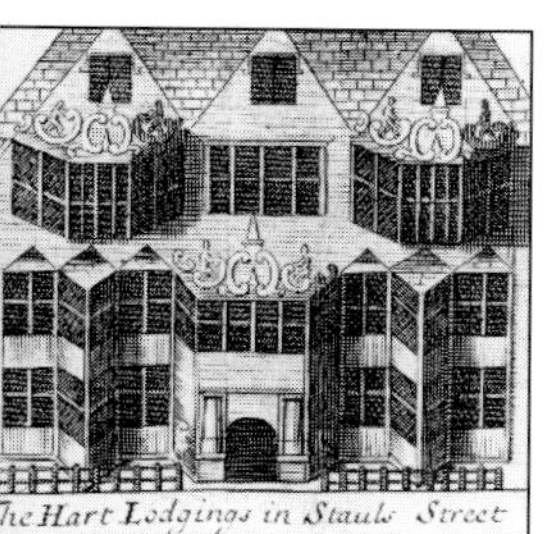

he Hart Lodgings with its rge glass windows belonged the influential Chapman mily and backed directly on the Queen's Bath

clients, to share in the pickings. Apothecaries too profited from pain and disease; almost any medical treatment involved drugs, and even simple bathing had to be preceded by a course of purging. The King's and Queen's Baths were the most frequented by wealthier visitors at this stage, for they were surrounded by convenient guest-houses that led directly to the slips by which the bathers reached the steaming waters. In a book to publicize the spa (1628) one local physician, Tobias Venner, criticized the too-often cosy arrangements between medical advisers and certain lodgings, and deplored the hectic touting for custom that took place when newcomers appeared. In theory each bath had different therapeutic qualities and should have been prescribed to suit the individual case, just as certain patients were ordered localized applications of hot water or mud treatments rather than full immersion. The baths were not the scenes of constant disorder and licence they have often been painted. It is true that private interests around the baths hindered complete control by the magistrates and that the custom of mixed, nude bathing, which survived attempts to suppress it in 1621–5, scandalized some. But regulation did become more effective in time. The Council appointed official attendants, laid down how often the baths must be refilled (daily from 1645), and maintained the fabric. By the standards of the day the baths and city as a whole were decently kept. A borough scavenger (or refuse collector) was appointed in 1615, and the dung heaps outside the gates eventually disappeared. Regular attention was paid to the cold water supply that fed the public drinking fountains from springs on Lansdown and Beechen Cliff. The streets were periodically re-cobbled. A bellman began to patrol the town at night. Stocks, a pillory, a ducking-stool and a lock-up 'cage', as well as the prison and workhouse, catered for offenders. In 1623 alehouses had come under tighter scrutiny.

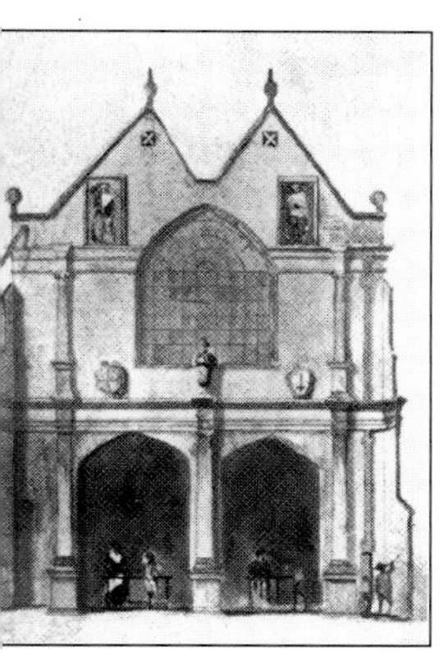

orth end of the Stuart uildhall with the open-sided arkethouse below. Symbolic gures in the gables presented King Edgar and e mythical King Cole

Such measures helped to promote the spa, as did effective medical propaganda in books by Tobias Venner, Edward Jorden and Thomas Johnson between 1620 and 1634. In spite of competition from Buxton, Tunbridge Wells, and in due course Epsom and Harrogate, Bath easily held its own in attracting wealthy patronage. A long list might be compiled of the courtiers, state ministers, church dignitaries, noblemen and gentry who made a stay. (Only rare visitations of bubonic plague seemed to halt the pilgrimage of health-seekers, especially in 1604 when a minor epidemic scared off the chief secretary-of-state, Lord Cecil, and in 1625 and 1636 when temporary pest-houses were set up on the town common.) The greatest catch of all was naturally royalty itself. And if Elizabeth failed to make her much awaited return trip in 1602, James I's queen, Anne of Denmark, atoned handsomely coming 'with a noble train' twice in 1613 and again in 1615, so establishing a happy Stuart precedent. To the queen and other influential guests the mayor gave presents, often of wine, sugar loaves, meat and poultry, in the hope of future favours. All the same, little of the expenditure by visitors flowed into the often impoverished city coffers. Most of the Corporation élite, by contrast, benefited very well personally by providing rooms, food and drink, medicines and other services. Keepers of bowling greens and royal tennis courts, organizers of bear baitings and visiting companies of actors (so long as these were tolerated) profited similarly.

All kinds of people headed for what Venner called that 'little well-compacted city . . . beautified with very fair and goodly buildings for receipt of strangers'. In 1605 several of the Gunpowder Plot conspirators gathered there. Sick state prisoners and Catholic recusants might be granted travel permits 'to the Bath'. The healthy came as well, curious to see the sights; a party of distinguished botanists, for instance, in 1634; or John Taylor, the poetic waterman, who sculled most of the way from London around 1641 to view 'the famous, renowned, ancient, little pretty city'. The ill and crippled poor who journeyed under licence for hot water bathing had a chance to stay at Bellot's Hospital, founded in order to lodge just such cases. Homeless vagrants on the other hand would have no such luck and risked being whipped out of town.

From the 1620s onwards the city authorities can be seen taking a severer line on social and moral deviance. Sanctions were applied against drunkenness, unruly behaviour, sexual misconduct and Sabbath-breaking. Performances of plays ceased to be allowed and noisy popular diversions were frowned on. Meanwhile preaching was encouraged by the institution of midweek sermons in 1627 and special feast-day sermons a few years later. Puritanism was fast gaining ground, not merely at Bath but through the whole region, fostered by local gentry such as John Harington of Kelston and the already much-persecuted William Prynne of Swainswick. Events in the 1630s gave Puritan thinking a more political slant. The Bishop of Bath and Wells's campaign to enforce the Laudian liturgy and to silence puritan preachers caused deep offence. Added to it was mounting resentment at the erosion of civil liberties, Charles I's suppression of Parliament, and his repeated demands for ship money. Bath paid its contributions, at least initially, but the level of anger at this extra tax burden was manifest at the 1638 summer assizes held in the city.

As the country polarized on the brink of civil war, Bath and Somerset tilted unquestionably towards the Parliamentary cause. That much became plain to the Marquis of Hertford when he appeared at Bath in July 1642 during the crowded assizes, since he failed to win control of the militia forces for the king and encountered a vast muster of Puritan opposition on the Mendips. Bath Corporation was none the less divided politically, for the ardent Parliamentarians headed by Matthew Clift were balanced by a group of Royalist sympathisers under Henry Chapman, while a large minority stayed uncommitted. Whatever their affiliations they could only watch as the national conflict drew closer. By spring 1643 a large contingent of Sir William Waller's Parliamentary forces was quartered at Bath, the military gateway to the strategic city of Bristol and the springboard for forays into the western counties. On 4 July, after a series of skirmishes and counter-marches, the Royalist army led by Sir Ralph Hopton encamped at Marshfield just north of Bath while Waller watched from the plateau of Lansdown, protecting the town to his rear. Battle was joined next day, a confused succession of bloody engagements, with cavalry, cannon, musketry and pikemen all struggling for control of the escarpment. By nightfall the Royalists had gained the edge of the down, but at such cost they had to beat a retreat next morning and allow Waller's tired but exhilarated troops in Bath to claim victory. It was a short-lived success. A week later Waller was overwhelmed on Roundway Down above Devizes leaving Bath undefended. Within days it was seized for the king.

The city now faced two years of compliance with Royalist occupation and exactions. It was placed on a full military footing. The defences were strengthened, sections of wall rebuilt, the gates blocked

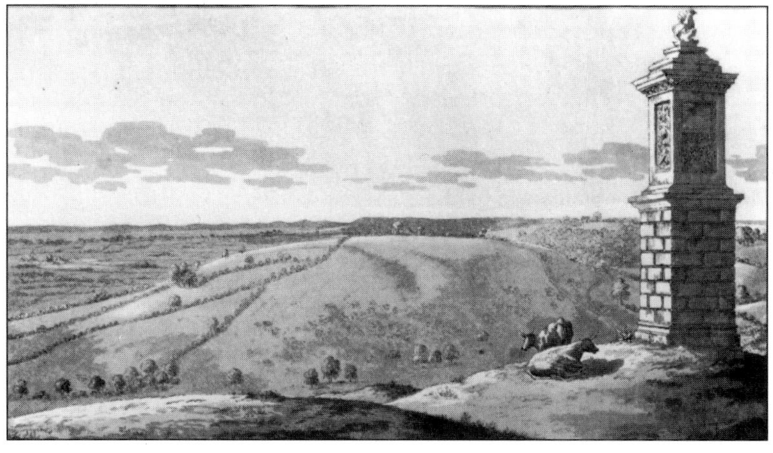

Ionument to the fallen oyalist commander, Sir Bevil renvile, at the site of the attle of Lansdown in July 643 (aquatint by T. Cadell, 793)

or barricaded, guards posted. Cannon stood on Gascoyne's Tower at the north-west corner. Forced to purchase ten barrels of gunpowder, the Corporation sank deeper into debt. Furthermore it had to house the governor, Sir Thomas Bridges of Keynsham, supply him with linen, humour him with gifts, and give free quarter to his garrison. The citizens found themselves paying arrears of taxes and extortionate new levies. When the king and queen made separate visits in 1644, presents of silver plate added to the expense. Only Bath's slim band of committed Royalists rejoiced under their leader, Henry Chapman, who now held the rank of captain in the regiment of militia. The Puritan opposition got on instead with symbolic protests. By ostentatiously celebrating the Fifth of November and the anniversary of Elizabeth's accession they at least asserted their religious and political allegiances. In mid-1645, heartened no doubt by the approach of Fairfax's Roundhead army, they took to voicing more open dissent, and at this moment Bath quite unexpectedly changed hands. A scouting party sent by Fairfax managed to gain entry at the South Gate on 29 July. Governor Bridges, mistakenly believing himself surrounded by the enemy, gave up the city and a mass of weaponry without a fight. All at once the Parliamentary majority held power again.

During the Royalist interlude Bath had suffered. An epidemic of plague or typhus in summer 1643 killed more than a hundred people in the two inner parishes alone. The billetings and movements of troops led to looting and damage to streets and buildings. Both the cloth and the spa trades were disrupted. Wounded soldiers used the baths. Nor did all this change for the better overnight. The Parliamentary side also imposed heavy taxes and expected free lodging for over 1,000 men until early 1646, when the garrison began to be run down. Nevertheless, as soon as the defences ceased to be a drain on civic finances, the neglected work of repairing buildings, highways and the bridge got under way. The former weekly sermons were reinstated. Fresh by-laws were drawn up. In a mood of reconciliation the City Council at first retained its Royalist members, but in December 1647 was compelled to carry out a Parliamentary order to expel Henry Chapman and six of his activist colleagues. At the same time William Prynne, now a national figure, became the city's recorder. The embittered Chapman took his revenge the following April. Backed by an influx of Royalist sympathizers from outside Bath, he defied the recorder, the mayor and the puritan rector by having the abolished prayer book openly read in St James's church, and by organizing bull-baitings just outside the city magistrates' area of jurisdiction. It was a foretaste of things to come.

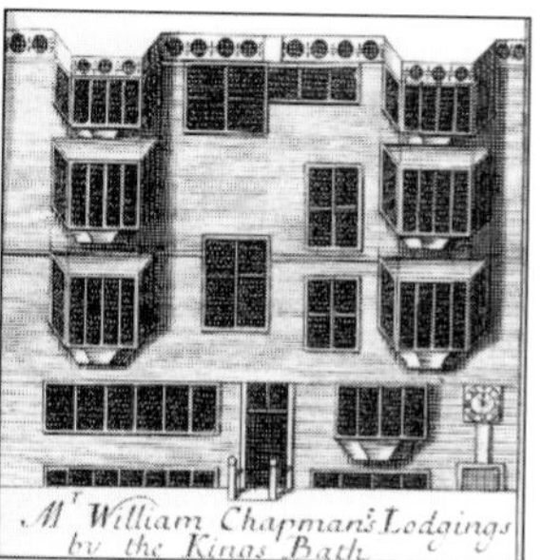

Another Chapman property, built in 1652 overlooking the east side of the King's Bath. Fireworks at the celebrations for Charles II's coronation in 1661 damaged its lead roof

The 1650s were a decade of slow recovery. Aware of the economic benefits of a navigable waterway to Bristol, the Corporation tried – as it had tried several times in the past – to obtain an Act of Parliament for the purpose, but was again defeated by vested interests. It was some compensation that the health traffic seemed to be returning, though the arrival of over 200 maimed soldiers in 1653, sent for treatment at government expense, brought a sharp reminder of the recent conflict. The diarist John Evelyn, coming a year later to 'trifle' and bathe, discovered a stone-built town (albeit with narrow unpleasant streets) and a King's Bath 'esteemed the fairest in Europe'. He was followed in 1658 by a more prestigious visitor, Richard Cromwell, the new Lord Protector himself, whom the Corporation duly fêted at the hurriedly refurbished Guildhall. But the city, like the nation, was now wearying of the Commonwealth. Even its mentor, the former rebel Prynne, looked forward to a monarchy.

If Bath was to live by its reputation as a spa and stay ahead of possible rivals, it had to court the favour of the good and the great, and to secure patronage at the highest level. This explains why it was the first place in the kingdom to proclaim Charles II and to submit a loyal address, and why it marked the coronation with such an effusive display of costumed processions, street decorations, bell-ringing, musket volleys, fireworks, bonfires and distributions of alcohol. All this, and a timely present to the king of £100 in gold, had its reward in 1663 when the royal pair bathed at the now fashionable Cross Bath. But the cost of loyalty may be seen in the financial retrenchments that followed, the cuts in officers' salaries, the selling of unwanted Corporation land, and the efforts to profit from supplying water or renting out the town common and the city's Mendip coalmine. When a new master was needed at the Grammar School, the cheaper applicant was preferred. Even so, revenue from municipal property (plus the granting of freedoms) barely matched annual outlay, and money still had to be borrowed at interest from wealthier citizens.

Meanwhile the membership of the City Council had undergone a dramatic transformation. The eight Royalists swept on to the Council by the Restoration were easily outvoted at the ensuing contest for Mayor. Puritan MPs were similarly returned at the 1661 parliamentary elections, notwithstanding a separate mock election staged by Henry Chapman with some support from the otherwise disenfranchised freemen. Chapman's two successful candidates (one of them the erstwhile governor of Bath, Sir Thomas Bridges) were inevitably rejected by the House of Commons. For the mayoral

Letter from William Prynne, Recorder of Bath, to the Somerset deputy lieutenant Sir Hugh Smyth complaining about the arrest of Bath councillors in 1661

election of 1661 Chapman and Bridges resorted to rather more desperate measures, having nine (then two more) puritan councillors arrested and taken before the Sheriff of Somerset 30 miles away. Speedily released for want of evidence, they rushed back to the Guildhall in time to overturn the vote taken in their absence. The thwarted Chapman, still openly scornful of the mayor and recorder, was ejected from the Council and even briefly imprisoned for debt. Affairs then took an ironical twist. Under the Corporation Act fourteen members of the Council, including seven aldermen, were

A
DISCOURSE
OF
BATHE,
AND THE
HOT WATERS There.
ALSO,
Some Enquiries into the nature of the
Water of St. Vincent's Rock, near Bristol;
and that of Castle-Cary.
To which is added,
A Century of Observations, more fully declaring the Nature, Property, and distinction of the BATHS.
WITH
An Account of the Lives, and Character, of the Physicians of Bathe.

By THO. GUIDOTT, M. B.
Physician There.

Virtute vincam Invidiam.

LONDON,
Printed for Henry Brome at the Gun in St. Paul's Church-yard, the West end, 1676.

Medical propaganda for the developing spa

purged from office as political and religious dissidents. Into the vacancies stepped Chapman and his fellow-Royalists, triumphant at last. Their old ally Bridges and two of the king's commissioners who had appointed them were rewarded with honorary freedoms, and the royal visit of 1663 provided the seal of Court approval.

The Restoration period saw Bath deliberately promoted as health resort and loyal city. The gradual ebbing of the cloth trade meant a greater emphasis on the spa – whose virtues were now promulgated in 1664 for the first time in a London newspaper. Strenuous, but ultimately ineffective, attempts were made in the 1660s to have the summer or Lent assizes permanently settled at Bath, for the county sessions always brought an influx of gentry. Of much greater moment for future prosperity, however, was the launch of mineral water drinking. In 1661 a drinking pump was installed at the King's Bath, so at last guaranteeing an uncontaminated source. From this small beginning a minor industry (already established at other spas) developed. By 1673 Bath water was being marketed in bottles and small casks at other West Country towns and in London. Within another generation the water cure had taken over from bathing as the dominant excuse for a trip to Bath. A whole mystique arose over how the waters should be prescribed, how they acted on the patient, and what their vital constituents were (the presence or absence of sulphur becoming the nub of many a learned argument).

It was plain to an eyewitness in the 1680s, Thomas Dingley, that Bathonians 'chiefly get their Bread by . . . the Baths', meaning also the ancillary activities of lodging and victualling people. He reckoned the city 'the prettiest of this Kingdom', small but attractive. The old patchwork of gardens and open spaces that once existed within the walled enclosure was more and more disappearing under new buildings. Samuel Pepys in 1668, like Evelyn before him, already had a sense of a mainly stone-constructed, narrow-streeted place. Some of the inns and lodging-houses looked especially imposing. Henry Chapman, always a doughty publicist for his native city, thought them almost palatial in 1673, and the seasoned traveller Celia Fiennes acknowledged in the 1680s that several recently built examples were well ornamented and furnished. The bathing establishments had likewise been improved, with pumps and spectators' galleries added at the Hot and Cross Baths, and the Cross and King's Baths adorned with new stone crosses. Other amenities demonstrated a care for visitors' leisure needs: a coffee house (before 1680), a fine bowling green for the nobility and gentry, pleasant walks laid out east of the Abbey Church, Kingsmead field with its cake-houses serving syllabubs and summer drinks, and a growing number of

THE EIGHT KING OF THE BRITAINS
FROM BRVTE, A GREAT PHILOSOPHER,
AND MATHEMATITIAN; BRED AT ATHENS,
AND RECORDED THE FIRST DISCOVERER,
AND FOUNDER OF THESE BATHES, EIGHT
HVNDRED SIXTY AND THREE YEARES
FIVE HVNDRED THIRTY FIVE YEARS
SINCE
ANNO DOMINI 1672

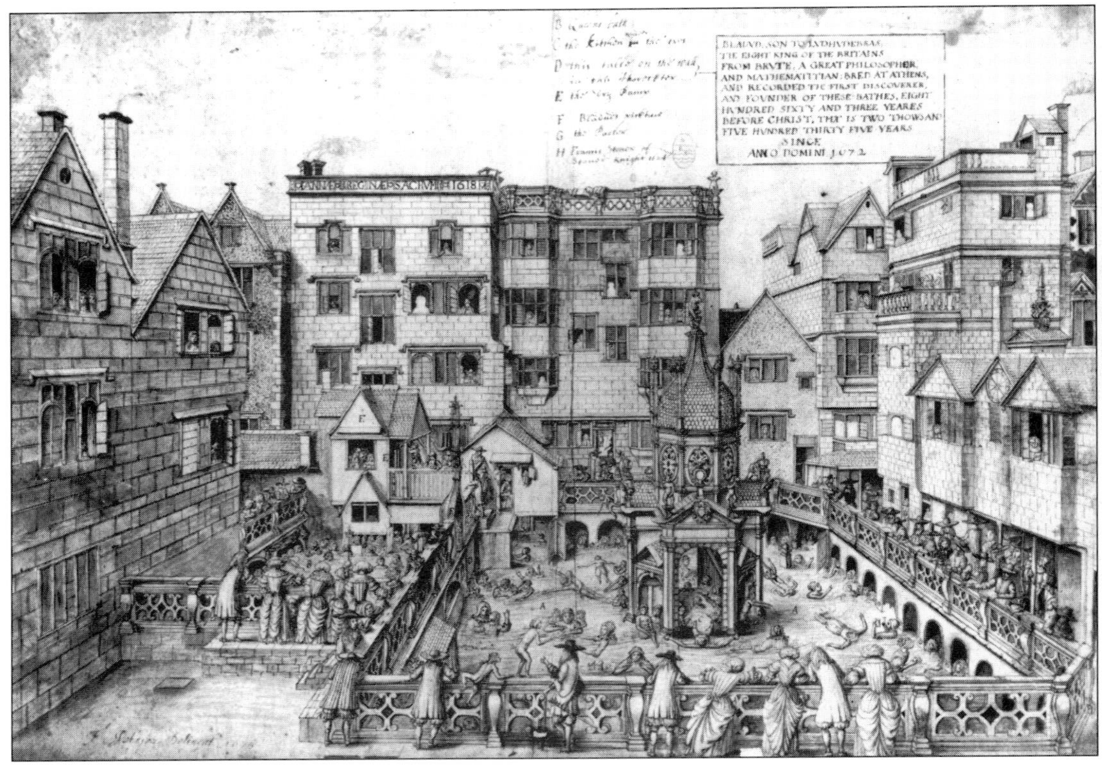

Hemmed in with lodging houses, the King's and smaller Queen's Baths seen from the east in Thomas Johnson's drawing of 1675

sedan chairs for hire. Eventually, in 1699, a riding area was fenced off on the Common. In Celia Fiennes' view the provisions market, plentifully supplied and inexpensive, constituted another advantage. Fuel and lodgings were the dearest items, she observed, 'but they give you very good attendance'. None of this, however, persuaded the Somerset gentry to remove the summer assizes to Bath from the cheaper and more central venue of Wells, which had the asset of a larger meeting room then the Guildhall at Bath offered.

This Guildhall was nevertheless the setting for much anxious deliberation by the City Council in the years running up to the 1688 Revolution. The Popish Plot and Exclusion Crisis around 1680 brought former divisions and animosities to the surface again, only this time focused more directly on the Catholic tendencies of the monarchy. The 'very loyal city' of Bath felt itself pulled two ways, especially over James, Duke of York, the Catholic heir to the throne. Small numbers of Catholics and Nonconformists (Quakers always

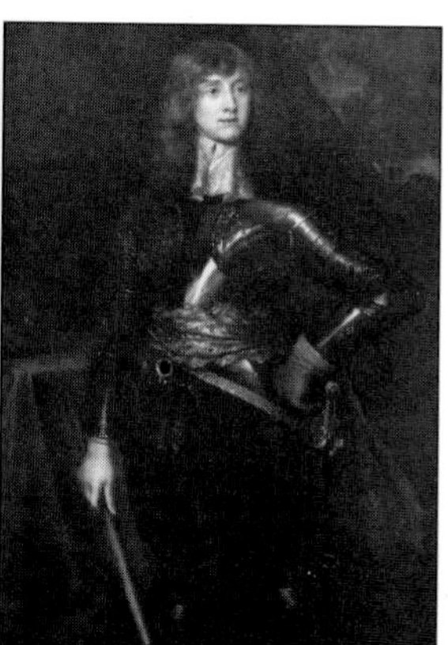
The Protestant Duke of Monmouth, once enthusiastically received at Bath but shut out during the western rebellion in 1685 (portrait attributed to John Riley)

excepted) had long been tolerated and indeed, as spa visitors, welcomed; but the Council, predominantly Anglican, split into Yorkist and anti-Yorkist camps. In this fraught atmosphere spies and informers flourished, and one alderman, loose-tongued in his criticism of the future James II, was denounced to Whitehall in 1679, forced into hiding, sentenced *in absentia* at the county sessions, only to be reinstated to the City Council scarcely two months later. Another influential Councillor, a 'most busy pestilent Presbyterian', survived until late 1684 before being ousted. Uncertainty and schizophrenia prevailed through much of the 1680s. In August 1680, a mere three months after presenting a fulsomely loyal address to the throne, Bath received the alternative heir, the Protestant Duke of Monmouth, with the greatest enthusiasm, a procession of 200 mounted gentry and citizens escorting him into town. The mood soon changed. Fearful of losing its Corporate privileges, the city conferred more and more honorary freedoms on potential protectors, but in December 1684 was obliged to surrender its 1590 Charter and pay expensively for a new one that gave the king unprecedented rights to overrule local wishes and pick his own nominees for civic office. The following February, on the death of Charles II, the intimidated Council declared for his Catholic brother James, so spurning its former patron, the rebellious Monmouth. Thus in July, when Monmouth's demoralized troops halted 'in bravado' outside Bath after their defeat at Sedgemoor, they found the gates firmly shut against them; and in the grisly aftermath of the uprising four of the rebels were hanged, drawn and quartered in the city.

Reluctant accomplice of a Papist monarch, Bath now became the unlikely instrument of his downfall. In summer 1687 the spa's reputation for curing female infertility prompted James II to bring the Queen, Mary of Modena, to try for an heir. Unlike her predecessor, Catherine of Braganza, Queen Mary conceived. Next June she bore a son – the future Old Pretender – and emissaries from Bath hastened up to Court with another assertion of unwavering devotion. But for many others in the country the prospect of a perpetuated Catholic dynasty was unthinkable. At the same time as the Anglican bells of Bath rang out to welcome Lord Waldegrave (the Catholic high steward just foisted on it), William of Orange was preparing his Protestant invasion. Within months James II had fled and William and Mary reigned. Having backed the loser Bath did what it could to make amends. It got rid of the Papist insignia and inscription set up at the Cross Bath only a short time before. It reinstated an Anglican master at the Grammar School, and at the

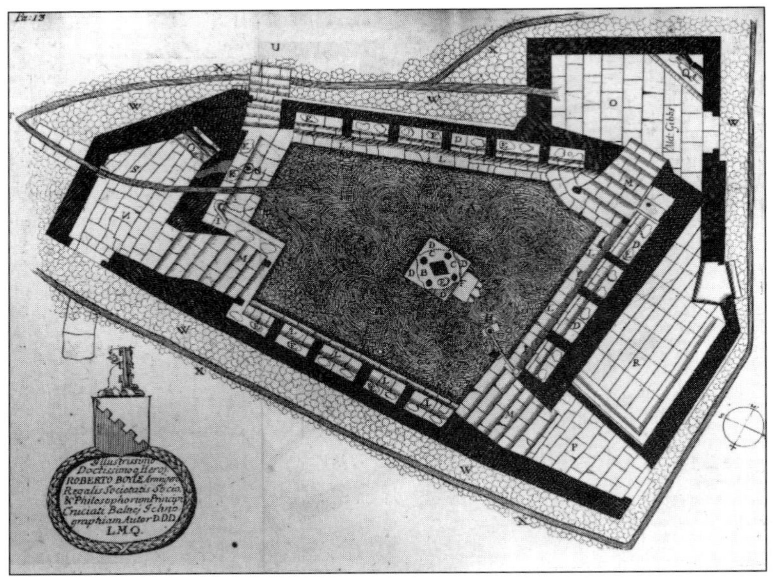

The fashionable Cross Bath from Thomas Guidott's *De thermis britannicis* (1691). After Queen Mary had bathed here in 1687 it briefly displayed Catholic symbols

Coronation festivities hymned a sovereign sent by Heaven to 'drive Rome's priests (those vipers) from our land'. Yet the taint of Jacobitism, once acquired, was hard to lose. Though Bath still had one royal ally in Princess Anne, she too fell under suspicion of desiring James II's return. When she visited in 1692, the mayor's endeavour to pay her the customary honours earned him a sharp rebuke from the queen. A government informer meanwhile reported on the princess's contacts and the crowd of notables her stay had attracted to Bath – enough indeed to force up the cost of lodgings.

Even without the draw of a royal guest the seasons were getting busier. Medical publicity played its part. Two Bath physicians, Robert Pierce and Thomas Guidott, issued separate accounts of the cures achieved by bathing and water-drinking. Their lists reveal that patients were travelling from as far afield as Scotland and Ireland, that they included children as well as adults, and that they made up a cross-section of the nation, from aristocrats and gentry, through the professional and commercial classes, to artisans and even paupers. Many were sent by their own physicians at home, though not always to Bath's gain, as Guidott came to recognize; the worthy but incurable poor were hardly more welcome than the 'scandalous Persons, Vagabonds and Cheats' who also congregated at the spa on the pretext of needing the waters. Others required no such excuse. 'Our city is very full and balls every

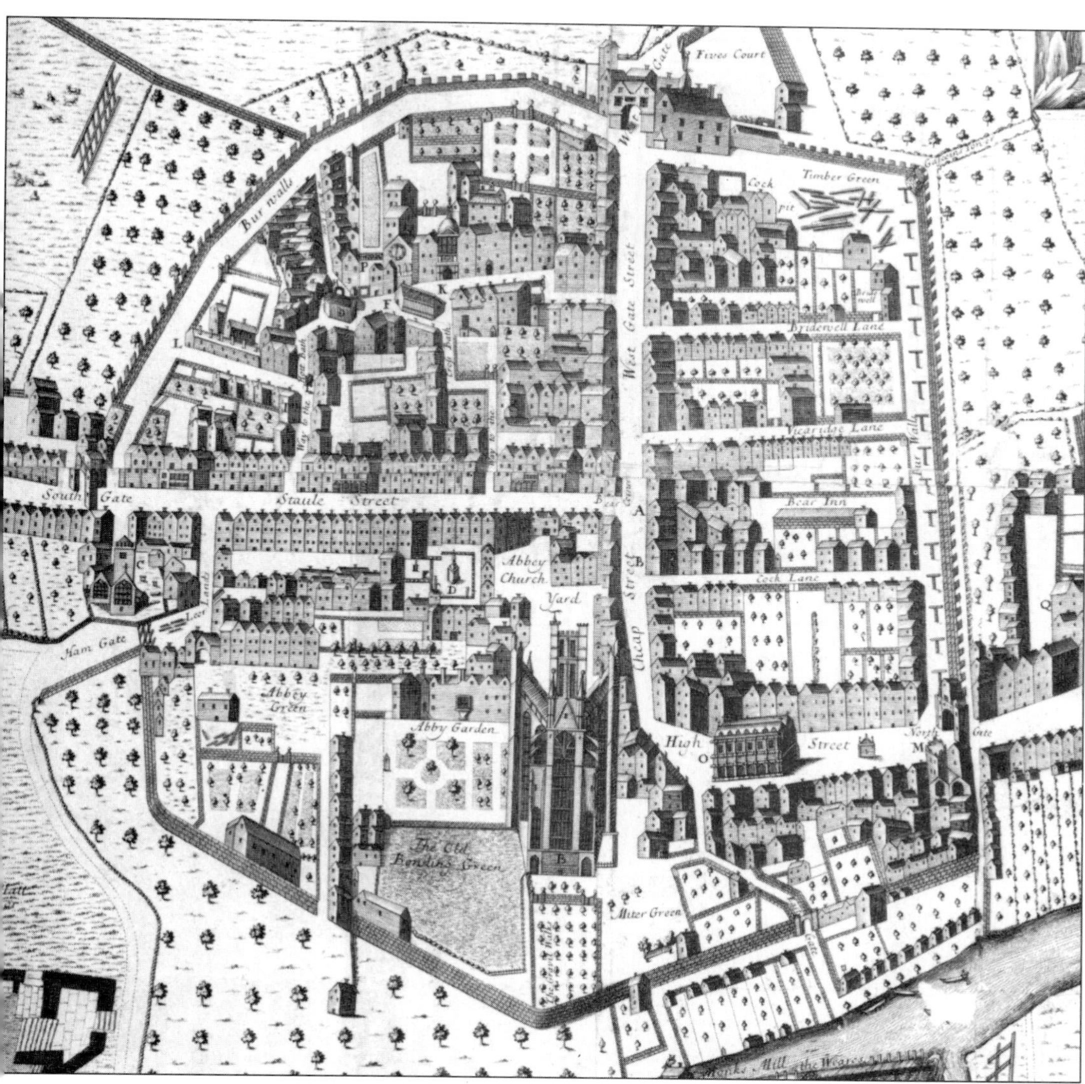

'he walled city in 1694, a
etail from Gilmore's map
vhich also publicized the chief
uildings and lodgings in
ignettes round the border
north is on the right)

night in the Town Hall,' ran one comment in 1696. In 1697 it was reported fuller still. Not all these people had come for their health. Another Bath was coming to the fore – the social rendezvous, the leisure resort, the magnet for adventurers. Gradually it would learn to capitalize on its splendid potential, but it would take time.

CHAPTER FIVE

Investing in the Company

In 1700 Bath showed little sign of the explosive growth that was to come. While its resident population had certainly increased from the 2,000 or so suggested by the Hearth Tax returns of 1664–5, it can still scarcely have exceeded 2,500–3,000 – a figure much swollen, however, in the summer months by invalids, pleasure-seekers, and crowds of servants. To contemporaries the town with its straggles of suburb appeared sunk 'in a bottom', overlooked by steep hills and awkward to approach. Market gardens, orchards and meadows closely hemmed the built-up area, and above them cornfields, pastures and woods rose to the open downs. From the raised walks on the town walls there were views of the river and more distant glimpses of hamlets, villages, and the half-dozen highways that converged on Bath. The fine scenic setting, the immediacy of the countryside, and the opportunities for pleasant airings and excursions had a pastoral charm for many visitors that would only increase.

All the land in and around Bath was corporately or privately owned, but the new security of tenure guaranteed by the political settlement of 1688 did not itself mean that holdings could easily be developed for profit. According to the West Country custom of letting land in fairly small acreages on lifehold tenancies, a property could not revert to its nominal owner until all three lives named on a lease were 'extinguished'. The landowner meanwhile received a very meagre annual rent, for his chief gains were reckoned to come from fees paid when leases were renewed or updated. It might take decades of reversion and amalgamation before an estate was worth granting, at much higher rents than before, to building developers. Once the conditions were right though, a title to land might be the key to affluence. The 329-acre Walcot Lordship, for example, which around 1640 hardly brought in £10 a year, had become 150 years later one of the richest pieces of real estate in the land. In the interval methods of raising capital, securing loans, and spreading development costs had been transformed into a fine art.

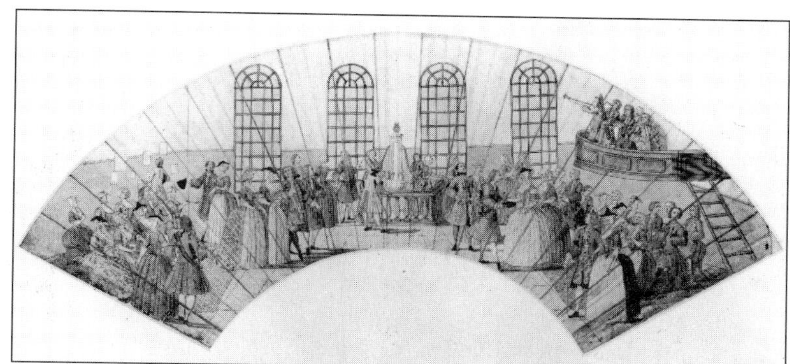

Morning rendezvous at the Pump Room of 1706. George Speren's fan picture also shows the simple musicians' gallery erected in 1734

The gratifying stay of Queen Anne and many courtiers in 1702, and again in 1703, had a catalytic effect on public and private investment. Recognizing perhaps that Bath was lagging behind Tunbridge Wells in its amenities, the Corporation took note of medical opinion by erecting an elegant Pump Room (1706), and also leased ground in the Gravel Walks for a row of smart shops fronted by a parade. Equally important, it obtained an Act of Parliament (1708) to repair the ruinous approach roads (so creating an early turnpike trust), to improve street lighting, cleansing and paving, and to license up to sixty sedan chairs. In another innovation George Trim, a city councillor, was allowed to breach the town wall on the north perimeter to give access to an extramural street of houses he began building in 1707. The same indulgence was not extended to an outsider, Thomas Harrison, who in 1709 put up a simple assembly room, without permission, abutting the exterior of the wall on the east, and then laid out a garden running down to the river. During the six years of legal wrangling that ensued, Harrison had the powerful backing of his clientèle against all the Corporation's efforts to assert its rights, for he was providing visitors for the first time with a place of their own, a club, gambling saloon, ballroom, private garden, where they could disport themselves without being subject to Corporation whim. For Harrison the motivation lay in the profits to be made out of the nationwide gambling fever that had spread from the Stuart court. By 1700 the royal official in charge of gambling, the groom-porter, was already orchestrating play at Bath, and in 1706 the descent of fifty professional gamesters sent a clear signal to Harrison to proceed with his venture. One such gamester, Richard Nash, had arrived around 1703 and soon became Harrison's vital associate in persuading the *beau monde* to flock to Bath and indulge themselves at the gaming tables.

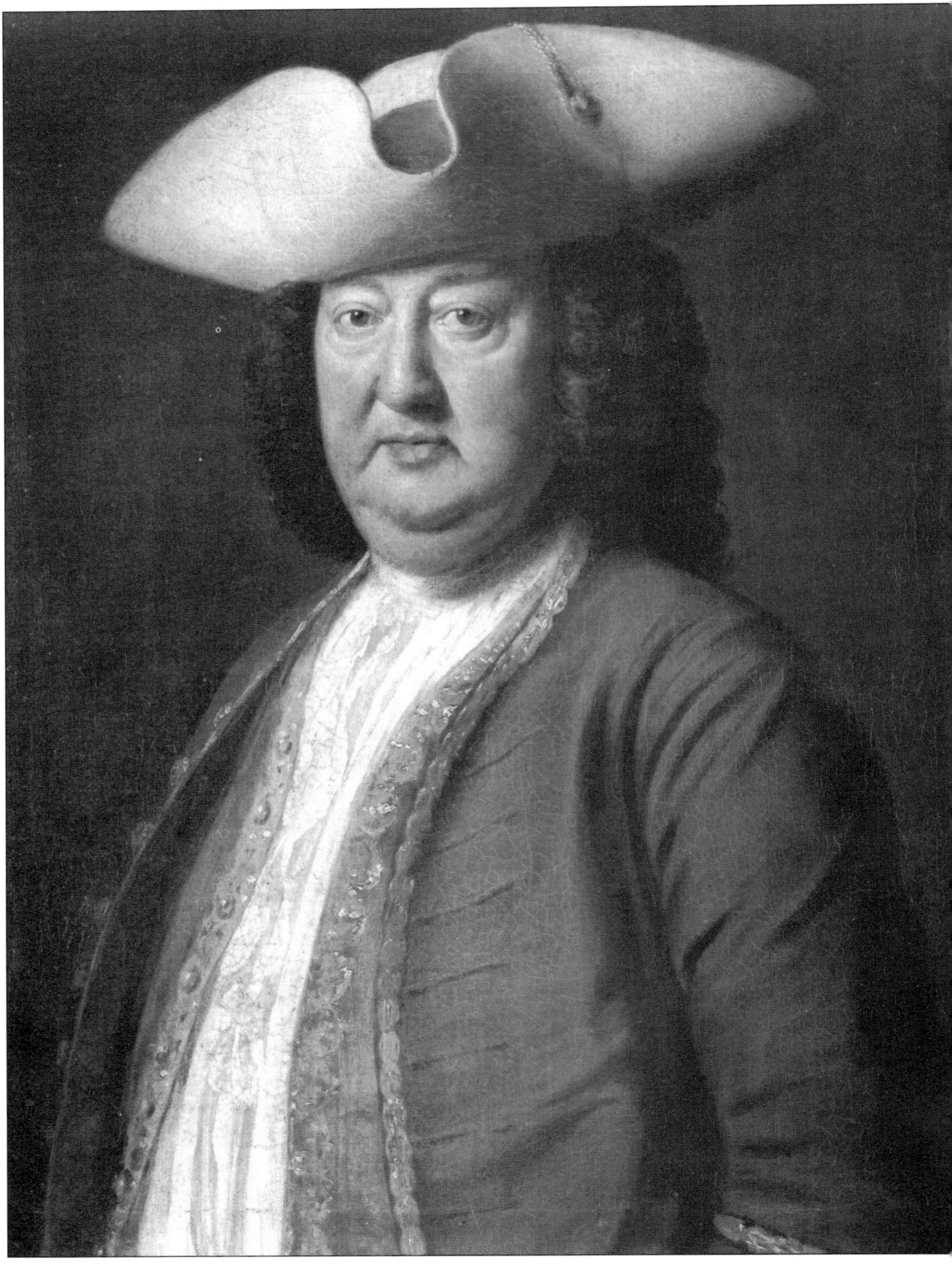

Out of cards and dice was spun Nash's astonishing fifty-year career as master-of-ceremonies. A mere commoner, but with formidable self-assurance, organizational flair, and a web of useful connections, Nash gradually rose to become the indispensable figurehead, the linchpin around which polite life revolved, the acknowledged King of Bath. His great achievement was in nurturing the idea of 'the company', encouraging the fashionable society that came to Bath to mingle and participate without too much ceremony, while at the same time maintaining due precedence on formal occasions (such as the performance of the high-status minuets at balls). His famous rules of conduct, his restraints on antisocial behaviour, his role as confidant and arbitrator, all served his purpose in promoting (as one of his many female supporters phrased it) 'a coalition of all parties and ranks'.

Without some spirit of spa bonhomie Bath might well have been damaged during the years of revived Jacobite activity and political strife. Nash the peacemaker, as well as Nash the propagandist for Bath, was surely recognized in the honorary citizenship he received in 1716. Ever since 1688 the city had been trying to live down its Jacobite reputation. By 1705 it seemed an entirely reformed place, reported Daniel Defoe in his guise of government informer. Thanks to Nash the company never split into antagonistic factions, as for instance the assembly did at York; nor did its exemplary Bluecoat charity school, opened in 1711, become a pawn in the in-fighting between Jacobite Tories and Hanoverian Whigs as happened elsewhere. On the other hand only muted joy was expressed at George I's coronation in 1715. By contrast the Somerset Jacobite, Sir William Wyndham, was loudly rung into town by the bells of the Abbey Church, whose rector turned out to be deeply implicated in plans for a rising in support of the Pretender. The plot may indeed only have been thwarted by a timely warning to General Wade, who discovered an arsenal of weapons in Bath and 200 ready horses. This reminder of old disloyalties must have been compounded by another seizure of arms in 1718 at Badminton, the seat of the Duke of Beaufort, a patron of Bath. Arrests of visiting Jacobite suspects continued: eight in 1718 and then in 1722 the Duke of Norfolk. In 1719 it was believed that a majority in the region still favoured the Pretender. In response the Corporation put its authority firmly behind the Hanoverian succession, made General Wade a freeman in 1716 and its MP eight years later. But only with the next reign would the city's name be properly cleared.

pposite: Richard Nash in his mbolic white beaver hat, inted by William Hoare 1749. Later MCs wore a dge of office donated by the siting company

Its notoriety for gambling and 'deep play' in which thousands of guineas might change hands was another matter. Women were as addicted as men, and it was no wonder that a publication of 1714

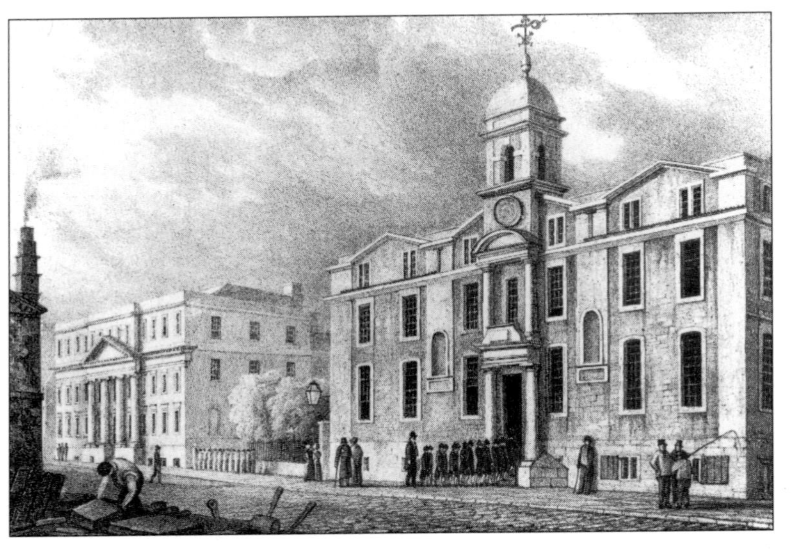

Around 1723 the Bluecoat School moved into new premises designed by William Killigrew. Beyond it rises the General Hospital of 1738–42 with a top storey added in 1793 (R. Woodroffe, *c.* 1830)

spoke of the 'great Gravity of the Countenances round Harrison's Table'. Although Harrison's proved sufficiently lucrative to merit the building of an extension in 1720, it held no monopoly on betting. More clandestine gaming houses existed and one was prosecuted at the Quarter Sessions in 1713. People wagered too on cockfights, and on games of billiards, bowls and ninepins. In 1722 the City Council leased a tract of Claverton Down and established horse-racing. Raffling shops might tempt the most genteel visitor into a modest flutter. According to one writer Bath was 'a perfect snare for all design'd', where card-sharpers, pimps and travelling prostitutes flourished. At a more respectable level it was a place for cementing alliances of every kind, political, social, financial and matrimonial. Nash's principle that it was a crime not to appear in public aided the process, since the company not only intervisited among themselves but repeatedly met at the Pump Room, on the walks, in church, at coffee houses and plays, among the audience for the Italian castrati singers or Powell's celebrated puppet shows, and in dozens of other encounters within the small compass of the town.

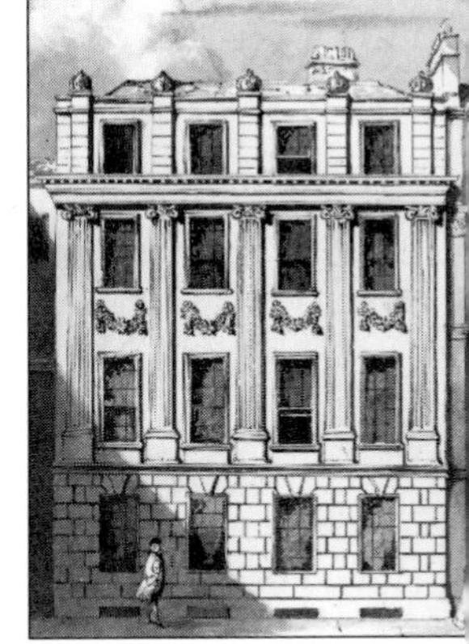

The Abbey Church Yard house of General (later Field-Marshal) George Wade, Bath MP and civic benefactor (H.V. Lansdown, 1855)

A social gulf, however, divided the company from the citizens of Bath despite the many everyday contacts between the two. The Mayor and Corporation, for all their scarlet and regalia and private property-holdings, were after all mostly tradesmen at heart. Nash could if necessary act as go-between, but otherwise both sides attended to their

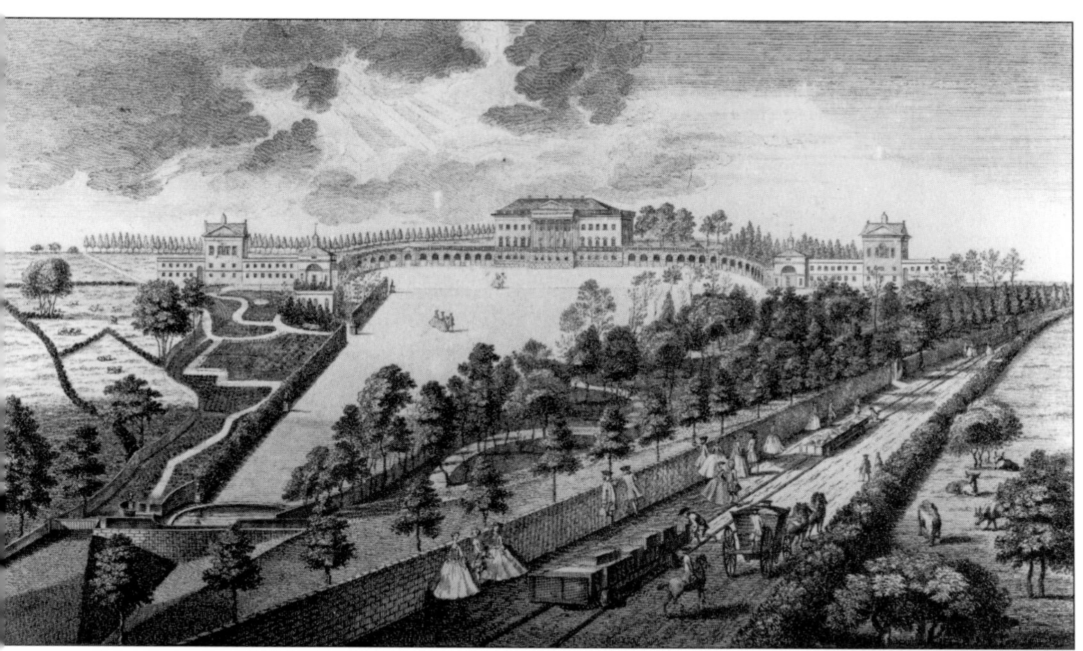

unning beside Ralph Allen's state of Prior Park, a railroad ansports blocks of freestone om Allen's quarries down to wharf on the Avon engraving by A. Walker, 752)

own affairs. The Corporation remained as much a restricted oligarchy as ever and the same family names recurred time after time in its membership (Atwood, Biggs, Bush, Chapman, Collibee, Gibbs . . .). Yet municipal advancement was far from closed off to meritorious newcomers, as the case of Ralph Allen would show. The young Cornish postmaster may well have been Wade's source of intelligence at Bath when the Western rising of 1715 was forestalled. At all events he was Wade's client and in due course secured advantageous government contracts for running much of the kingdom's cross-country mail service, making himself rich in the process. Looking to further ventures he and his family took five of the thirty-two available shares in the Avon Navigation. The Act that Bath finally obtained in 1711 to canalize the river to Bristol met such residual opposition that in 1724 the city was glad to hand over the £12,000 project to a private company masterminded by a Bristol timber merchant, John Hobbs, and with Allen one of the treasurers. When in December 1727 the first cargo passed through the six locks to Bath, it signalled a transformation in the supply of building materials and other heavy goods to a place ripe for physical development. It held a special promise for Allen; the limestone quarries he had recently acquired on

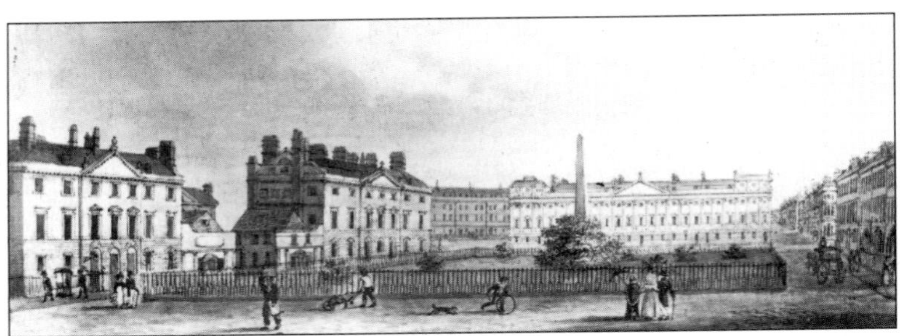

Anonymous view of Queen Square looking north (*c.* 1790?). The central building on the west side was set back and the space not infilled until 1830

Combe Down could now be exploited not only for use in Bath but wherever in the country water transport penetrated. By 1731 he had constructed an innovative railway to bring blocks of ashlar from his hill-top quarries down to his stoneyard on the Dolemeads riverside.

The Corporation was in no position to finance speculative building, even if it did own three-quarters of the property within the walls and had boosted its income from water rates and the Pumper's rent. True, it modernized and extended the Guildhall (1718–25), obtained a fresh Improvement Act (1720) for its streets and turnpikes, and began a campaign of sewer-laying from 1718 onwards. But major works were left to private enterprise. It was capital investment from Bristol and London that stimulated three projects of the 1720s: Beauford and Kingsmead squares beyond the West Gate, and a second suite of assembly rooms, Thayer's, opposite Harrison's. The designer of these new rooms, John Wood, had returned to his native city by 1727 with grandiose schemes for remodelling it on correct classical lines. In Chandos Buildings he introduced the Palladian style to Bath, but his really adventurous move came with Queen Square. Chandos Buildings had been financed by a single tycoon duke. Queen Square demonstrated a quite different way of capitalizing a project by bringing the joint contribution of many smaller speculators to bear on a unified development. For part of the Barton Farm estate north-west of Bath, unencumbered by tenants, Wood came up with an unprecedented plan – an elegant square of houses on the grandest scale, with symmetrical classical façades that attained an almost palatial splendour on the north side. But the beauty was also in the economics. Between 1728 and 1734 the landowner, Robert Gay, cautiously released the ground in half a dozen plots for a total rent of £137 a year; Wood then granted building leases for each house, which fetched him in turn rents of £305 a year; the individual builders raised mortgages on the strength of their leases and eventually sold or sublet the finished buildings for their own profit.

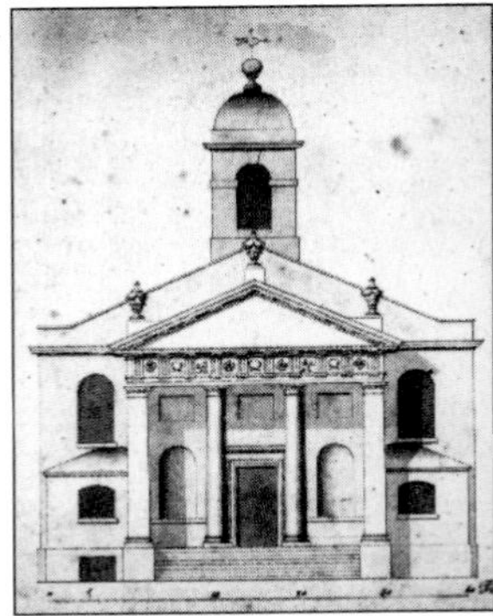

The elder Wood's front elevation for St Mary's chapel, Queen Square, the first of some half-dozen private subscription chapels at Bath

Provided the chains of credit held, the risks were safely distributed. It was one of those cost-sharing, risk-limiting mechanisms on which the expansion of Georgian Bath depended. Another, more suited to public buildings, was the device of a share-holding consortium that Wood preferred for Queen Square chapel (consecrated 1734), the first of the exclusive proprietary chapels in which pew subscriptions paid both the stipend of a fashionable preacher and the dividends of shareholders.

The name Queen Square was chosen purposely for its royal resonance. In 1727 the accession, coronation and birthday of George II had been celebrated with unusual fervour, thanks largely to the entertainments and ox-roastings organized by an ultra-loyalist jeweller, Thomas Goulding, who wished to silence once and for all accusations that Bath was 'a disaffected place'. Success followed at once, for Princess Amelia, the first royal visitor since Queen Anne, made a long stay in 1728, advertized the new river transport by taking a wherry trip to Bristol, attracted a crowd of sightseers, and left promising her patronage. Again Goulding shone, and the Bath actors scored a popular hit with *The Beggar's Opera*. A precedent had been set and every important royal anniversary was henceforth accompanied by rejoicings. Nash, at the height of his influence, was in his element. He commemorated the Prince of Orange's successful cure in 1734 with a symbolic obelisk in Orange Grove (the rechristened Gravel Walks) and marked the festive visit of Frederick, Prince of Wales, in 1738 with an even taller obelisk in Queen Square.

The anti-gambling legislation of 1738–9 and 1745 none the less dealt Nash a severe blow. Despite the crowded seasons of 1738 and 1739 the two assembly rooms on which he relied financially must have lost revenue, and one of them was fined a substantial £500 for operating illegally. For a time several new games supplanted dice, hazard, pharaoh and other banned favourites. Nash imported EO, a species of roulette, from Tunbridge Wells, but though this prospered briefly until its suppression in 1750, it appears that Nash was cheated of his expected share in the takings. Eventually, with his pocket and reputation both suffering from his revealed business with the rooms, he found even his honest custody of public subscription money for the balls and Pump Room music under attack.

Before serious gambling was driven underground, the famous diversions of Bath were already settling into a bland routine of 'busy idleness' and the constant 'doing of nothings' that some complained of: morning gatherings at Pump Room and coffee houses, services at the Abbey Church, parading in the Grove and Harrison's gardens, calls at milliners' shops or Leake's gossipy circulating library, carriage

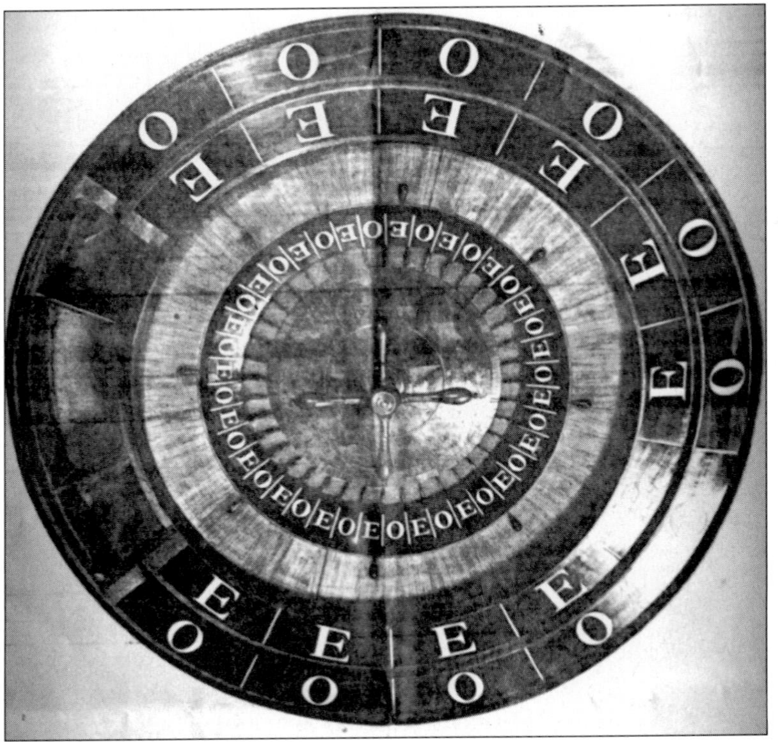

An EO table, a device introduced to evade the prohibition on card and dice gambling

outings and rides on the downs; then later the private visiting and the careful preparations for evening parties, balls, concerts and plays. More and more the subscription system was helping to underpin the investment in leisure and entertainment. Having been welcomed by reward-expectant bell-ringers and musicians, new arrivals ran a whole gauntlet of subscription demands before they could enter the full circle of the polite company, just as they faced an excess of tipping and bill-settling on their departure. Yet while a stay at Bath involved expenditure enough, it was not an intrinsically dear place for the well-to-do to visit: the tariff for lodgings had been standardized at 10s. a room per week in season (5s. for servants' garrets); food prices at the well-supplied market were generally moderate; and subscriptions, once paid, did represent fair value.

For their part, Bath traders and providers wanted no obstacle to tapping the five-month season for all it was worth. The City Council persistently tried to stop non-freemen trading within the Bath liberties. It also tackled public nuisances that might deter business, shutting

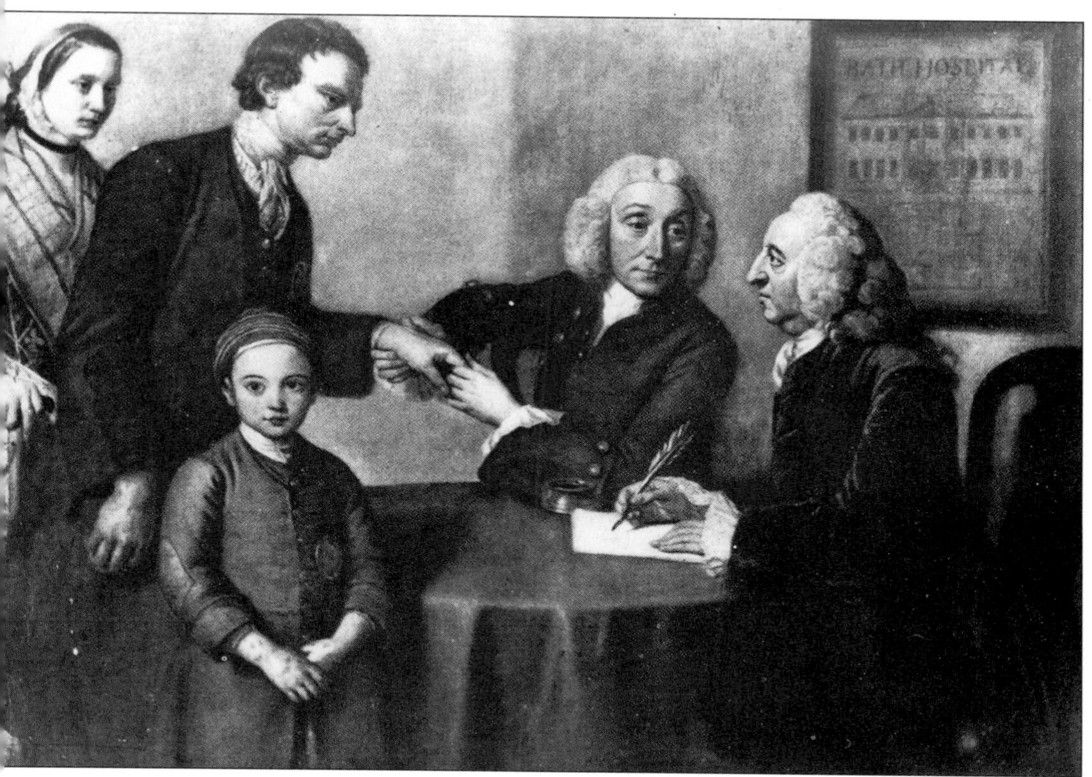

The physician William Oliver and surgeon Jeremy Peirce examine patients. This propagandist canvas by William Hoare also displays Wood's architectural design for the Hospital

disorderly ale-houses, getting the town crier to hound beggars off the streets, repairing the gaol, and appointing a night watch. As late as 1727 it employed the pillory to punish two notorious brothel-keepers, for although the chances of sexual adventure (and the availability of pornographic literature) no doubt attracted some custom to Bath, on balance it did the spa's image no good. More positively the Corporation levelled and replanted Orange Grove, where the most desirable lodgings were now to be found, and discussed enlarging the increasingly inadequate Pump Room – if not by John Wood's elaborate plan then at least by constructing a musician's gallery to give extra space to the thronged morning assemblies.

A more complex institution, the long-mooted General Hospital, began building in 1738 on the former theatre site and opened in 1742. Its terms of admission, however, reflected not so much pious philanthropy as a desire to restrict access to the carefully vetted few. Local residents were excluded on principle, and 'cripples and other indigent strangers' from a distance required convincing testimonials,

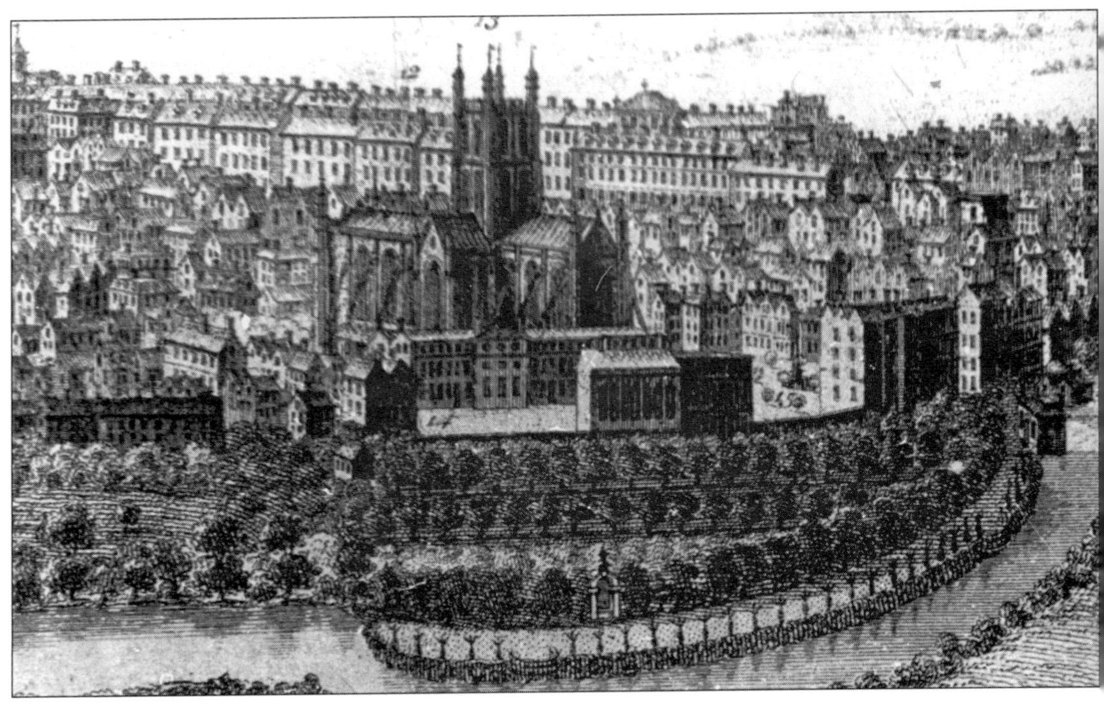

Looking across the river and Harrison's gardens to the two assembly rooms in Terrace Walk before the building of the Parades (S. and N. Buck, 1734, detail)

as well as their return fares, before they were admitted for treatment. The hospital served in fact as Bath's alibi. In theory it permitted the nation's deserving poor to receive the bounty of the hot springs; in practice it also gave the authorities a fine excuse to get rid of undeserving vagrants. Still, altruism played some part in the enterprise and to be associated with the hospital brought credit to its benefactors and governors, prominent among them Ralph Allen, who donated the building stone, and that indefatigable fund-raiser Richard Nash, treasurer to the hospital almost up to his death. Collections at church services helped significantly towards the £25,000 raised in the period 1738–50, though this sum barely covered building costs and the fairly austere regime of care for some one hundred patients at a time. All the same the hospital was a glowing advertisement for Bath. The citizens may not have enjoyed its direct benefits, but its very existence proclaimed the potency of the waters and the charity of the inhabitants.

The completion of Queen Square in 1739 must have given Wood's financial backers the confidence to participate in his next scheme – once at least it had been reduced from the visionary concept of a

94 *Anno Regni duodecimo*

the Top of Kingsdown-hill, *and the City of* Bath; *and for amending ſeveral other Highways leading to the ſaid City; and for cleanſing, paving, and enlightening the Streets, and regulating the Chairmen there; and for keeping a regular Nightly Watch within the ſaid City and Liberties thereof.*

Preamble, reciting the Acts 6 Anne,

Whereas by an Act of Parliament paſſed in the Sixth Year of the Reign of her late Majeſty Queen *Anne*, intituled, *An Act for repairing, amending, and enlarging the Highways between the Top of* Kingsdown-hill, *and the City of* Bath, *and alſo ſeveral other Highways leading to and through the ſaid*

A succession of local Acts of Parliament gave the authority for improving approach roads, city streets, and policing

Royal Forum bridging the river to the more manageable project of the Parades. The low-lying Ham site by the river may have been marshy but it had signal advantages – fine rural prospects, proximity to the rooms and other amenities, and ease of transporting building materials by water. It enabled the 2nd Duke of Kingston to realize part of his Bath estate, and satisfied the Corporation preference (aided by its policy of differential charges for sedan chair hire) to focus new building in the lower town. Once work on the Parades had begun, however, Wood was obliged to lay aside his designs for splendid frontages in favour of cheaper, utilitarian façades insisted on by his sub-lessees, perhaps because of the costs already incurred in building foundations on marshy ground. Even so, Ralph Allen's five houses cost him a good £10,000. The development took ten years, capital being hard to raise in the 1740s, but it found favour with visitors who especially appreciated the broad, clean, pennant-stone pavements where they could stroll and rendezvous. Promenading was an occasion for self-display, and Grand Parade ('one of the noblest Walks in Europe') made a fitting climax to the fashionable route from the Pump Room through shop-lined Wade's Passage, Orange Grove and Terrace Walk. If it overlooked Harrison's garden and spoiled its former seclusion, at least a new retreat had been called into existence – Spring Garden, a ferry ride away across the Avon.

By now Ralph Allen dominated civic affairs. He continued to cultivate friends in high places, and at his new mansion of Prior Park entertained not just writers like Pope and Fielding who could laud his philanthropy in print, but a wide circle of acquaintance, even in 1750 the heir to the throne. The events of 1745–6, the Young Pretender's march on London and the threat of a French invasion, gave Allen another opportunity to display his loyalist credentials. In an atmosphere of intense local patriotism he raised his own uniformed troop of volunteers, marched and drilled them around Bath, and kept them under arms until 1749. Nash meanwhile purchased a set of twenty-one cannon from Bristol, which added notably to the din of musket-volleys, fireworks and bell-ringing during the incessant acclaiming of victories and royal anniversaries. On the death of Field-Marshal Wade in 1748, Allen quickly saw to it that Wade's successor at the Ordnance, Lieutenant-General Ligonier, should also accept his Bath seat in Parliament.

All the excitement drew an extra flood of visitors. Up to 5,000 were arriving each autumn, and some families overwintered, a fresh influx joining them in spring. In summer they repaired to other spas. A new pattern had emerged. The more Bath invested in its leisure

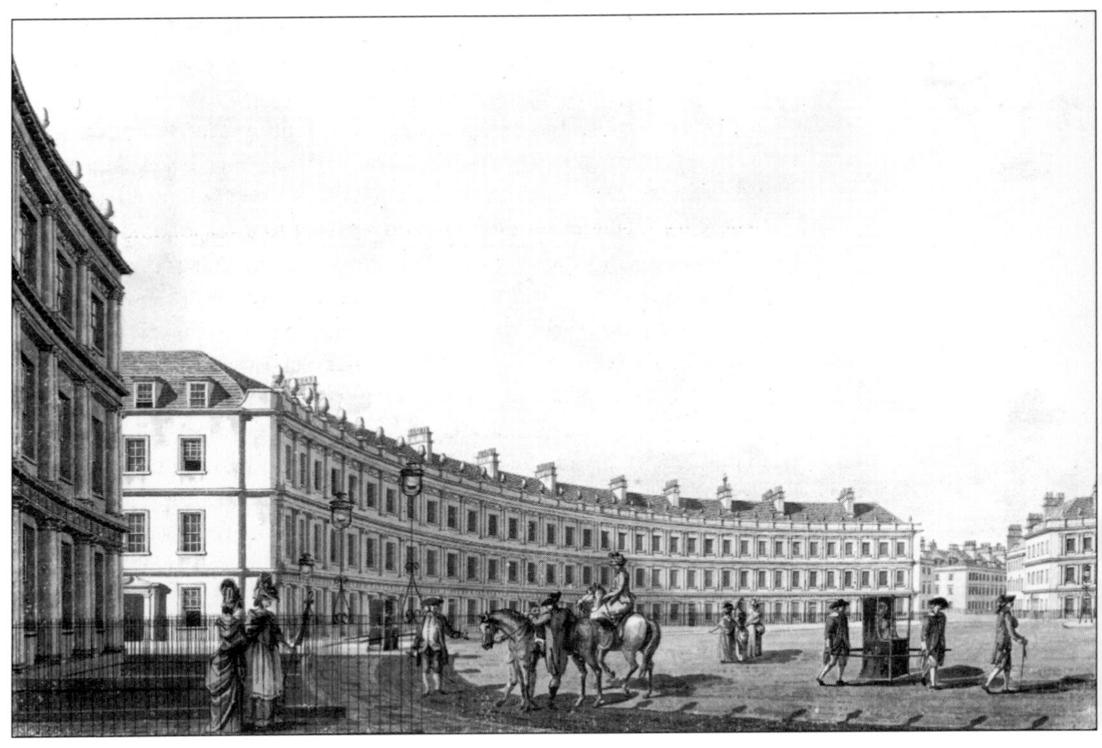

Thomas Malton's watercolour of 1784 creates a typically elegant vision of the Circus, built 1754–66

industry, the more it expected a lengthy season pay-off. As long as it enjoyed good business from September round to May, it could willingly sacrifice the summer to its lesser rivals, nearby Clifton Hotwells and up-and-coming Cheltenham among them. None could match the magnetism of Bath. Its principal coffee house, Morgan's, had 300–400 subscribers every season. Around 700 attended the formal opening of the grand ballroom at Simpson's (previously Harrison's) in January 1750. Only a fortnight before, the *Bath Journal* was boasting of the nineteen peers and peeresses then in town, and more visitors than ever known in midwinter. In spring 1750 the Prince and Princess of Wales stayed on South Parade.

The confident interlude before the Seven Years' War began to sap investment saw a marked upsurge in building. In the quarter south of the Abbey Church more houses went up on the Kingston estate, and in the clearance of ground here for new private baths a section of the Roman *thermae* was uncovered. Beyond Queen Square the irrepressible John Wood began building Gay Street up the slope to lead into his most remarkable invention, the richly ordered Circus with its provocatively angled exit streets suggesting expansion still to come. Overseen by the younger Wood on his father's death in 1754, the first of the three crescent-shaped segments rose swiftly, but the drying up of credit delayed completion of the entire residential plan until 1766, when the next spurt of growth was already under way.

The City Council, having reduced its debt to a reasonable £1,000, was at last able to look beyond humdrum matters of street cleansing and market administration to undertake projects of its own. In 1750–2 it extended the Pump Room. In 1752–4 it salved the civic conscience by erecting a proper Grammar School after two centuries of misappropriating the funds intended for its benefit. It pulled down the North and South gates and widened the old bridge to assist the flow of traffic. It made grants towards a new dairy-house on the Common and the construction of St Michael's church tower. It turned land speculator itself, leasing a plot belonging to the city estates on Lansdown for a terrace to be named after another royal personage, the city's mythical founder Bladud.

By 1760 the residential population may have reached 10,000, domestic servants helping to account for the decided excess of females. A thriving economy was attracting so many outsiders to try their luck that the Corporation moved to protect freemen's interests by reviving the trading companies. From 1752 seven new companies, banners flying, joined the still-surviving guilds of tailors and shoemakers in the mayoral processions. Their legality was nevertheless challenged successfully in the courts, and in 1765 they marched for the last time. On the eve of its great boom period Bath was once again open to all-comers.

CHAPTER SIX

'Emporium of Elegance and Taste'

The accession of George III in autumn 1760 came at a time of high success in the war with France. The following June, as Bath proclaimed its patriotic loyalty with a grand illumination and fireworks, it could take pride in its two MPs – the elderly Field-Marshal Ligonier, commander of the armed forces, and William Pitt, the minister principally responsible for prosecuting the war. Pitt's bellicose policies soon forced his resignation from government, however, and he was still opposing the peace terms in 1763 when Ralph Allen wrote on behalf of the Corporation approving them. Pitt was outraged at this disloyalty from the man who had secured his Bath election in 1757, and Allen perhaps came to regret his own high-handedness. He soon resigned his influential alderman's office and died in 1764. Pitt retained his parliamentary seat until 1766, but then compromised his local reputation by accepting an earldom.

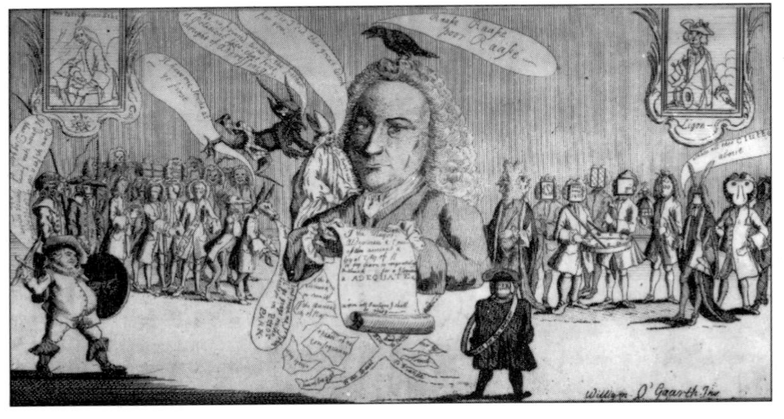

'The Knights of Baythe, or The One-Headed Corporation a satire of 1763 by 'William O'Gaarth' on Ralph Allen's role in the Pitt affair

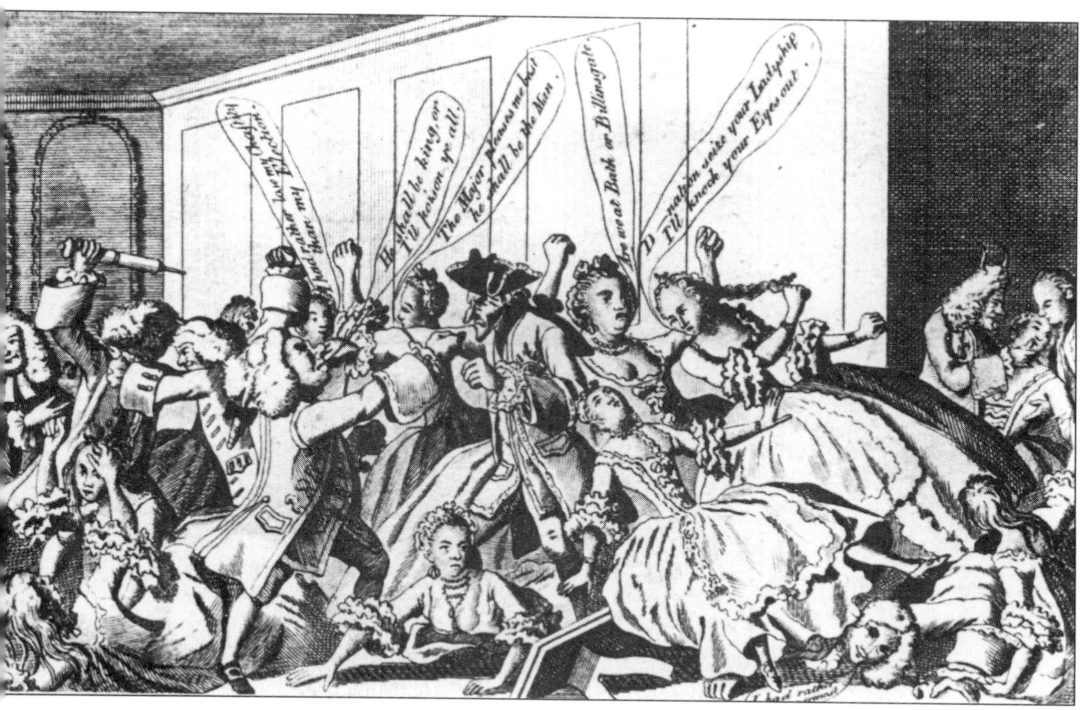

he *beau monde* riot over the ioice of the next master-of- remonies in 1769

In the short term the war had not served Bath's interests; investment had dried up and the cost of living had risen. In 1764 the lodging-house keepers cited inflation as the reason for extending high-season charges to nine months of the year, September to May. In 1765, with food prices soaring, the city authorities warned profiteers about the penalties for interfering in the free market, at the same time making preparations to swear in the sedan chairmen as special constables in case of food rioting. The danger passed, however, and social unrest was averted. When rioting did break out in 1769 it was from an entirely unexpected quarter.

Beau Nash had died in 1761, embittered, impoverished, but maintaining his 'tyranny' over the polite assemblies almost to the end. The Corporation paid his funeral expenses, six aldermen supported the coffin, the managers of the assembly rooms made fitting mourners, and the obituarists dwelt on his humanity, his civilizing mission, and the massive benefits he had brought to Bath. Such a gap was hard to fill. Nash's successor resigned within two seasons after repeated opposition to his rulings. Samuel Derrick then survived six difficult

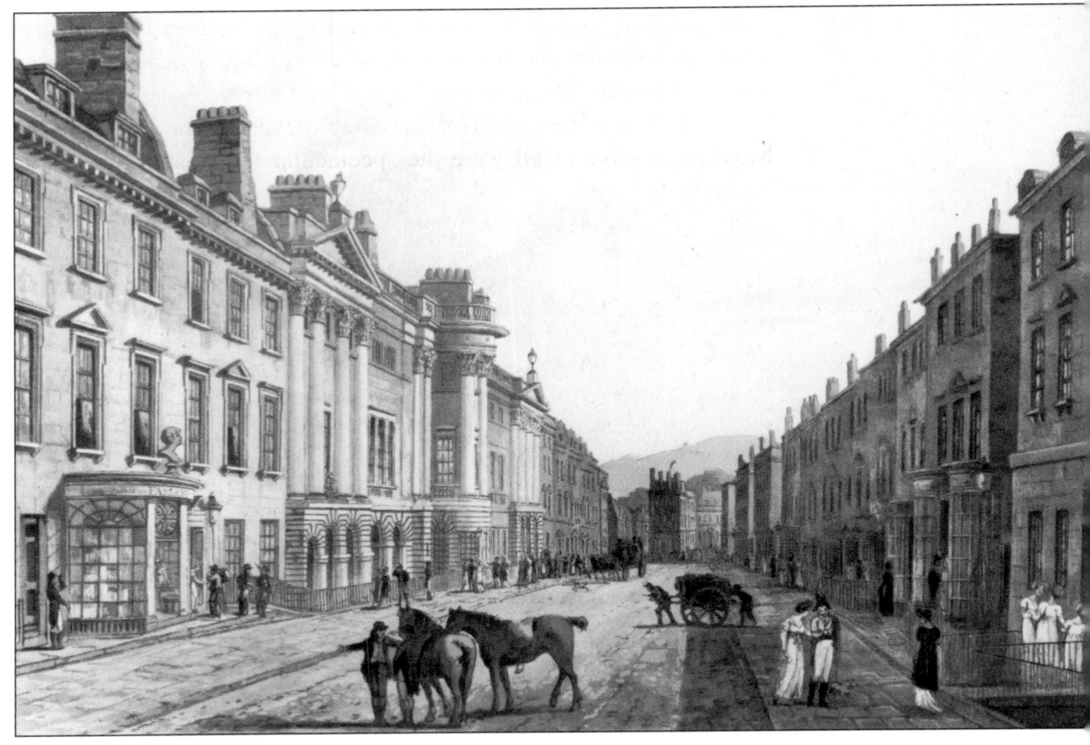

Laid out in the early 1760s to connect upper and lower towns, Milsom Street soon attracted a range of high-class shops (aquatint by J.C. Nattes 1805)

years in the post, before his death in 1769 unleashed a most unseemly power struggle over who should take office. For two unprecedented weeks the easy cameraderie of the spa was shattered. The company split; each side vociferously supported its own candidate, and held its own partial election, and the affair culminated in a violent confrontation at one of the rooms when the hastily summoned mayor had thrice to read the riot act. It was a shocking but sobering episode and ended in a compromise choice, the suave and well-connected William Wade. Harmony, for a time, was restored.

Not all the 600-odd subscribers entitled to vote for the master-of-ceremonies had been temporary visitors, for the increase in resident gentry was becoming noticeable. Bath's clientèle was changing in other ways too, as the upwardly mobile middle classes – the parvenus and 'impudent plebeians' so gleefully characterized in Smollett's novel *Humphry Clinker* – responded to the spa's attractions and undoubted snob appeal. The greater the influx, the more was investment encouraged. In a single ten-year burst of speculative building (1765–75) a considerable upper town mushroomed in Walcot, lower Bath spilled across the Ambury and Kingsmead, and upper and lower towns were linked by Milsom Street. Meanwhile a second river crossing, shop-lined Pulteney Bridge, pointed to the eventual development of Bathwick. Most impressive of all were the spectacular terraces and dramatic locations on Lansdown, boldly engineered along the contours and up slopes only just negotiable by carriages. Already 'rich in Pediments, Pillars, Porticoes', Bath gained its finest set-piece yet in the Royal Crescent, the younger John Wood's great sickle-shaped block of prestigious houses, set just within the city's open north-west boundary where the new desiderata of 'airy situation' and extensive outlook were ideally met. Wood's Upper Assembly Rooms (financed by a group of shareholders and lavishly inaugurated in 1771) were soon framed by streets of uniform classical houses, while Belmont and the Paragon and other terraces rose in similar pattern-book style nearby.

The threat to the lower town in this shift of gravity northwards was quickly apparent. Within weeks of the launch of the Upper Rooms one of the old assembly rooms closed for good. Simpson's too lost custom and began to plan a new ballroom to revive interest. Commercial activity had already started spreading from the traditional centre into Milsom Street. Too much was at stake for the Corporation to ignore. In 1766 it had promoted a local Act with far-reaching consequences. Responsibility for environmental and policing matters was taken away from the four parishes (where a previous Act of 1757 had ineffectively placed it) and vested in a body of twenty property-owning Commissioners with substantial powers of control, the first step towards a modern style of local government. Funded by a consolidated city rate, the Commissioners energetically set to work to impose order, improve street lighting and remove encroachments – including the clutter of hanging shop signs. A key section of the Act concerned the clearance of the market from High Street, where it impeded traffic and caused a litter nuisance. This in turn brought up the future of the dilapidated Guildhall, which sat on top of the market-house. The resulting project to redevelop both market and Guildhall in the space between High Street and the river turned into a struggle among property-owning and building interests that lasted well into the 1770s, yet finally produced a splendid civic headquarters surrounded on three sides by one of the best-appointed provisions markets in the country. With its chandeliered and richly stuccoed banqueting room the Guildhall was undoubtedly intended as a municipal riposte to the Upper Rooms from which the city dignitaries were socially excluded. When the Corporation began hosting its own status-conscious

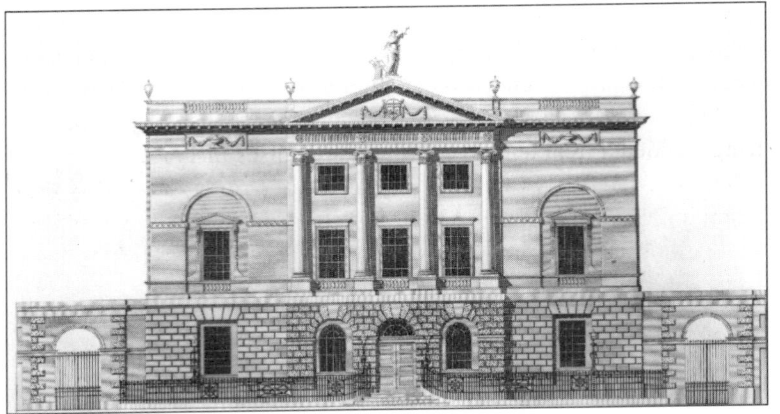

Thomas Baldwin's splendid Guildhall fronting High Street was completed in 1777. John Palmer's alternative plan would have sited it overlooking the river

assemblies, presided over by its own master-of-ceremonies, the symbolism was complete.

As Bath grew, its partly planned, partly accidental townscape struck contemporaries with a sense of wonder. Guidebooks, town plans and topographical prints documented every addition to the urban scene, while countless printed and private descriptions enthused about its elegance and novelty. Year by year the sights and amenities seemed to multiply. Two more proprietary chapels had opened: the luxurious Octagon in Milsom Street (1767) and Margaret Chapel near the Royal Crescent (1773). Opposite the Paragon stood the Countess of Huntingdon's private preaching chapel (1765), home to a Calvinistic strain of Methodism that both fascinated and repelled Bath society. Its moral crusading at a place notorious for 'sauntering frivolous dissipation' (indeed 'Satan's throne' in John Wesley's blunt description) was nevertheless a portent of the future.

'Frivolous dissipation' took many forms. By 1770 at least six circulating libraries were in existence. Portrait painters of the calibre of Gainsborough and William Hoare earned a good living. Plays and music had enthusiastic followings. The Orchard Street theatre, the first outside London granted a royal patent, would soon be regarded as a prime nursery of talent for the metropolitan stage. Concerts under Thomas Linley and William Herschel were programmed throughout the season, and in the summer months took on an *al fresco* character at Spring Garden. The need for exercise and the delights of Bath's countryside sent people walking, riding and driving on to the downs or to neighbouring beauty spots such as Prior Park grounds or Lyncombe Vale (where a secluded pleasure garden, King James's Palace, was now being promoted). Horse-racing drew immense crowds: 800 carriages and 20,000 spectators were said to have attended on Claverton Down in 1777. Two riding schools taught equestrianism, and one of them, on the city's northern fringe, added a 'real tennis' court to its premises in 1777.

The pull of the upper town remained strong. One sign was the migration of genteel promenading from the Parades in the lower town to a new 'mall' in the meadows below Royal Crescent. The upper-lower division was exacerbated by the public quarrel that erupted in 1774, ostensibly about the conduct of the master-of-ceremonies, William Wade, but in fact turning on the rights of the Upper Rooms shareholders to protect their £23,000 investment by dictating how the assemblies should be run. After weeks of argument, vituperation and mutual boycotts that polarized opinion between Upper and Lower Rooms, further damage to Bath's good name was prevented only by reinstating Wade as representative of the *whole* body of subscribers. It had become evident, though, that no single person could reconcile such conflicting interests. On Wade's resignation in 1777 separate MCs were appointed to each of the Rooms, the expectation being that they would co-operate as far as possible to avoid friction or divergent rulings on dress and conduct.

The peace was more alarmingly shattered in June 1780. Spurred on by the Gordon Riots in London, a mob of 300–400 burned down the newly finished Roman Catholic chapel and adjacent buildings. The Bath Royal Volunteers endeavoured to stem the violence and the sedan chairmen patrolled the streets overnight until dragoons and militia arrived from Devizes and Wells. One man was killed and seventeen suspects were arrested before the scare was over, and by then many visitors had fled – a veritable public relations disaster for a resort that cultivated an image of decorum and security. Prompt measures were needed to calm the anxieties of property owners and the spa trade alike. Sufferers received compensation, the forces of law and order were rewarded, and troops remained stationed at Bath for some time to come. In August the rioters' ringleader was publicly executed. But a nervous fear of popular disorder lingered on. The journeymen tailors, shoemakers and carpenters had been agitating for better wages. Poor families from outside Bath, attracted by the prospects for unskilled labour, were swelling the numbers already living near the breadline in slum areas like Avon Street. Applicants for parish poor relief were on the increase, and beggars and ragged street urchins as ever marred the spa's glossy image.

One remedy was seen in the Sunday schools, introduced from 1785

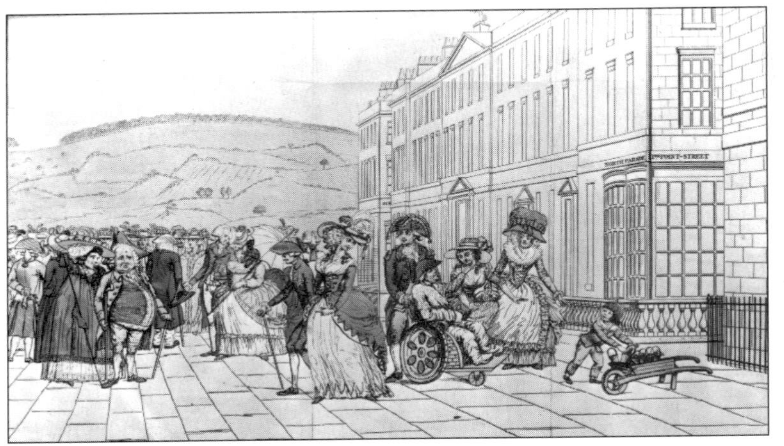

Though children are a forgotten social dimension of Georgian Bath, one appears in this scene as does an early form of wheelchair (attributed to Humphry Repton, *c.* 1787)

under close clergy supervision, in the hope of inculcating habits of deference while teaching the rudiments of Anglican doctrine and basic literacy. By 1789 thirty Sunday schools across the city claimed a weekly attendance of around seven hundred poor children, the afternoon sessions always ending with the pupils being shepherded to a service at the Abbey Church. A separate School of Industry fostered the work habit through spinning, knitting, sewing, netting and garment-making, activities that also produced sales income. Like the Bluecoat School the Sunday schools depended largely on charity, but Bath was known as well for its single-sex fee-paying schools where girls learned needlework and polite accomplishments, and boys followed a practical syllabus to equip them for careers in commerce or the armed forces. Teachers of music, drawing, dancing and foreign languages abounded, and the Grammar School under the Revd Nathanael Morgan offered a classical education of real distinction. For adult audiences various lecture series provided instruction and rational entertainment, especially in the sciences. Several courses given in the later 1770s by the itinerant chemist John Warltire and the resident lecturer John Arden inspired the formation of the Bath Philosophical Society in December 1779. This shared its secretary, Edmund Rack, with an agricultural improvement society founded two years before (the future Bath and West Agricultural Society), but its most productive member was the music master and astronomer William Herschel, who in 1781 announced to a society meeting the first sighting of the planet Uranus.

Medical practitioners figured prominently among the Philosophical Society's membership, as they did on the City Council

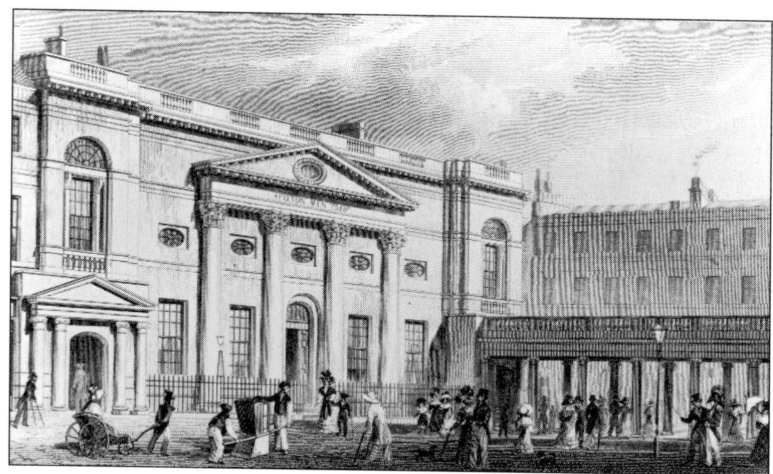

he Pump Room of 1791–5 y Thomas Baldwin, modified y John Palmer) was on an together more heroic scale an its predecessors (aquatint y David Cox, 1820)

and in many other Bath affairs. Hydrotherapy and other treatments supported more than fifty physicians, surgeons and apothecaries (without counting occasional visiting quacks), and in 1788 and 1792 a Casualty Hospital and an Infirmary improved medical provision for poorer citizens. Except for a brief alarm in the 1750s when the hot springs were shown not to contain the magic ingredient sulphur after all, the value of water drinking, in carefully monitored doses and for an astonishing catalogue of complaints, went almost unquestioned. The quantities consumed at the source and the widespread demand for bottled Bath water (supplied under the city seal) can be guessed from the rent that the Corporation was able to charge the Pumper, rising from £300 in 1760 to a considerable £840 thirty years later. The water cult perhaps reached its zenith in 1795 with the completion of the impressive new Pump Room, with its permanent advertisement in gold letters to the virtue of the springs. In the interim, from the mid-1770s onwards, bathing facilities came under scrutiny after years of comparative neglect. The Hot and Cross Baths were successively rebuilt and new private baths, under Corporation supervision, were added to the King's Bath complex.

Partly to neutralize the influence of the mushrooming suburbs the Corporation had engaged on an expensive campaign of inner-city renewal. A further Improvement Act (1789) authorized the raising of funds from turnpike tolls to make possible the removal of a swathe of properties, the widening and re-fronting of Cheap Street and parts of Stall Street, and the construction of Bath Street and other thoroughfares.

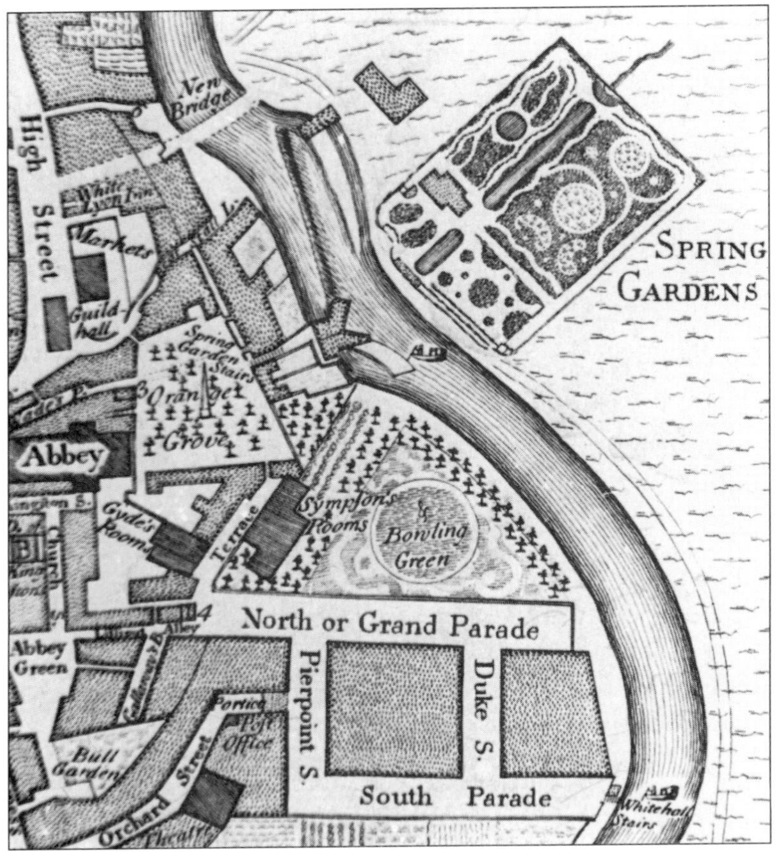

Spring Garden was served by ferry until the completion of the 'New Bridge', i.e. Pultene Bridge, in 1774

By 1795 the Commissioners' plans had been largely realized. The former cramped, old-fashioned-looking centre had given way to colonnades, regular façades and elegant spaces. Only a protracted dispute over compensation for the Bear Inn delayed the long-desired connection between the revitalized core and the busy artery of Milsom Street.

Bold though the transformation was, contemporaries marvelled even more at the centrifugal pressure on the city margins, the renewed 'shooting out' of roads and buildings into green fields and across hillsides. The ending of the American War of Independence in 1783 rekindled speculative enthusiasm and released land and capital in every quarter. Around 1790 the building frenzy made Bath one of the fastest-growing places in Britain. Local architects, builders, businessmen and attorneys spearheaded most of the construction projects: Green Park and Norfolk Crescent in the south-west,

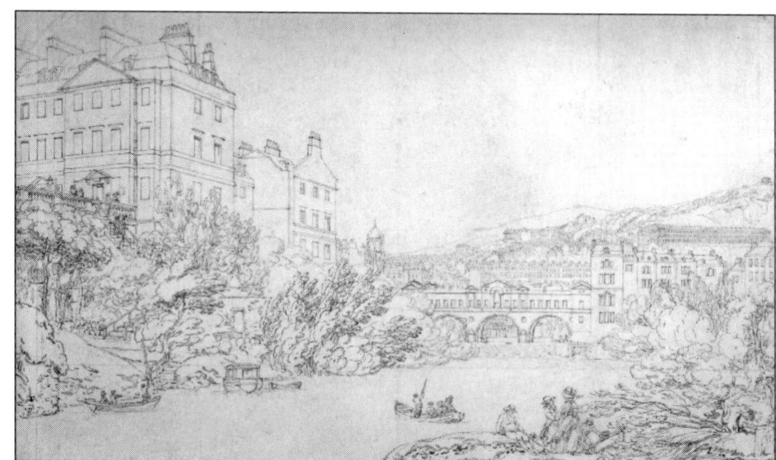

.obert Adam's Pulteney
ridge became the eventual
ey to the development of the
athwick estate in the great
uilding boom around 1790
sketch after Thomas Hearne,
. 1790)

Marlborough Buildings against the western boundary, and a dozen or more major developments in outer Walcot beyond the city limits, including Burlington Street, St James's Square, Somerset Place and Lansdown Crescent (accompanied by All Saints' proprietary chapel), prestigious Camden Crescent, and a ribbon of growth eastwards along the London road as far as the ambitious rows of Kensington and Grosvenor. Little wonder that the city freemen, who had historic rights to profits from the Common, were demanding that it too should be developed for their advantage, even filing a Chancery suit against the unwilling Corporation to this effect. Across the river a still grander design was taking shape under the guidance of William Johnstone Pulteney, chief trustee of Bathwick manor. For fifteen years his costly bridge spanning the Avon led only to the watermill and small cluster of Bathwick, a patchwork of market gardens, the city prison (1774), and the rival pleasure grounds of Spring Garden and Bathwick Villa (opened 1783). Lifehold tenancies on the estate had been eliminated, and though he had been thwarted in his attempt to link the bridge by a turnpike to Bathford, Pulteney was well placed in 1787 to benefit from the boom by granting leases to build. The master plan by the city architect, Thomas Baldwin, envisaged an entire neo-classical suburb of gracious streets, open spaces and Adamesque façades, with a spacious pleasure garden to replace the two that would be swept away. Well before 1790 the extensive foundations necessary for the low-level site were under construction, and Laura Place with the long spine of Pulteney Street was visible on the ground.

Bath was being overbuilt, a nostalgic few complained, but the majority thought otherwise. The city was attaining the status of an icon, an aesthetic masterpiece, 'the most admired city in Europe'. To Fanny Burney it looked 'beautiful and wonderful throughout . . . a city of palaces, a town of hills . . .'. Artists depicted it from every angle, finding even in the stone-blackening smoke a picturesque effect. Idealized prints proclaimed its beauties. Travel literature spoke of its charms. Two minutely detailed town models were separately crafted in cabinet-work and exhibited in London, tourist promotion *par excellence*. Indeed, removable buildings from one model were shown invitingly to George III at Weymouth, but neither this nor the mayoral delegation that waited on him at Cheltenham in 1788 persuaded the king to visit Bath. No reigning Hanoverian ever did.

Yet by now it hardly mattered. The resort had a momentum of its own and in any case enjoyed the patronage of the Prince of Wales and Duke of York. The stream of visitors had turned into a flood. An estimated 25,000 arrived in 1791 alone, a statistic presumably excluding others merely in transit or the numerous day-trippers and shoppers for whom Bath was a regional centre. They came on horseback, in private vehicles, or by the network of scheduled coaching services – and over much improved turnpike roads, good enough by 1784 for John Palmer to launch his thirteen-hour mailcoach run to the capital. Most carriage and wagon routes terminated conveniently at the larger inns such as the White Hart or the York House Hotel (opened in the upper town in 1769). The number of lodging- and boarding-houses

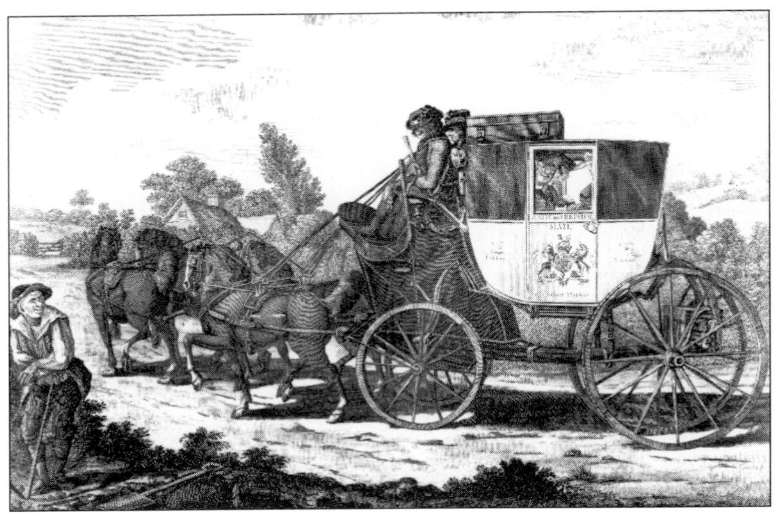

An early publicity image for the fast mailcoach service between London, Bath and Bristol. Bath's links with both cities were crucial to its growth

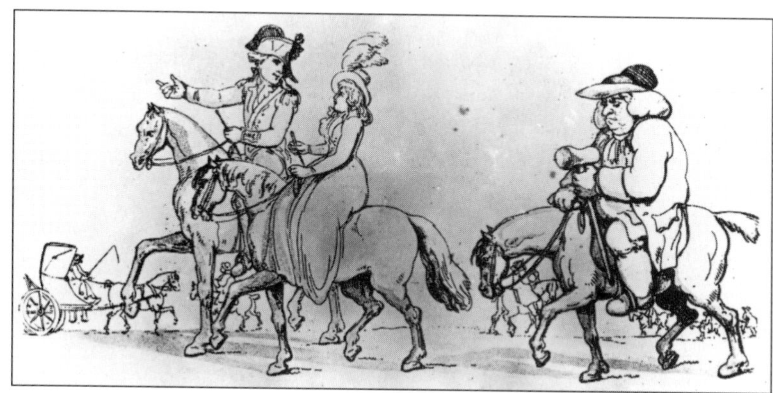

Riding was encouraged for health reasons, but Rowlandson's caricature is a reminder of the importance of horse transport generally in the spa's economy

appears to have matched demand and surpassed 450 by the end of the century, while the stabling for horses must also have been substantial. Besides the 170–200 licensed sedans, invalid wheelchairs were becoming a common sight in the flatter parts of the city. Wheelchair manufacture was in fact a minor local industry, along with furniture-making, coach-building, metalworking and brewing (with water-powered weaving mills and brassworking just downstream at Twerton). Although most manufactured goods on sale at Bath originated in the workshops of London, the Midlands and the North, the bespoke clothing trade provided considerable employment for both men and women (in tailoring, dress- and staymaking, shoe-making and millinery), as did retailing in general and domestic service, for women the biggest employer of all. The luxury shops at Bath, especially the fashion 'warehouses' and dazzling gift shops, were unrivalled outside London's West End, but many humbler traders down to pawnbrokers and street hawkers played essential roles in the spa's economy.

In March 1793 that economy was brusquely jolted. The outbreak of war with France undermined financial confidence and two of Bath's five banks collapsed, over-extended by the speculative mania. Construction work all over the city ground to a halt. Creditors called in their loans. A string of bankruptcies ravaged the building trade. All round Bath, for years to come, shells of unfinished terraces and crescents would stand as melancholy witness to the disaster. Only a fraction of the Bathwick scheme was ever completed, but that did include the Sydney Hotel and pleasure garden, just as the Grosvenor pleasure garden was salvaged out of the many projects halted along the London road. Splendid gala evenings at both gardens with illuminated walks, music and fireworks, helped brighten the closing years of the century.

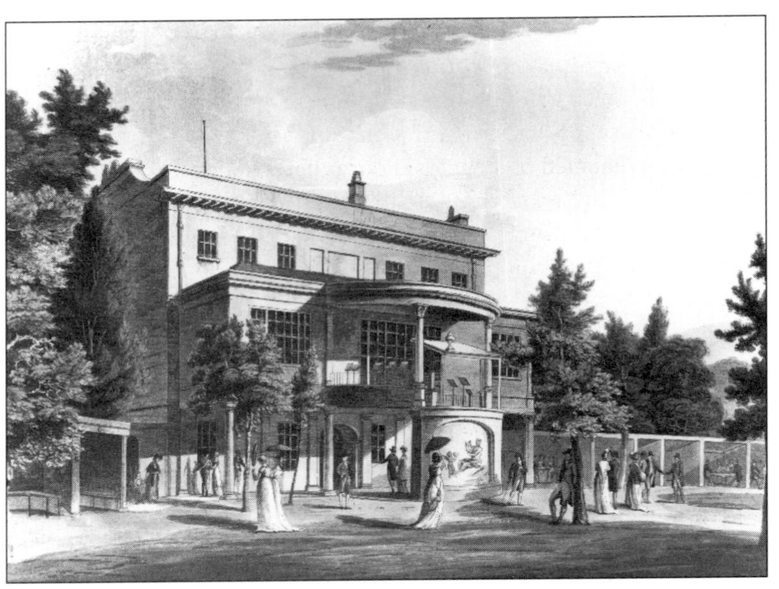

Sydney pleasure garden and its bandstand at the rear of the Sydney Hotel (aquatint by J.C. Nattes, 1806)

Depression and the reduced demand for labour came at a bad time for the poor, already suffering from high prices. The city magistrates (increased from two to nine by the renewed Charter of 1794) had reason to fear disorder, remembering the Gordon Riots of the recent past. Reformist and radical groups in the city posed a constant risk of subversion; 'seditious' literature circulated, and the many *émigrés* taking refuge at Bath were a daily reminder of the bloody events across the Channel. Once again loyalist instincts came to the fore. In late 1792 the Bath Loyal Association was formed 'against Republicans and Levellers'. Backed solidly by property-owners the Association collected thousands of signatures of support at the Guildhall and had a symbolic effigy of Thomas Paine burnt on Beechen Cliff. By 1793 the Corporation was paying bounties to the unemployed and others who enlisted for naval or military service, and several radicals were prosecuted by way of example. But anxieties resurfaced during the near-famine year of 1795: a Provisions Committee hastily began supplying the needy with cheap foodstuffs, and the well-off had to give up their white bread and pastries until the danger of violence passed. Five years later the possibility of dearth and disorder again sounded alarm signals, and another large relief operation was mounted. Even so, arsonists burned down a brewery and the volunteer militia had twice to be

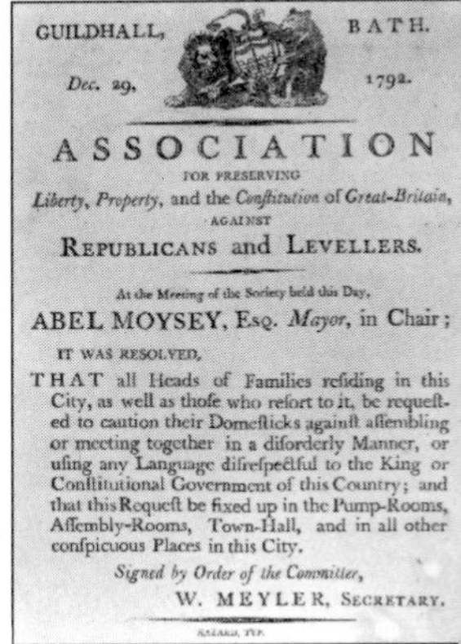

GUILDHALL, BATH.
Dec. 29, 1792.

ASSOCIATION
FOR PRESERVING
Liberty, *Property*, and the *Conſtitution* of *Great-Britain*,
AGAINST
REPUBLICANS and LEVELLERS.

At the Meeting of the Society held this Day,
ABEL MOYSEY, ESQ. *Mayor*, in Chair;

IT WAS RESOLVED,

THAT all Heads of Families reſiding in this City, as well as thoſe who reſort to it, be requeſted to caution their Domeſticks againſt aſſembling or meeting together in a diſorderly Manner, or uſing any Language diſreſpectful to the King or Conſtitutional Government of this Country; and that this Requeſt be fixed up in the Pump-Rooms, Aſſembly-Rooms, Town-Hall, and in all other conſpicuous Places in this City.

Signed by Order of the Committee,
W. MEYLER, SECRETARY.

Loyalist broadside issued during the 1790s hysteria against radical reformers called on to disperse hungry protesters. Acts of petty crime, theft and vandalism soared at this period in spite of every effort of the Bath Guardian Society, an organization established to protect property and to bring prosecutions at the inconveniently distant assizes. The streets were haunted by beggars. Poor relief had never cost more.

The moral and economic plight of the working-class and pauper population could not be ignored. Sunday schools, the much-praised mutual benefit societies and a motley group of charities (the Monmouth Street Society of 1805 being particularly active) all did useful work. Hannah More's edifying Christian tales, printed at Bath, were distributed in huge numbers. Concern about the scandalous lack of provision for the poor in Anglican churches led to a Free Church (Christ Church) being erected in the heart of Walcot for respectable families and servants unable to afford the usual pew rents. But these were palliatives and scarcely bridged the yawning social divide so apparent to anyone passing from the more affluent neighbourhoods to the insanitary, overcrowded slums about Avon Street and the Quay, or across the river in Holloway. The 1801 census revealed a total population exceeding 33,000, half of whom lived in bloated Walcot. In less than a century Bath had been transformed from a country spa into one of the dozen largest cities in England.

Architectural showcase or urban sprawl, this was also Jane Austen's moneyed, leisured Bath, with its polite air of conspicuous consumption, its well-swept pavements and constant passage of carriages and sedans, its seductive shops, discreet gaming houses, gentlemen's catch clubs, brilliant concerts under the impresario Rauzzini, and opulent new theatre in Sawclose (1805) starring London performers. If the hectic round of private evening parties often deprived the public assemblies of support, big occasions like the master-of-ceremonies' balls drew glittering attendances; even the vulnerable Lower Rooms held its own until its admired MC, James King, moved in 1805 to the plum post at the Upper Rooms. Like most of his predecessors King officiated in the out-of-season summer period at one of the other watering-places, in his case the flourishing Regency resort of Cheltenham. But neither the rise of Cheltenham, Leamington and other spas that followed the Bath model, nor the competition from thirty-or-so seaside resorts, nor even the lure of Continental travel once peace returned in 1815, seemed to dim Bath's popularity. Milsom Street – 'the very centre of attraction' – thronged as ever with modish visitors, and the stays of Louis XVIII in 1813, Queen Charlotte in 1817, and the Duke of Sussex with his masonic brethren in 1819, created particular stirs of excitement.

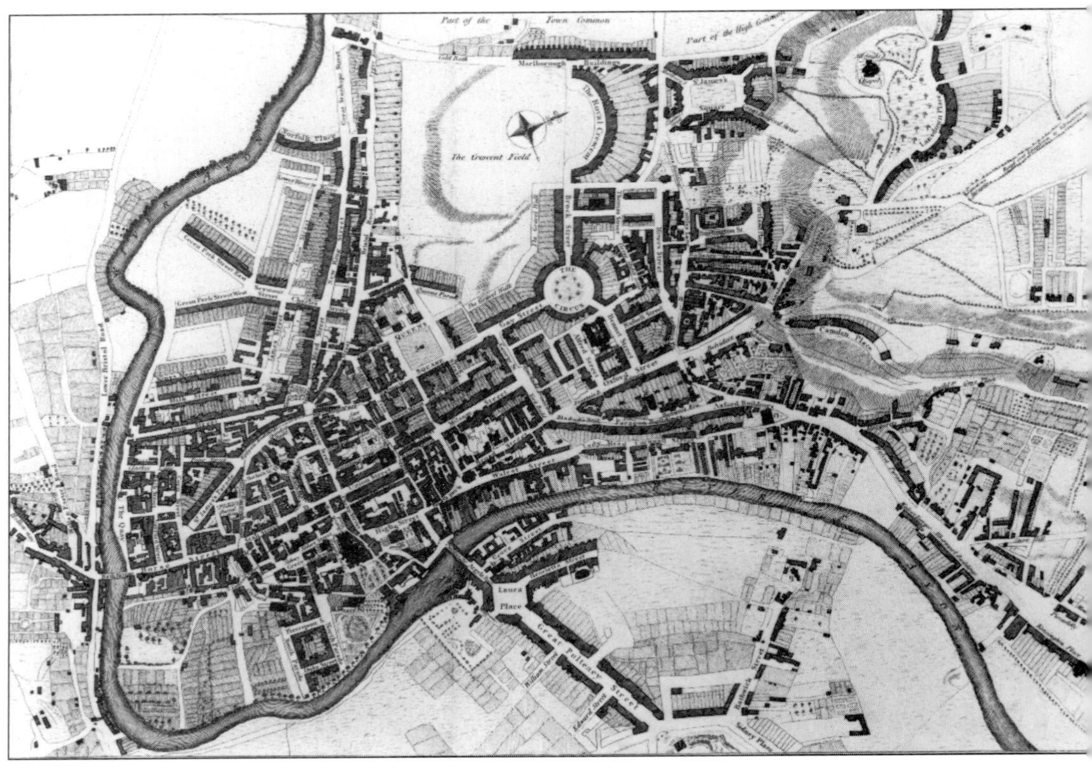

The Harcourt Masters map of 1801 reveals the extent of urban development beyond the original core still evident in the street plan (north is on the right)

And yet, with hindsight, a clear shift of balance can be detected. Gradually the spa's economy was becoming less dependent on the seasonal trade and holidaymakers, more on permanent residents – the lesser landed gentry, pensioned naval and military officers, ex-colonials, retired merchants and clergy, widows and unmarried gentlewomen, and chronic invalids, all of them appreciating the large stock of desirable houses and so many 'concentrated conveniences and comforts'. Much of the new building after 1800 appealed to this market: the stylish terraces and crescents of Bathwick, Widcombe and Lansdown with their spacious windows and exterior ironwork, and from the 1820s the detached residences and Italianate villas set in private gardens well up the slopes of leafy suburbia. But rows of artisan housing were being built too as the population leapt by another 50 per cent between 1801 and 1831. The greatest surge, in Lyncombe-Widcombe, followed the cutting of the Kennet and Avon Canal, which by 1802 carried a packet-boat service to Bradford-on-Avon, and in December 1810 was open its entire length from Bristol to Newbury

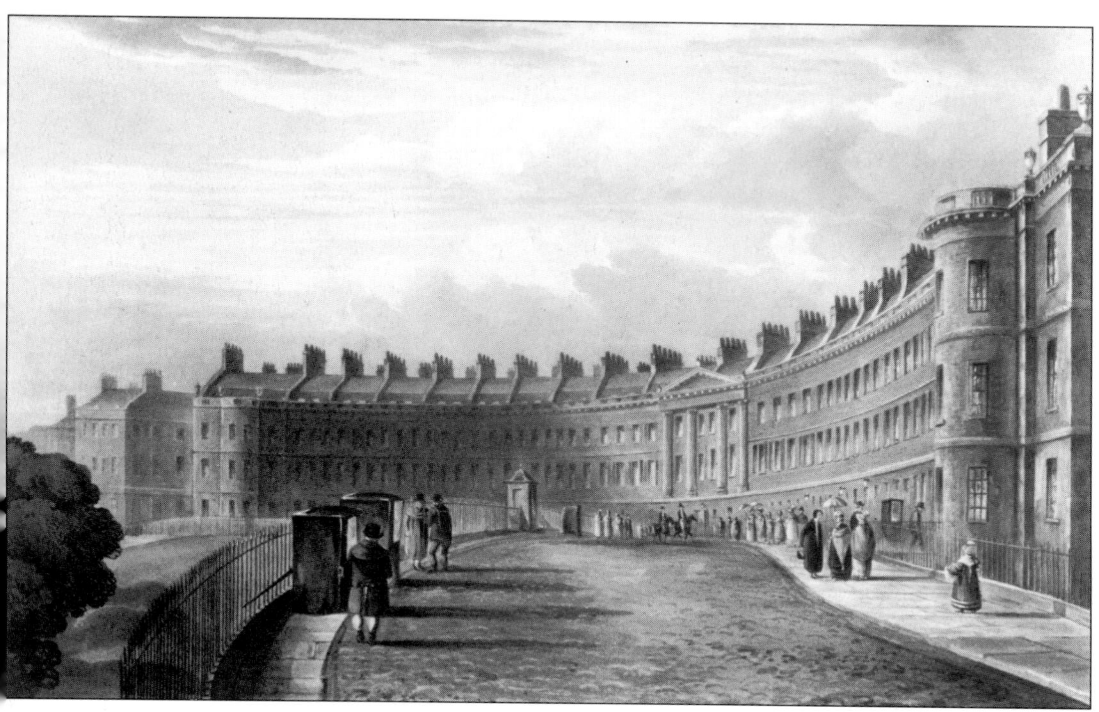

Lansdown Crescent of 1789–93 used the higher contours and commanded spectacular views. Note the sedan chair stand and the stone watch-house (aquatint by David Cox, 1820)

via the Avon Navigation and the seven-lock flight at Widcombe. A junction with the Somerset Coal Canal meant that Bath could be supplied with the cheap coal it relied on. This in turn encouraged the use of steam power for brewing and engineering, the city's main industrial processes next to the Twerton textile manufacture.

Between 1805 and 1810 movement in and around the centre was eased by street widening and the making of Union Street, New Bond Street and York Street, the latter intended as the key to restoring the fortunes of the Lower Rooms (to which a grand Doric portico was added in 1809–10) and developing the whole Manvers (formerly Kingston) estate on the Ham. All this scheming came to little. Manvers Street and the adjacent area evolved piecemeal, and the Rooms, gutted by fire in 1820, became the home of a sedater enterprise, the Bath Literary and Scientific Institution, opened in January 1825.

Takings at the baths and pumps had been declining steadily, for Bathonians used the establishments less than visitors. In response the Corporation reduced the Pumper's rent from £840 to £630 in 1816 and to £500 in 1820, an income it must have been loath to lose as it struggled to liquidate the massive debt incurred in the 1790s rebuilding. Even with the Commissioners to delegate to, the Corporation was overburdened by the administration of an expanding community and by the responsibilities thrust on it for water supply, sewerage, fire precautions, health, street amenities, public nuisances, policing, justice in the petty courts, markets and fairs, weights and measures, licensing alcohol sellers, regulating sedan chairs (and from 1829 hackney cabs), and managing its many properties and the institutions under its wing (almshouses, baths, Grammar School and gaol, for example). From time to time fresh powers were obtained. In 1805 the local Court of Requests gained the right to try cases of debt up to £10. The Policing Act of 1814 brought the city liberties in line with outer Walcot and Bathwick, which had obtained their Acts in 1793 and 1801. On the other hand powers could be lost, as in 1819 when a private company introduced gas lighting in the teeth of opposition from the Commissioners. In the continuing feud with the freemen over building on the Common, the Corporation repeatedly stalled: as late as 1827 detached houses were being proposed for the site, but all that evaporated in the flush

Extract from the *Bath Chronicle*, 4 April 1805. Newspapers were an indispensable means of circulating advertisements and, increasingly, local news and opinion of enthusiasm to lay out an exclusive area for recreation, Victoria Park, in 1829–30, one of the earliest public parks in the country.

Certain problems proved less tractable. Periodic flooding of the poorer districts near the river, the wretched Dolemeads especially, focused attention on the obstructed course of the Avon, but the remedial work recommended by the engineer Thomas Telford in 1825 would have cost £50,000, and his proposals were shelved. The markets provided better news. The coal market in Sawclose, though a nuisance to theatregoers, made a steady profit; the Walcot Street corn and cattle market opened in 1810; and the central market, with 438 stallholders in 1818, yielded handsome returns to the rotating pair of bailiffs who farmed the lease. Such profitable sinecures, the prevailing culture of favour and influence, the monopoly of voting and the lack of accountability, all fuelled arguments for municipal reform. National campaigners like John Cartwright and Henry Hunt discovered fertile ground when they came to Bath. The result of the parliamentary election of 1812, decided as usual by a mere thirty aldermen and councillors, was violently contested by a

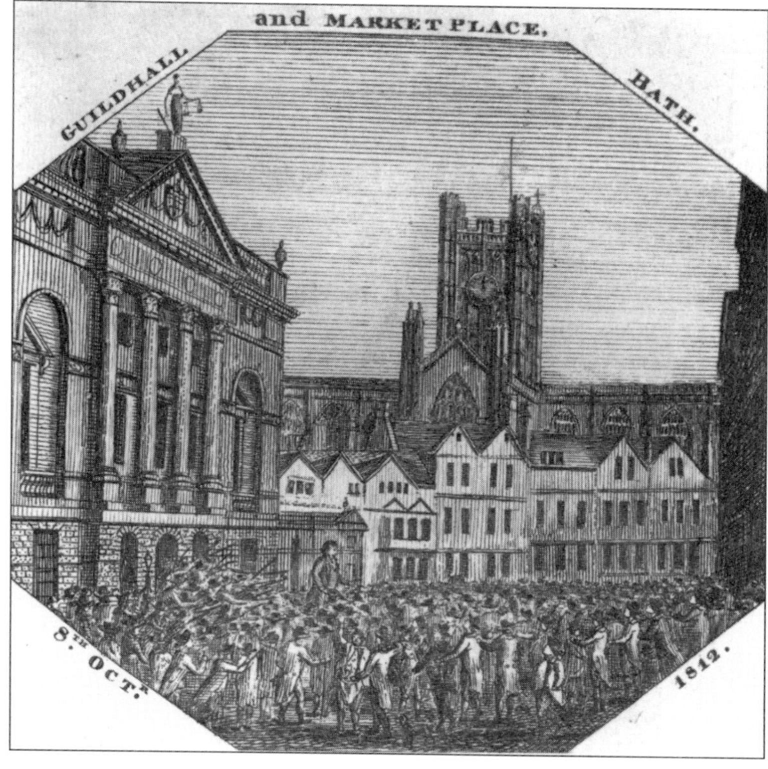

gitation in 1812 for emocratic reform was led by ohn Allen, a propertied Bath eeman (from C. Hibbert, *View of Bath*, 1813)

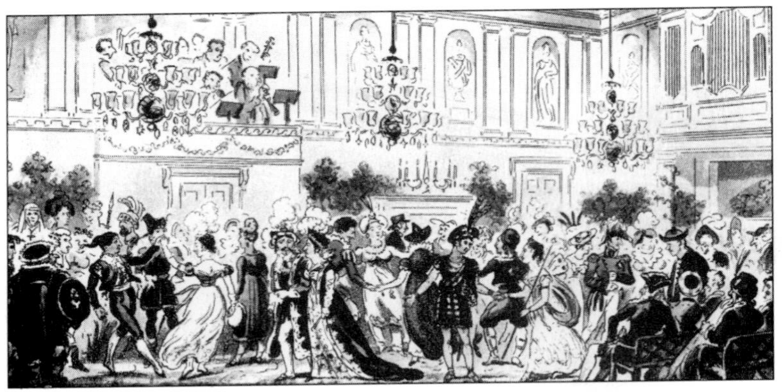

In the 1820s entertainments were still well patronized – Robert Cruikshank's impression of a fancy-dress ball at the Upper Rooms, 1825

party of freemen demanding their right to vote, and some years later a reform society took proper root.

Many initiatives, however, were largely independent of the Corporation unless perhaps for grants of land. Among these were the setting up of large monitorial schools from 1810 (notably the non-sectarian Bath and Bathforum School and the Anglican 'National' School at Weymouth House), and the merging of the Casualty Hospital with the Infirmary and Dispensary in 1826 to form the Royal United Hospital in a new building in Beau Street. The religious denominations strove to keep pace with potential congregations. Another free church, Holy Trinity, was consecrated in 1822. A handsome Methodist chapel (1815–16) and St Saviour's out at Larkhall (1829–31) attested to the ceaseless growth of Walcot. In Bathwick, where the Independent preacher William Jay still drew a devoted congregation and the proprietary Laura Chapel had its own fashionable following, St Mary's was built in 1817–20 at a strategic point of residential expansion up the hill. Meanwhile the exploding population of Lyncombe-Widcombe had its echo in St Mark's church, consecrated in 1831. Every new church meant another opportunity for evangelical preaching, and evangelical preaching was an assault on the frivolity of Bath, an antagonism that would shortly assume greater proportions.

CHAPTER SEVEN

Keeping Up Appearances

Once the trend-setting national spa, the pioneering holiday resort and the prototype retirement town, Bath faced relative decline after 1830. Unable to forget its Georgian heyday it struggled to adapt to reduced circumstances while preserving an air of faded gentility and physical charm that still endeared it to devotees. But the polite veneer concealed disturbing facts. The average life expectancy of fifty-nine years for affluent Bathonians compared with a mere thirty-one years for families of artisans and labourers. Epidemic disease struck disproportionately at the poor; deaths in the cholera and smallpox outbreaks of 1832 and 1837 were confined almost wholly to squalid, impoverished neighbourhoods. A report of 1842 painted a damning picture of the 'dens' of Avon Street, overrun with prostitutes, thieves, beggars and illegitimate children. The Dolemeads had an equally unsavoury reputation. Indeed, the travelling showman George Sanger, who witnessed the drunken wrecking of Lansdown Fair in the 1830s, considered that the Bath slums at that time harboured 'the most brutish and criminal mob in England'. These were discomfiting realities for the reformed City Council to contemplate.

Middle-class activists and the more politically conscious workforce had long pressed for reform. By October 1831 the movement was strong enough to stage a huge rally in Bathwick before the Sydney Hotel, but while rampaging rioters put Bristol to the torch, violence at Bath was limited to a skirmish in the Marketplace. In November a Political Union was formed, and the following spring 50,000 supporters of this and other district unions marched through Bath in a convincing demonstration of feeling. The succeeding Reform Act increased the borough's parliamentary electorate from 33 to 2,835 at a stroke. Previous ballot-box certainties could no longer be relied on. For decades the Council oligarchy had regularly balanced a Tory member against a Liberal/Whig. At the ensuing election (due in the main to voters of the three central parishes and Lyncombe-Widcombe) the Tory candidate was rejected in favour of an out-and-out Radical, J.A. Roebuck, with the popular standing MP, Charles Palmer (son of the former mailcoach operator), re-elected on the Liberal ticket. In modern terms it represented a lurch to the left. Roebuck stood for the dismantling of the whole hierarchy of power and privilege, for undermining the very social structure on which Bath had been built. Putting an outspoken revolutionary into Parliament seemed to traditional voices a decidedly unhelpful advertisement for a respectable spa.

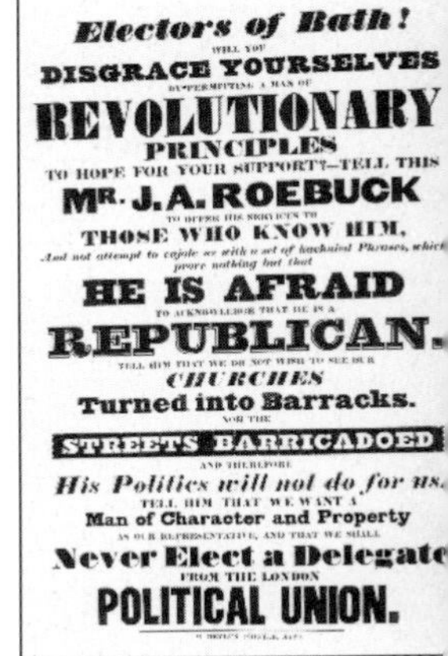

Despite fierce opposition the Radical candidate Roebuck won one of the city's two seats at the 1832 general election

The Municipal Reform Act and the re-vamping of the Poor Law resulted in further sweeping changes. The government commission that investigated Bath in 1833 was scathing about corrupt practices – the way the Corporation had long 'twisted' the Elizabethan Charter to its own ends, denied the freemen their rights and misappropriated public funds. By 1830 it was almost £56,000 in debt, an increase of 75 per cent over the past thirty years. The city still lacked the authority to try felonies and it was inconsistently policed, having separate arrangements for inner Bath, Walcot and Bathwick, and none at all for Lyncombe-Widcombe. Worst of all, the Council was incestuous and self-perpetuating. The new legislation changed all that, giving ratepayers a direct say at last in local government. In December 1835 they duly elected forty-two councillors, six for each of seven wards. Only six members out of the old Corporation survived, but the Tory-minded *Bath Chronicle* took comfort that no more than sixteen of the incomers could be classed as 'downright radicals'.

The Council's first speedy initiative was to set up a twenty-four-hour police force of 144 men covering the entire borough, a coercive measure in the eyes of the poor but one appealing to property-owners, who must also have approved the arrival of quarter sessions in 1837 and the construction of an up-to-date prison at Twerton in 1842. Responsibility for the destitute had meanwhile passed from the individual parishes to a centralized Board of Guardians, whose object was a more cost-effective means of relief that would exclude the work-shy and 'undeserving'. Existing poorhouses in and around Bath were replaced by a single Union workhouse, which opened at Odd Down in 1838 to cater for some six hundred able-bodied paupers from twenty-four district parishes. At the same time outdoor relief was restricted to the most needy cases of age and infirmity. The consequence was an immediate reduction of 40 per cent in the Bath poor rates, but at the cost of a harsher regime. Only the work of thirty or more charities, including several dispensaries and the notable Bath Friendly Society, helped to stifle protest and alleviate the worst hardship.

A split between Radical and Liberal factions had cost Roebuck his

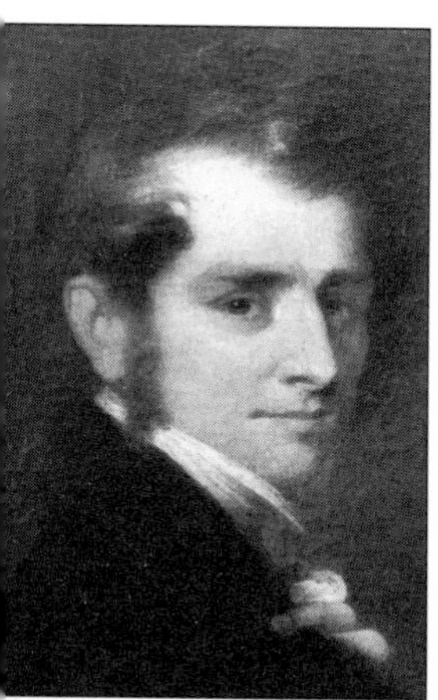

.A. Roebuck served some leven years as a member for Bath, 1832–7 and 1841–7 portrait attributed to James Green, detail)

seat at the 'drunken election' of 1837, but he swept back in 1841. For a time middle-class Radicals made common cause with the Bath Working Men's Association to advance Chartism. A large rally was permitted at Bath in 1838 when contingents from Bristol and Wiltshire came to hear the rousing Henry Vincent, but after the more inflammatory meetings at Trowbridge and elsewhere the magistrates took fright, banned a follow-up rally at Bath in 1839, and forced it to be diverted to Midford, spoiling its effect. The Chartist and allied causes nevertheless received much local support into the 1840s, but by 1847 the Radical fervour had evaporated, and in a bitter electoral contest Roebuck was finally ousted after losing the backing of Dissenters. Bath's flirtation with progressive politics was effectively over.

Although some blamed political wrangling and the taint of Radicalism for Bath's sharp decline in the 1830s and 1840s, there were other reasons. Ever since 1830, when a treatment bath had been installed at the Mineral Water Hospital and a swimming pool adjacent to the Hot Bath, the bathing establishments had been a rather neglected asset. With the number of regular bathers down to scarcely twenty-five a week, the Council in 1841 appointed two private managers to modernize the facilities. Yet the spa was out of medical fashion, and even the upgrading of the Hot Bath complex to Continental standards failed to attract the expected custom. It was part of a pattern. The visitors were drying up and the wealthier residents leaving. As once-stylish streets began to empty, rents fell and humbler folk moved in. Luxury shops saw a falling-off in trade, concerts and balls languished, the theatre played to thin houses. Had clients tired of Bath at last? Did other resorts now have more to offer? Or did the cause lie more at home? For some observers the real culprits were the evangelical clergy.

Evangelical preaching had long roots at Bath, but alarm about its infiltration into Anglican churches was not voiced until the 1820s. From then on it was a relentless process: the installing of evangelical ministers at Kensington and All Saints' proprietary chapels, the purchase of the Bath Rectory benefice in 1835 (with the right to appoint at St James's and St Michael's) by the Simeon Trust, the dismissal of more traditionalist curates. By 1840 a majority of Bath pulpits were under evangelical control and overflowing congregations were imbibing a severe puritanical message that consigned lovers of worldly pleasures to eternal damnation. Plays, dramatic fêtes, balls, card-playing, racing, even sacred oratorios and the crowd-pulling horticultural shows (started in 1834), all came under the lash. The public diversions, central to the spa's

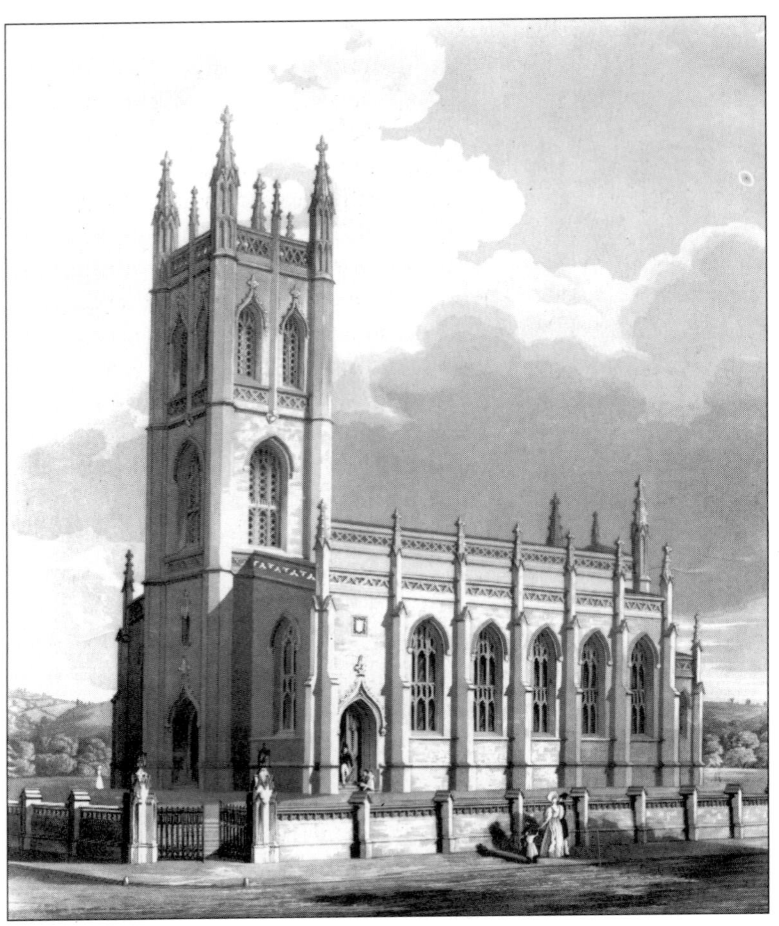

St Saviour's church, built 1829–31 to the design of John Pinch in the growing suburb of Larkhall

attractiveness, had never before been so damagingly attacked, and the crusade was accompanied by an onslaught on orthodox clergy and other denominations, especially the Catholics now ensconced at Prior Park. The controversy impinged too on education as evangelical diehards battled with fellow Anglicans to set their stamp on elementary schooling in the city, and crystallized again in 1847 over the merits or otherwise of a charity ball to raise funds for the poor in a hard winter. The impact of evangelicalism in the 1830s and 1840s seemed drastic enough to contemporaries; whether it did serious harm to the local economy can only be guessed at.

Hopes of a revival in civic fortunes briefly centred on the Great Western Railway, which reached Bath from Bristol in 1840, and from London in 1841. Not only did the trains fail to disgorge the visitors hoped for, however, but the competition from steam gradually affected the old coaching and inn trade and the profits of the turnpike and canal companies. A body set up in 1843 to promote the spa suggested alternative enticements – more villas, smarter hackney cabs, a public library, an art gallery, cafés and tea-gardens, promenade concerts, a zoo – but to little avail. There were more urgent concerns. Worries about water supply and sanitation in 1846–7 prompted inquiries by the Bath Health of Towns Association and led to extra reservoirs being constructed near Batheaston. The river remained badly obstructed and polluted. Cholera in 1849 (played down as usual by the Bath press) caused ninety deaths in the locality. Alcoholism was rife, over 200 beerhouses and taverns giving the nascent temperance movement much to contend with. Increasing numbers of vagrants, victims often of the agricultural depression in the late 1840s, begged in the streets or sought shelter at the overstretched Union workhouse.

Yet for the better-off this was still a seductive city – where Louis Napoléon stayed in temporary exile, where the fastidious William Beckford lived out his days, where Bath's other man of letters, W.S. Landor, entertained his literary friends. If the streets looked a little shabby and the riverside dilapidated, some sectors of the economy quietly prospered. Bath was still noted for high-class retailing, for bespoke tailoring and shoemaking, for medical and other professional services. Its breweries had perhaps the largest output in the west of England. The Twerton mills specialized in fine fabrics and several firms manufactured quality furniture, coaches and invalid chairs. The firm of Stothert & Pitt, already renowned for steam-engines, pumps and farm tools, was beginning to build the cranes for which it would become world famous. Stone extraction survived on Combe Down, but the discovery of superb freestone reserves during railway construction had removed much of this lucrative industry to Box and Corsham, just out of Bath. On the other hand commercial printing had recently become important with the setting up of the Pitman press. Altogether forty-six exhibitors from Bath showed at the Great Exhibition of 1851, a creditable performance for a town that the guidebooks liked to pretend was practically devoid of industry.

After decades of booming population growth the curve had flattened out. The 1851 census revealed Bath rapidly slipping down the demographic league table, with an increase of only 3,440 residents (to a total of 54,240) in twenty years, mostly in the southern suburbs. Its gender ratio was more skewed than ever, especially for adults: women outnumbered men seven to four thanks mainly to the opportunities for female employment (as domestic servants, washerwomen, milliners and seamstresses) and the exodus of younger males in search of work elsewhere. Another census of 1851 indicated the strength of religious attendance. Seating capacity for over 30,000 in twenty-eight Anglican churches and in thirty-three meeting-houses of other denominations was more than adequate for the population, and included a high 45 per cent of free places. Ecclesiastical building had gone on apace since the early 1830s: in central Bath St Michael's had been completely, and St James's partly, rebuilt; in the suburbs the Anglicans gained Holy Trinity (Combe Down), St Matthew's (Widcombe), and St Stephen's (Lansdown); and the Jewish, Catholic, Methodist, Swedenborgian, Moravian, and (in 1854) Independent congregations all put up new buildings.

A townscape punctuated by churches and chapels was matched by a river spanned with bridges. The arc of development from Bathwick round to outlying Twerton produced five new crossings of the Avon in eleven years, among them the substantial Cleveland (1827) and the North Parade (1835) bridges. Around 1840 Brunel added two more for the GWR. Another noticeable change to the city scene came with the opening up of the lower Marketplace in the mid-1830s, when Wade's Passage and the huddle of properties against the Abbey Church were finally demolished.

Even at its lowest ebb in the 1840s and 1850s the economy did not

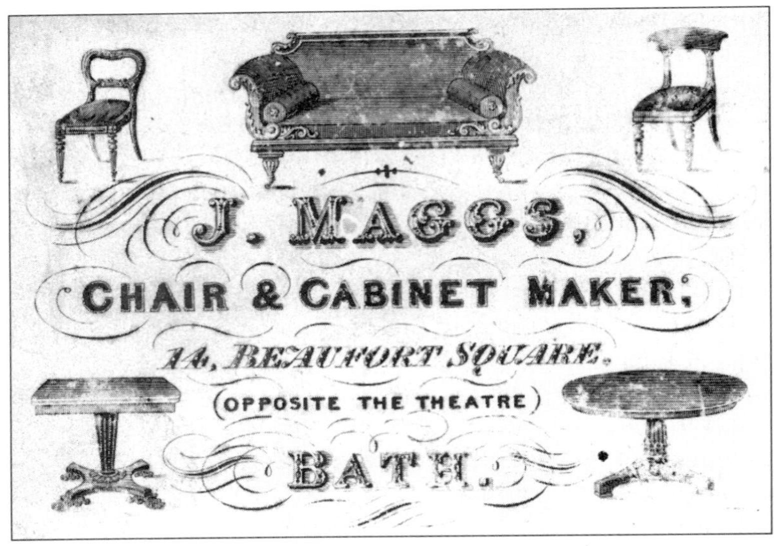

Trade-card of John Maggs, in business at various addresses in the decades around 1830

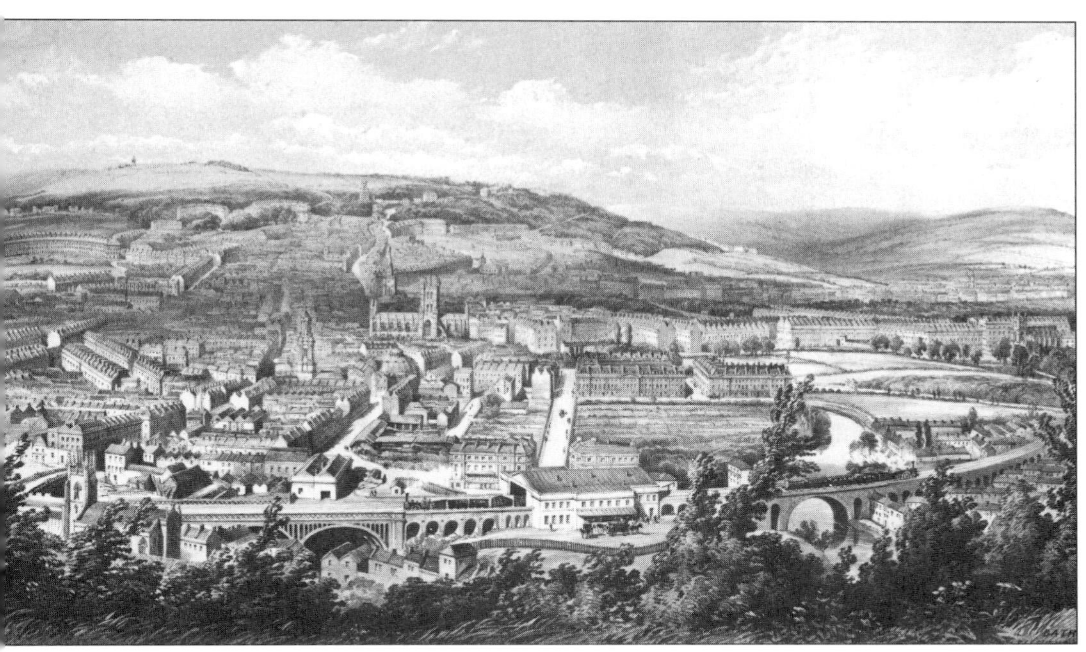

ath in 1846 with the GWR ne prominent in the oreground and newly built t Stephen's in the far distance arking the spread of esidential building up ansdown (lithograph by Syer)

stagnate. Forced to adjust to the marked drop in seasonal visitors Bath remained an important regional hub, the home of many small-to-medium businesses, and a desirable place of residence – inexpensive, attractive in ambience, and still not destitute of amusements. Social and cultural life was never entirely polarized between church and assembly room. A variety of private clubs and societies, the political parties, charitable bodies and organizations (such as the Athenaeum, the Commercial and Literary Institution and the Bath Literary and Scientific Institution) all absorbed much talent and energy. During the 1850s, furthermore, Bath reinforced its claim to be a centre of education. The Wesleyan Kingswood School (transferred from the outskirts of Bristol) and Lansdown Proprietary College (soon to be supplanted by the Royal School) both commissioned imposing new buildings from the busy local architect James Wilson. In the same period Sydney Proprietary College, aimed at the upper professional classes, set itself up in the former Sydney Hotel, but suffered a rift in 1858 when some of its staff founded the rival Somerset College in the Circus. The Grammar School was going through a long bad patch, beset by argument over its curriculum (classical versus commercial) and by the requirement to take a quota of non-paying pupils. The Bluecoat School, by contrast, was thriving and rebuilt its premises in 1860. The advent of a School of Art and the revival of the Bathforum elementary school in Monmouth Street, both in 1854, were other hopeful signs. Nearly fifty public day schools, the majority under church or chapel management, and over a hundred smaller private establishments, provided schooling for a respectable 75 per cent of the city's children. First of several 'industrial schools', the Sutcliffe School concentrated on rehabilitating young social rejects.

The linked problems of public health, poverty and crime were issues throughout the 1850s and 1860s. The wide-ranging Bath Act (1851) gave the Council full powers to tackle health matters, but it was private initiative that led the way, with the Society for Improving the Conditions of the Working Classes investigating the slums, the Baths and Laundries Society promoting hygiene, and other organizations attempting to keep visible misery off the streets by supplying essential relief. Calls for more positive action were stoked by adverse national publicity about the spa's comparative death rates and by the frequent epidemics of scarlatina, typhus, smallpox and other diseases. Following criticism voiced at the 1864 British Association congress held at Bath, and renewed during the severe water shortages of 1864–5, the Council appointed its first medical officer, C.S. Barter. His was a delicate task: to reassure the public and avoid alarmism while facing up to the gross abuses that did exist – 4,000 houses either without a water supply or reliant on polluted

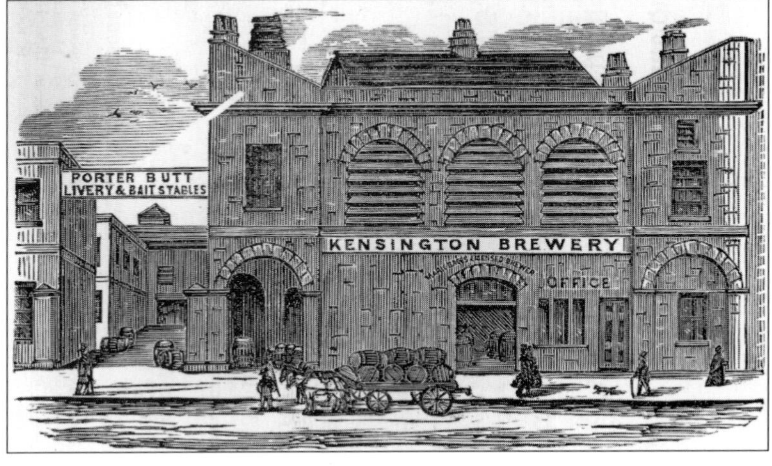

The city's breweries supplied a wide area round Bath; dark Bath porter was even traded overseas

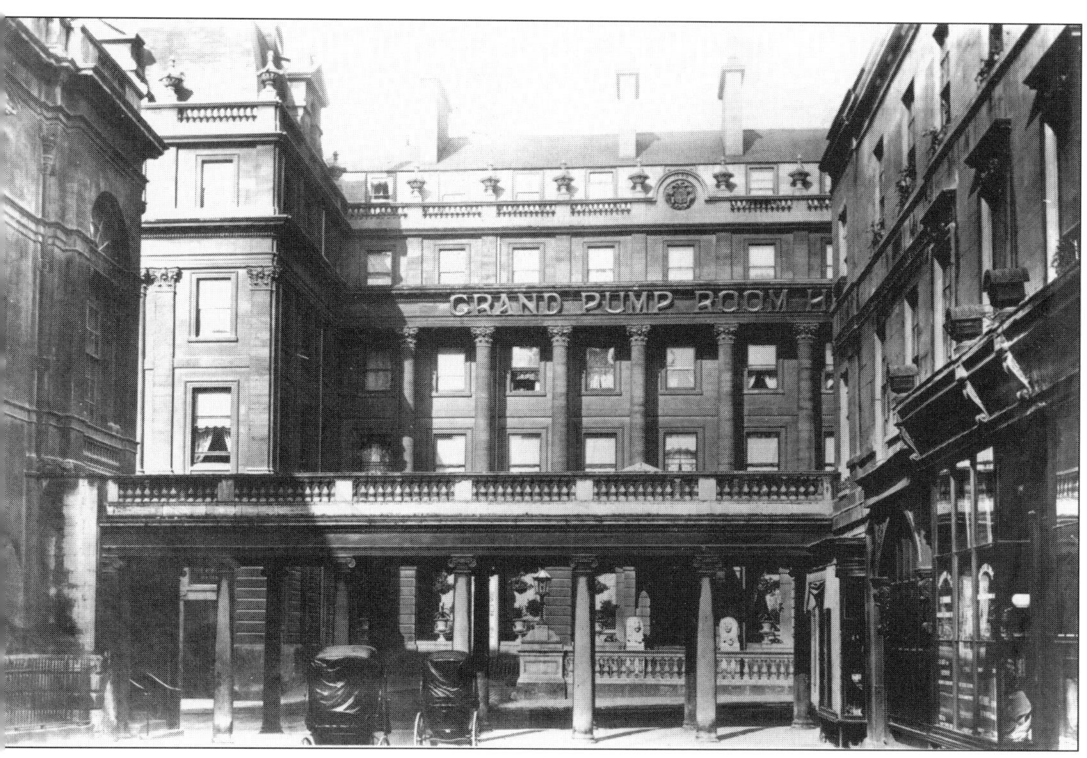

'wo invalid chairs wait
pposite the Grand Pump
oom Hotel, built by Willcox
: Wilson in a burst of mid-
'ictorian confidence

wells, a river fed by all the city sewers, many unregulated cheap lodgings, and fifty-three ill-sited slaughterhouses – to say nothing of numerous backyard pigsties. Some progress was made, but Bath's habitually stingy ratepayers had already thrown out the plan for a new reservoir. The chance of ensuring a clean water supply for every citizen had to await the 1870 Water Act, the buying out of the various private water companies and the creation of Monkswood reservoir. In the interim any talk of high mortality figures at a *health* resort could be countered by pointing to the uncommon numbers of invalids and elderly persons (women in particular) from other parts of the country who chose to spend their final days at Bath.

Though a scheme for a crystal palace in Victoria Park, to contain a music hall and winter garden, came to nothing in 1857, there appeared a growing determination to revitalize the spa and woo back the tourist trade. The Mineral Water Hospital, recently a haven for wounded soldiers from the Crimean War, added a new wing in 1861 and Turkish baths two years later, the railway having extended its catchment area for patients. The Royal United Hospital similarly expanded. Another show of confidence was a major redevelopment in the heart of Bath. Spurred on by Jerom Murch, former Unitarian minister and a great advocate of civic regeneration, an investment company working alongside the Corporation pulled down the once famous but now decrepit White Hart inn and erected instead a château-style Grand Pump Room Hotel. On the north side of Bath Street the Corporation simultaneously built a sumptuous suite of private baths, incorporating a ladies' swimming pool and connected to the hotel by a hydraulic lift. When these New Royal Baths were grandly inaugurated in 1870, the spa had palpably regained some of the ground lost to foreign competitors. Moreover it had a new theatre, rebuilt by subscription after its predecessor burned down in 1862, a new provisions market with an attractive domed hall and spacious avenue at the rear of the Guildhall (1863), and a new police station looking out on to Orange Grove (1865). Among the latest crop of churches St John the Divine in South Parade stood prominent; its 222-ft spire (1867) asserted Catholicism to a degree undreamt of since the Reformation, and remained Bath's tallest landmark until G.G. Scott responded in 1879 with the Anglican steeple of St Andrew's in Julian Road. Scott's most conspicuous work in the city, however, was the drastic restoration and fan-vaulting of the Abbey Church, carried out in 1864–73 at the inspiration of the rector, Charles Kemble, and at a cost of £37,000. The same years saw the small but influential Baptist congregation also raising its profile with new chapels in Vineyards and Manvers Street.

The effort to relaunch Bath coincided with the achievement of a north-south railway link in 1874, when the expensively tunnelled Somerset and Dorset line met the Midland Railway branch of 1869 at a terminus adjoining Green Park and Sydenham Field sports ground – the latter soon to be obliterated by goods and engine sheds. By the mid-1870s an 'Attractions Society' was actively marketing the spa, placing hundreds of advertisements in the London, provincial and overseas press. Usage of the bathing establishments rose sharply and income once more began to exceed expenditure. In addition to regular concerts in the public gardens and Pump Room, the programme included a stream of special events: art exhibitions, archery contests, lawn tennis tournaments (from 1881), the annual floral fêtes, medical meetings, the huge Church Congress held in 1873, the centenary of the Bath and West Agricultural Society in 1877 (an occasion marred, though, by the fatal collapse of the Widcombe footbridge under the weight of excursionists to the show). Unlike their Georgian forebears visitors seldom took rooms

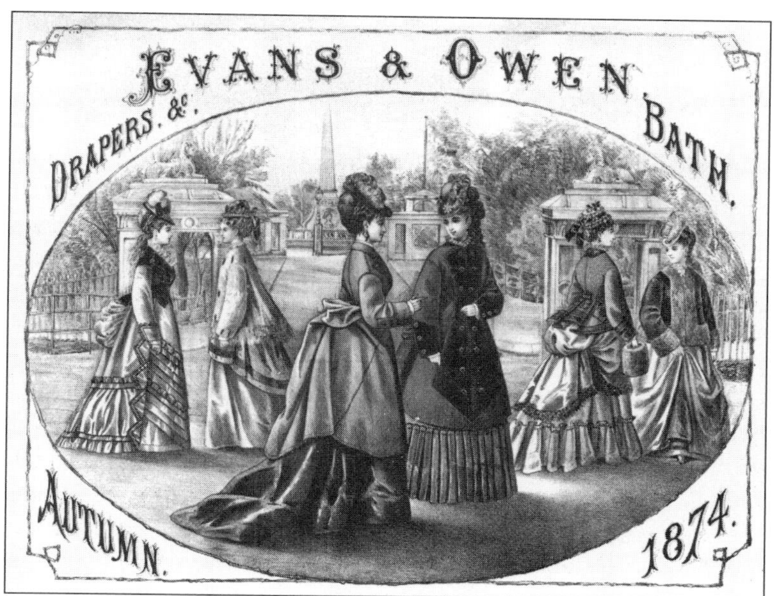

One of the new breed of department stores, Evans & Owen pose their fashion models against a backdrop of Victoria Park

any more in lodging-houses, which were now in terminal decline, but opted instead for hotel-style accommodation in the updated inns, the purpose-built Royal and Argyle hotels opposite the GWR station, or the Grand Pump Room Hotel itself.

Bath was as much a magnet for shoppers as ever, especially with the growth of department stores, Colmer's in Union Street, Jolly's in Milsom Street, and Evans & Owen's by the Assembly Rooms. Specialist products such as Bath Olivers, Sally Lunns, Pooley's malt bread, and polony sausage (claiming an annual sale of up to 40,000 lb) enjoyed a national reputation, and from 1880 the distribution of 'Sulis Water', bottled and aerated in the Pump Room vaults, called renewed attention to the mineral springs. The provisions market on the other hand continued to fade, the 1860s rehabilitation having failed to halt the draining of trade to a multitude of suburban food shops, street vendors, and the popular costermongers' market that filled Westgate Street every Saturday evening. Stallholders would shortly be reduced to sixty, a mere 15 per cent of the number two generations earlier. The beast and corn markets were likewise moribund, defeated by railways and by animal health regulations.

Social conditions for the worst-off had somewhat improved since the mid-century. Certainly many areas of squalor and deprivation remained: the Dolemeads (or 'Mud Island') still faced periodic

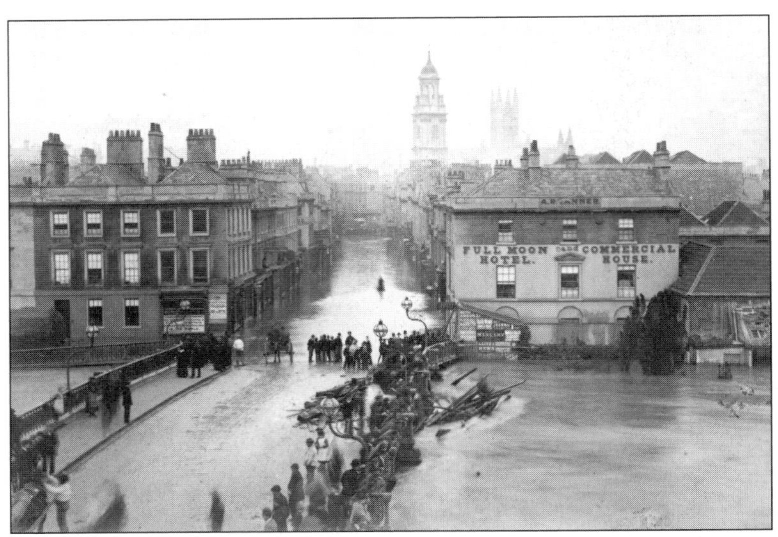

The uncontrolled river continued to wreak havoc: the area near the old bridge flooded in October 1882

inundation, and over a hundred artisan houses were lost in the Hedgemead landslips of 1875–85. A campaign waged by the vicar of St James's in 1881 against the pub-and-brothel culture of his parish met only limited success, but overall the incidence of drunkenness was down, a victory for temperance tracts, coffee rooms and Bands of Hope over the demon drink. Most children now attended elementary school: only four additional Board schools were needed under the 1870 Education Act, existing provision being largely adequate for a static or falling population. The prevalence of church schools, because of their separate financing, was reckoned to save 2d. in the pound on the rates – which in any case stayed unusually low from the ratepayers' notorious unwillingness to support a public library, museum, or any other avoidable charge on Corporation funds. All the same a deal had at last been struck with the surviving thirty-two freemen, whereby they sacrificed their interest in the Common in return for £25 annuities; the city subsequently purchased the remaining freehold portion of Victoria Park so that the whole became municipal property open for public enjoyment. The laying out of the botanic garden (1887) and the creation of Hedgemead, Henrietta and Alexandra parks soon followed.

Counting in the villages of Twerton and Weston, which strictly stood beyond the city boundary, the population hovered around 60,000 for the three decades 1851–81 before rising to almost 67,000 by the end of the century. These totals mask a dynamic movement out of central Bath, the ancient core, into the southern and western margins. Between 1851 and 1901 residents of the three inner parishes fell by 40 per cent from 11,647 to 7,141, whereas Lyncombe-Widcombe, Twerton and Weston almost doubled to 31,397. Twerton's unprecedented growth after 1881, encouraged by industrial development in the Avon valley, left it merging into Oldfield Park – the whole south-western agglomeration becoming a significant counterweight to once-dominant Walcot. Given the expansion, transport took on added importance. Horse-drawn tram and omnibus services (from 1880 and 1887 respectively) gradually connected Twerton to Bathford, Bathwick to Upper Weston. The streets were busy with broughams and landaus, hackney cabs and delivery carts, and more and more bicycles. Electric arc lamps, first introduced with incandescent lighting at Evans & Owen's store in 1882, superseded gas lamps in the main thoroughfares in 1890, about the time that trunkline telephones were also spreading through the region. Hoping eventually to profit from supplying electricity, as it had from its monopoly on water, the Council bought out the operator and improved the Dorchester Street generating plant at huge cost.

Indeed the Council had embarked on a late Victorian spending spree. It began in 1880 with the discovery and subsequent exposure of

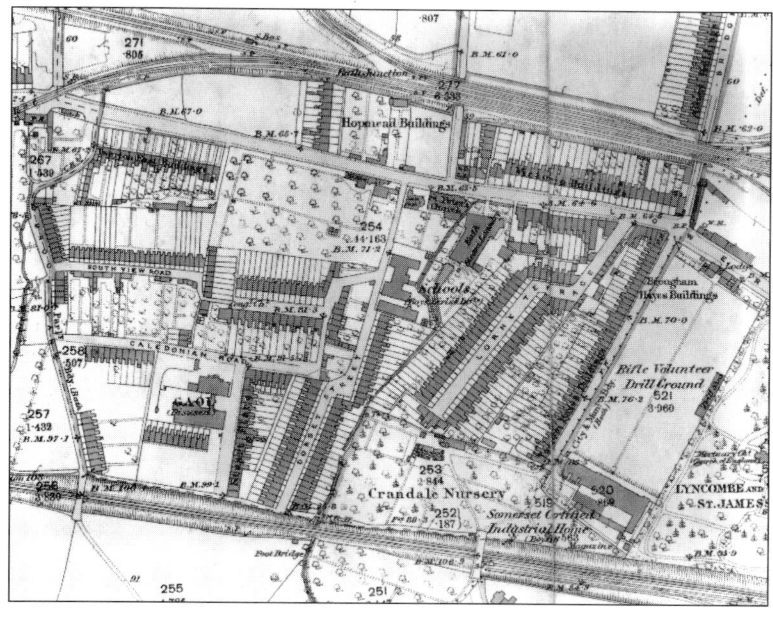

art of Twerton, sandwiched etween railways, in the late 880s but not yet incorporated ithin the city boundary

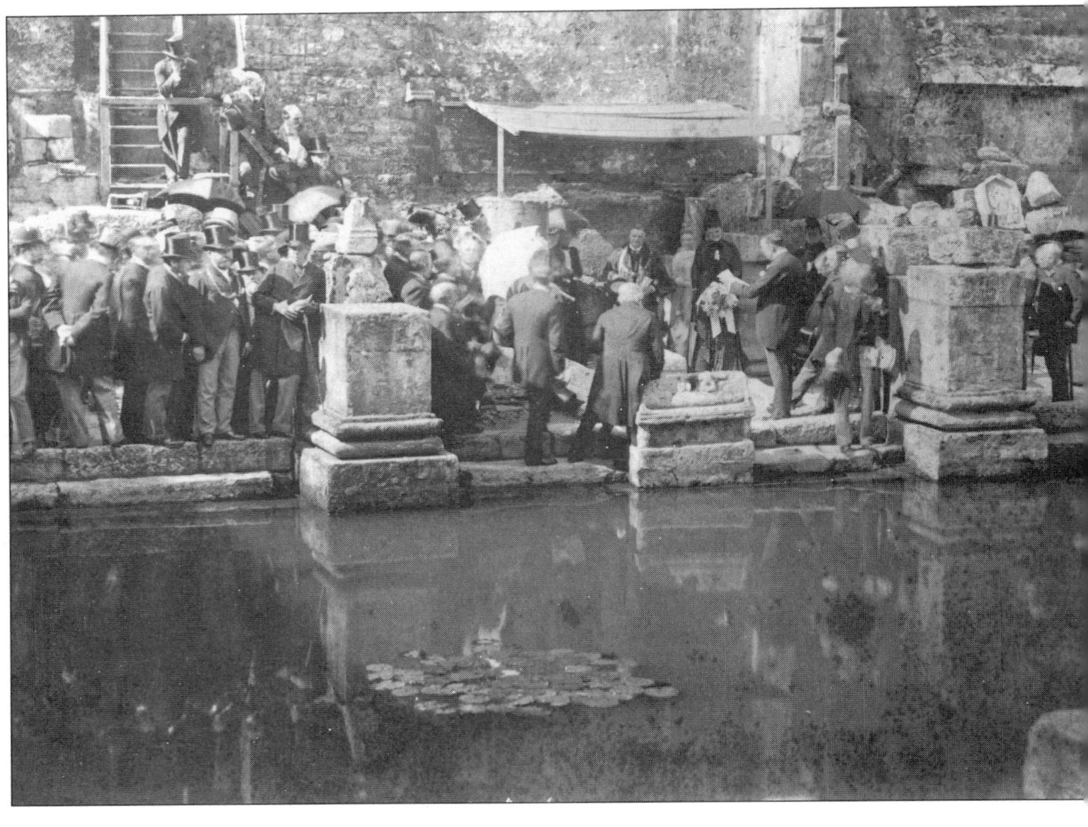

The discovery of the Great Roman Bath was significant not only for archaeology but for Bath's tourist industry

the full Roman baths complex by the borough surveyor, Major C.E. Davis, and the construction of a new medical treatment wing, with every Continental innovation, on the site of the demolished Queen's Bath. Publicized by scale models exhibited in London, the archaeological finds aroused enormous national interest and drew a flood of visitors, including another British Association conference in 1888. Owner of a range of bathing establishments now considered second to none in Europe, the Corporation found its annual revenue from this source alone exceeding £6,000, comparable with the income of £10,400 from property rents. The impetus carried forward into the major projects of the 1890s, three of them designed by the London architect J.M. Brydon: bold extensions to the eighteenth-century Guildhall to house municipal offices on one side and the united art and technical schools on the other; the domed concert hall immediately east of the Pump Room; and the Victoria Art Gallery to mark the royal diamond jubilee. All these ventures could be regarded as a fitting

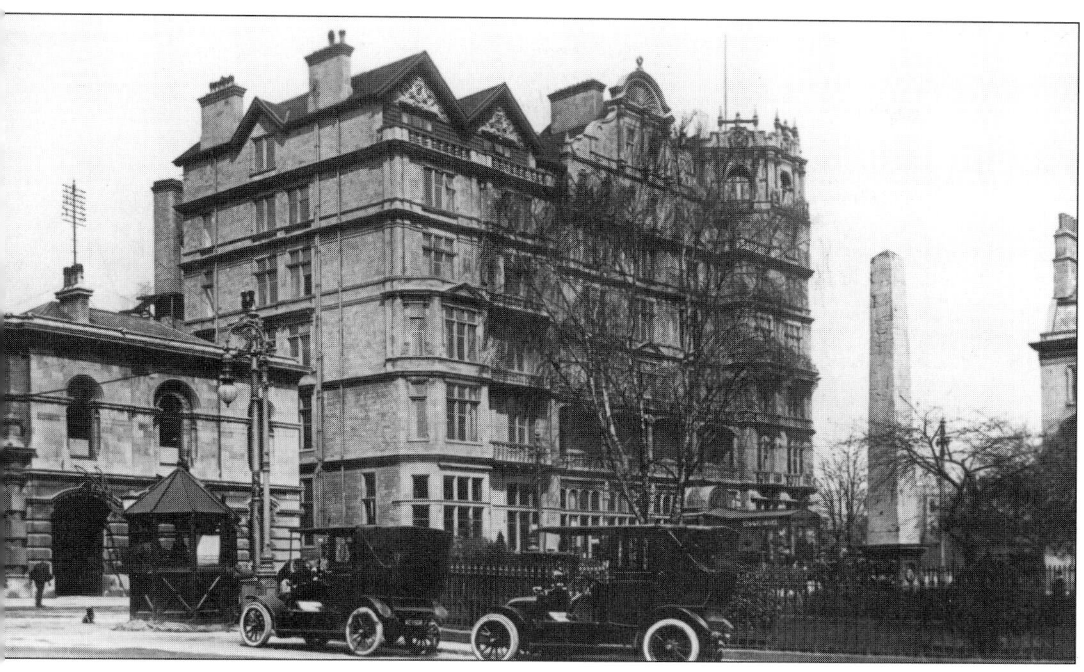

he construction of the Empire otel and Grand Parade ompleted the nineteenth-entury transformation of range Grove, once a shionable Georgian oasis

memorial to Bath's leading citizen and seven times mayor, Jerom Murch, who died in 1895 before any of them was quite completed.

By the end of the century the outlook seemed encouraging. The visitors were being persuaded back, not only the comfortable British middle classes but 'the rich and noble, the Colonist, and the American, in ever increasing numbers'. Manufacturers were doing well, with the city's engineering firms (e.g. Stothert & Pitt and Horstmann) and furniture-makers known worldwide. The amenities could stand comparison with any rival's. The borough supported nine banks and published seven newspapers. To its entertainments it had recently added a handsome Lyric Theatre in Sawclose. In Bath College it even had a prestigious public school. As the century closed the final touch was imminent, the opening of the Empire Hotel, the largest yet, planned by the controversial Major Davis and financed by a hotel chain whose other establishments were all at coastal resorts – a timely gesture of confidence in the prospects of an inland spa. Beside it ran the expensive riverside parade joining Pulteney Bridge at last with Orange Grove, the Corporation's ultimate contribution to the *fin de siècle*.

CHAPTER EIGHT

Pageant to Pizza-Hut: Twentieth-Century Realities

In 1902 the city joined the rest of the nation in celebrating the Coronation of Edward VII in streets garlanded with decorations and thronged with revellers. Other more local events closed the door on the old century and heralded the new; the last horse-drawn tram route ceased that year, while in Sydney Gardens a hot air balloon ascent, celebrating the centenary of a similar flight from the pleasure gardens in 1802, launched a tradition of aviation pioneering in the city. The event was organized by Patrick Alexander, who since the 1880s had conducted experiments in flight at his home in Batheaston. The next day Alexander staged a demonstration of unpowered flying machines on Lansdown which included Samuel Cody's man-lifting kites. In 1912 R.E. Bush built the 'Bath and London Motor Plane' in only three weeks at premises in Manvers Street, and on 21 May the same year, to demonstrate the potential of flight for the conveyance of post, B.C. Hucks flew from Hendon to the Bath Aviation Meeting at Combe Down with a consignment of the morning newspapers and a letter from the Lord Mayor of London to the Mayor of Bath. In less momentous ways Bath's public transport system was also developing. Electric trams were introduced in 1902, and in 1905 motor buses arrived in the more outlying areas to feed the tram network.

The buoyant years of the 1890s and early Edwardian period culminated in the Bath Historical Pageant of 19–24 July 1909. Planned at relatively short notice, the pageant proved a triumph of civic confidence; streets and buildings again displayed bunting and streamers and thousands of people set about building and painting sets, sewing costumes, and learning their parts and dances. Pigs were recruited for the Bladud scenes, horses to accompany Cavaliers and Roundheads. Before throngs of spectators in Royal Victoria Park eight tableaux played out the story of Bath from Roman times to the

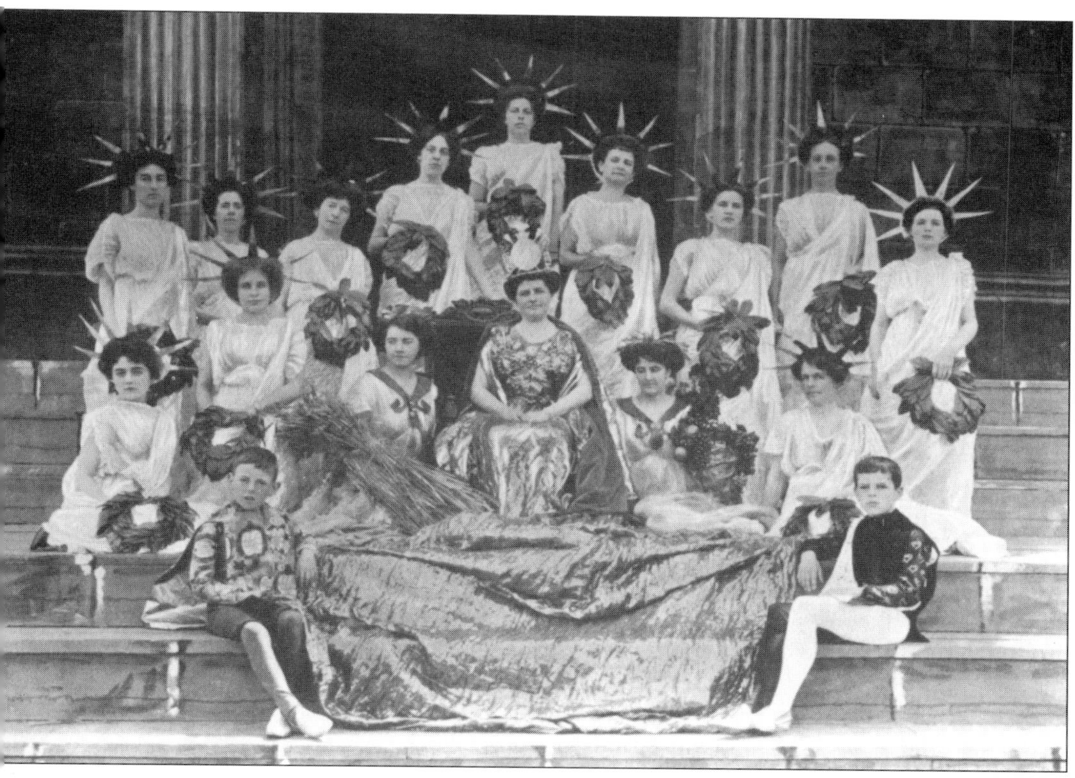

e Bath Historical Pageant, 09; Ladye Bath on the steps the Roman temple, attended maidens representing towns med Bath in America and nada

early nineteenth century, finishing with a grand march-past of the entire cast on the final day. This pageant, with its strong element of nostalgia, attracted critical acclaim from as far afield as America; Bath had celebrated its illustrious past and looked forward to a bright future.

By 1914 this hope had evaporated. The nation again plunged into conflict. Aviation in Bath ceased to be an adventure and became a deadly means of waging war. The Bristol Aircraft Company used the Assembly Rooms for building wings, and opened its Flight Works on the Lower Bristol Road for aircraft production. Fear of attacks by enemy aircraft led to the introduction of the first blackout precautions. Industrial firms like Stothert & Pitt were put to the production of munitions and other war work and, when manpower became short, women took on many new roles. Wounded servicemen were ferried back from France in ever-increasing numbers; in 1915 the Royal Mineral Water Hospital closed to civilians and the following year a new war hospital opened at Combe Park. Casualties were bussed into

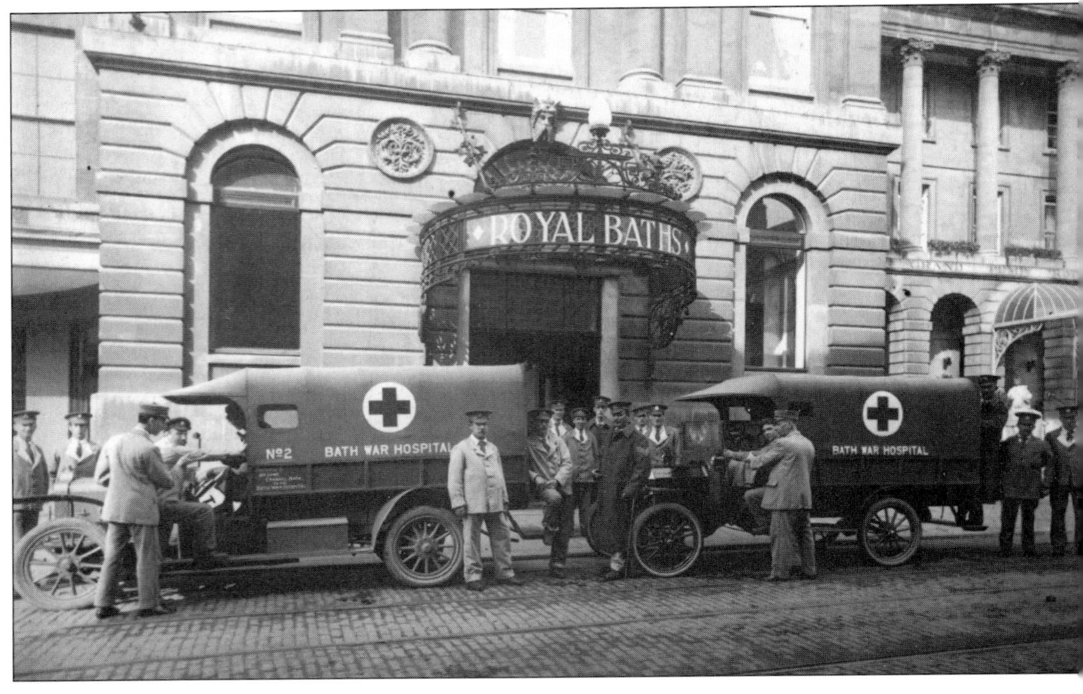

Transport for wounded servicemen from the War Hospital outside the Royal Baths entrance in Stall Street The Grand Pump Room Hote is on the right

the city to drink the spa water in the Pump Room and immerse themselves in the recently refurbished New Royal Baths.

The years following the First World War saw numerous improvements at Bath despite a national background of unemployment, hunger marches and the 1926 General Strike. Away from the heavily depressed areas of South Wales and the industrial north, and buoyed up by the popularity of the spa, Bath fared better than most cities. There was even some industrial expansion, with major companies like Stothert & Pitt and Pitmans extending their premises, and the Flight Works going over to furniture making, a prominent industry in Bath. William Harbutt, a Royal School art teacher who had invented plasticine in 1897, continued to manufacture at his Bathampton works, while the Horstmann Gear Company expanded its manufacture of precision control and switching equipment. The Moorland Brick and Tile Works benefited from the excessive cost of Bath stone, while other well-established local trades such as milling, clothmaking, bookbinding and, of course, hotel and domestic service, all provided employment for local people.

For their spare time there was plenty to keep Bathonians occupied.

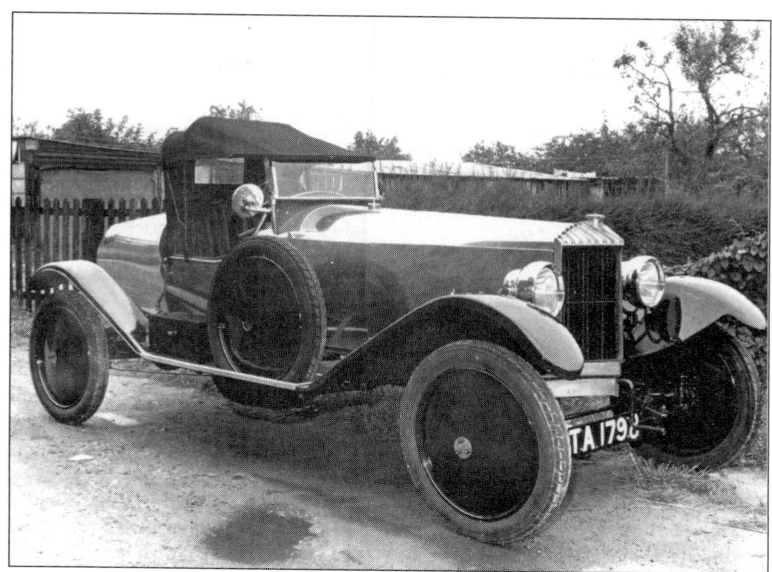

2 litre open two-seater car anufactured in Bath around 25 by the Horstmann ompany

Bath race meetings continued on Lansdown and a permanent fair stood on Broad Quay beside the river. The 1920s saw a boom in cinema and, in the absence of proper facilities, an enormous screen was installed in the Ball Room of the Assembly Rooms, where packed audiences enjoyed the latest films including *Monsieur Beaucaire* with Rudolph Valentino, and Bebe Daniels in *The Maltese Falcon*. Later the Bath Electric Theatre Company's Picturedrome opened in Southgate Street, followed by the impressive Forum Cinema on St James Parade and the Beau Nash cinema in Westgate Street. Everywhere in the city centre, in the hope of a hatful of coppers, street performers went through their paces.

The 1920s was a decade of considerable progress in education. The Bluecoat School and the Bathforum School closed, but only after grammar schools for boys and girls had been built in Oldfield Park to serve the needs of the growing suburbs south of the river. The former Industrial School occupying Prior Park was turned into an independent boarding school by the Irish Christian Brothers in 1924. The Bath Act of 1925 gave the Corporation new powers to control and direct improvements in the city. It could now buy and release the toll bridges across the river, provide parking spaces, tackle the growing traffic problems and regulate building styles and construction materials; ironically it had itself in 1901 rebuilt the Dolemeads estate in incongruous red brick. The Act allowed for strategic intervention in planning matters and gave the Corporation the opportunity to clear more riverside slums. Much of the notorious Avon Street had been demolished in 1908 and in 1932 further slums disappeared to make way for the building of the Kingsmead Flats, the first major housing redevelopment close to the city centre and one which countered the trend for building housing estates devoid of social facilities in the remoter suburbs. The Church responded to the outward spread of the city, erecting St Barnabas, Rush Hill (1903), Emmanuel church, Newbridge (1909) and St Bartholomew's church, Oldfield Park (1938); the fine neo-Byzantine St Alphege's Roman Catholic church at Moorlands was added in 1929. City centre improvements included the construction of new offices and showrooms for the Electricity Company in 1932, the demolition of the Royal Literary and Scientific Institution in 1933 to improve traffic management, and the Forum Cinema in 1934. The Electricity Company and the Forum Cinema both responded to corner locations with curving classical façades, perhaps inspired by Brydon's Guildhall extensions of 1895. Using a different approach the Post Office won widespread acclaim for its neo-Classical main office of 1925 on an awkward corner site between New Bond Street and Broad Street. Due to financial constraints many ambitions sparked by the 1925 Bath Act went unrealized but in 1937 a new Act brought fresh powers and new opportunities. For the first time buildings of architectural

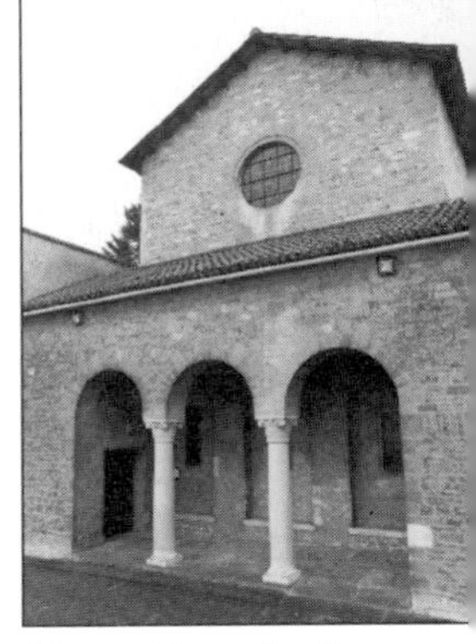

The neo-Byzantine Roman Catholic church of St Alphege in Oldfield Park, built by Sir Giles Gilbert Scott in 1929

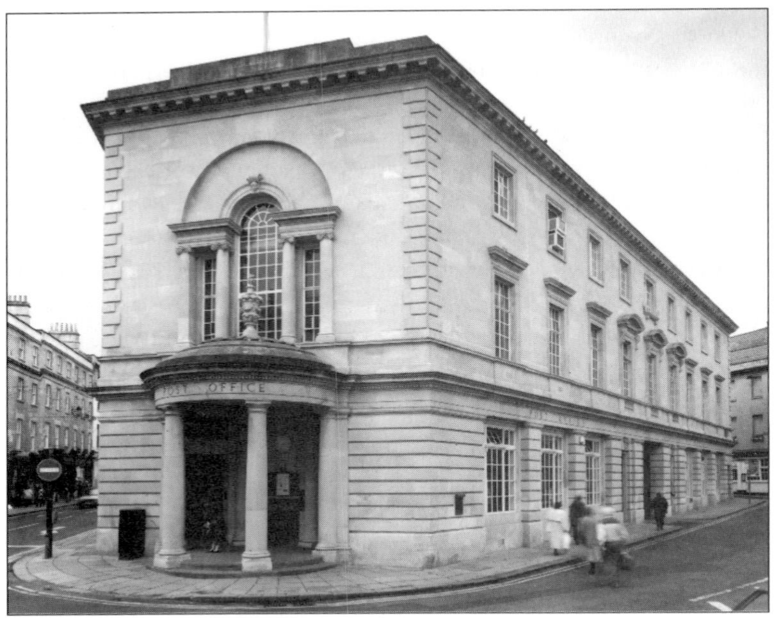

The new Post Office erected in 1925, one of the better neo-Georgian buildings of the inter-war years

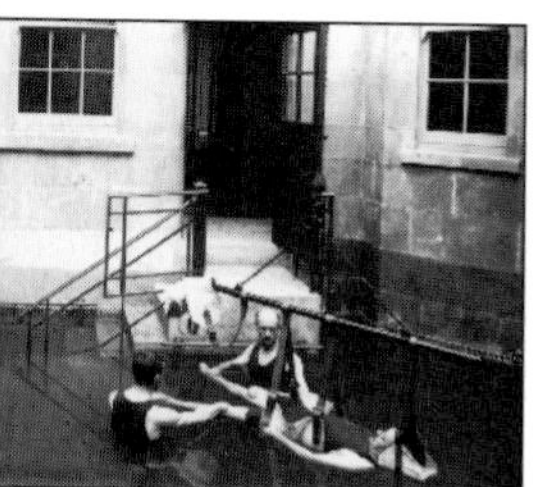

pa water immersion treatment
John Wood's Hot Bath pool
eing demonstrated by
embers of the staff

importance pre-dating 1820 could be listed and then not altered without Corporation approval.

In 1911, when the urban boundary was extended, the city's population increased to around sixty-nine thousand. The Town and Country Planning Act (1932) established a Planning Area of Bath and much of the neighbouring district, in an attempt to prevent the city's green-fringed horizon being swamped by suburban housing developments. The boundaries were further expanded in 1950 and again in 1965 to their present position; the city is now around eighty-five thousand strong.

Despite the hiatus caused by the First World War, the spa continued to attract visitors. Bath boasted four hotels of five-star quality – the Empire, Spa, Pulteney and Grand Pump Room hotels, the latter enjoying the convenience of internal access to the New Royal Baths behind it. The waters were either taken by drinking or used in a variety of immersion, douche, inhalation or mud-based processes. The medical establishment was evidently concerned that greater curative powers were attributed to spa water than it was capable of delivering. During the 1930s the Royal Mineral Water Hospital broke with tradition and introduced medically accepted treatments for arthritis, becoming the world leader in the treatment of arthritic and rheumatic diseases. In 1935 it became the Royal National Hospital for Rheumatic Diseases and was arguing for a new building worthy of its international reputation. By 1939 an appeal had raised £138,000 and a site for the new hospital was prepared in Avon Street. Eight days before the Queen was due to lay the foundation stone, war broke out and the project was abandoned.

As if to mark the end of an era and the start of a new and darker episode, a number of familiar institutions vanished in 1939. The Pump Room Orchestra was disbanded on grounds of economy, and the electric trams were withdrawn from service; remarkably, the same forty vehicles had remained in use since 1902. The Bath chairs that had lined the Abbey Church Yard all but disappeared from view. Numerous buildings were requisitioned by the Admiralty, relocating from London for reasons of safety; the Empire and Grand Pump Room Hotels were occupied, among others, and, to complement them, hutted encampments sprang up on the fringes of the city. The floating 'Mulberry' harbour used in the D-Day landings is said to have been designed at Kingswood School, its name inspired by a tree in the grounds. Airfields were hastily built on Lansdown, Charmy Down and at Colerne, while the city factories again augmented the war effort. All available land was used for food

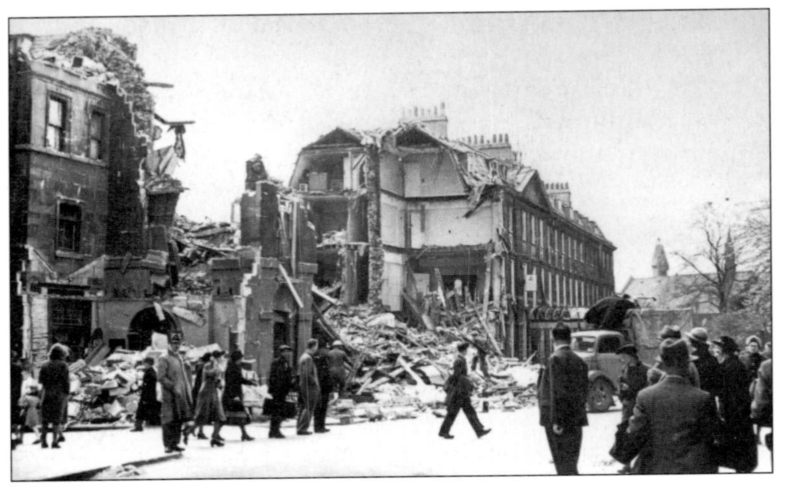

The Francis Hotel in Queen Square the morning after a bombing raid in April 1942. The hotel has since been rebuilt

production; even the park in front of the Royal Crescent was not immune – it was dug up for allotments.

On the nights of 25 and 26 April 1942 Bath was heavily bombed, one of the 'Baedeker Raids' on historic cities in reprisal for the Allied bombing of Rostock and Lübeck. Four hundred and twenty-one citizens lost their lives and over 1,000 buildings were destroyed or severely damaged. The National Fire Service worked tirelessly to prevent the fires spreading while the Queen's Messengers mobile emergency canteens attended to the survivors and homeless. The Assembly Rooms were gutted by incendiary bombs; Abbey Church House was all but destroyed, and severe damage was done to Queen Square, the Mineral Water Hospital, and houses in the Paragon, Circus and Royal Crescent. Most loss of life occurred in densely populated suburbs like Kingsmead, Holloway and Oldfield Park, but other residential areas such as Green Park and Julian Road also suffered. The east window of the Abbey was blown in but, remarkably, none of the other city centre monuments was hit. When the devastation wrought by bombing in Plymouth and Coventry is considered, Bath escaped relatively lightly.

Post-war reconstruction was slow and often countered by planners who, in a savage blitz of their own, cut a swathe through many eighteenth- and nineteenth-century streets and properties. Bombed-out shells were replaced by bland, oversized blocks of shops and offices, which paid no heed to the medieval street plan of the city centre. Traffic congestion and atmospheric pollution had now become issues that Professor Abercrombie's *Plan for Bath* in 1945 and two studies

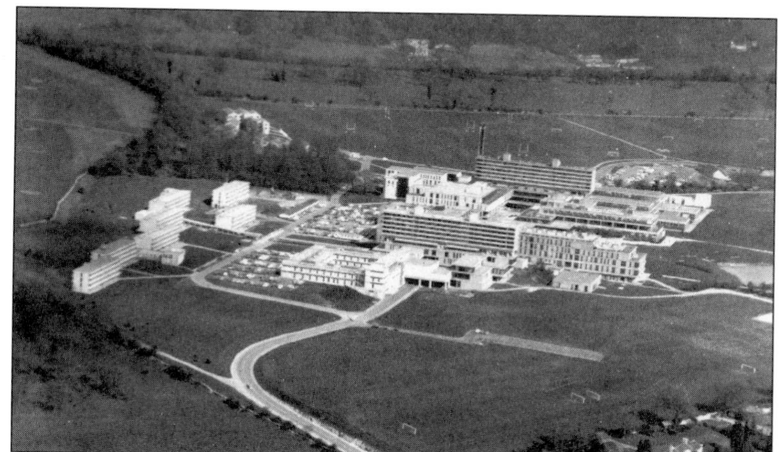

The University of Bath on Claverton Down; the annual rent of one peppercorn is ceremonially presented to the City Council each year

by Colin Buchanan in the 1960s sought to address. Despite some ambitious schemes, few of the proposals to deal with traffic were implemented. From 1955 Council grants were available for cleaning and repairing the blackened face of the city and by the 1980s much of the grime had been removed. By this time, however, the Council had lost many of its powers to the new county of Avon, created in 1974.

The war was a turning point in the fortunes of Bath as a spa. The loss of the major hotels to the Admiralty effectively cut off the flow of visitors and the spa centre went into terminal decline, closing in 1976. The Grand Pump Room Hotel reopened for a time as a railway hotel but did not succeed and was torn down in 1959. The Ministry of Defence remained as the largest single employer in the city. People now came to Bath for reasons other than health. Retailing had for centuries been a mainstay of the local economy and became a draw in its own right as Bath developed as a regional shopping centre. New cultural attractions emerged; the Bath Festival was inaugurated in 1948 and in 1963 the city acquired the prestigious Museum of Costume. Young people came to study; the Bath College of Art at Corsham rose to national prominence in the 1950s and in 1964 the existing college of advanced technology was upgraded to full university status.

Meanwhile reconstruction of another sort was taking place. The importance of ties with other countries had been recognized as early as 1909 in a Bath Pageant tableau depicting Ladye Bath attended by fourteen maidens from towns named Bath in the United States and Canada. In 1945 Bath forged its first twinning link, with Alkmaar in Holland, the result of personal contacts maintained through the dark years of war.

Subsequent ties were made with Braunschweig (West Germany), Aix-en-Provence (France) and Kaposvar (Hungary). By the 1980s Bath had taken its place on the world stage as a destination for international tourism and in 1987, in recognition of the city's urban landscape as one of the outstanding achievements of mankind, the name of the City of Bath was inscribed by UNESCO on the World Heritage List.

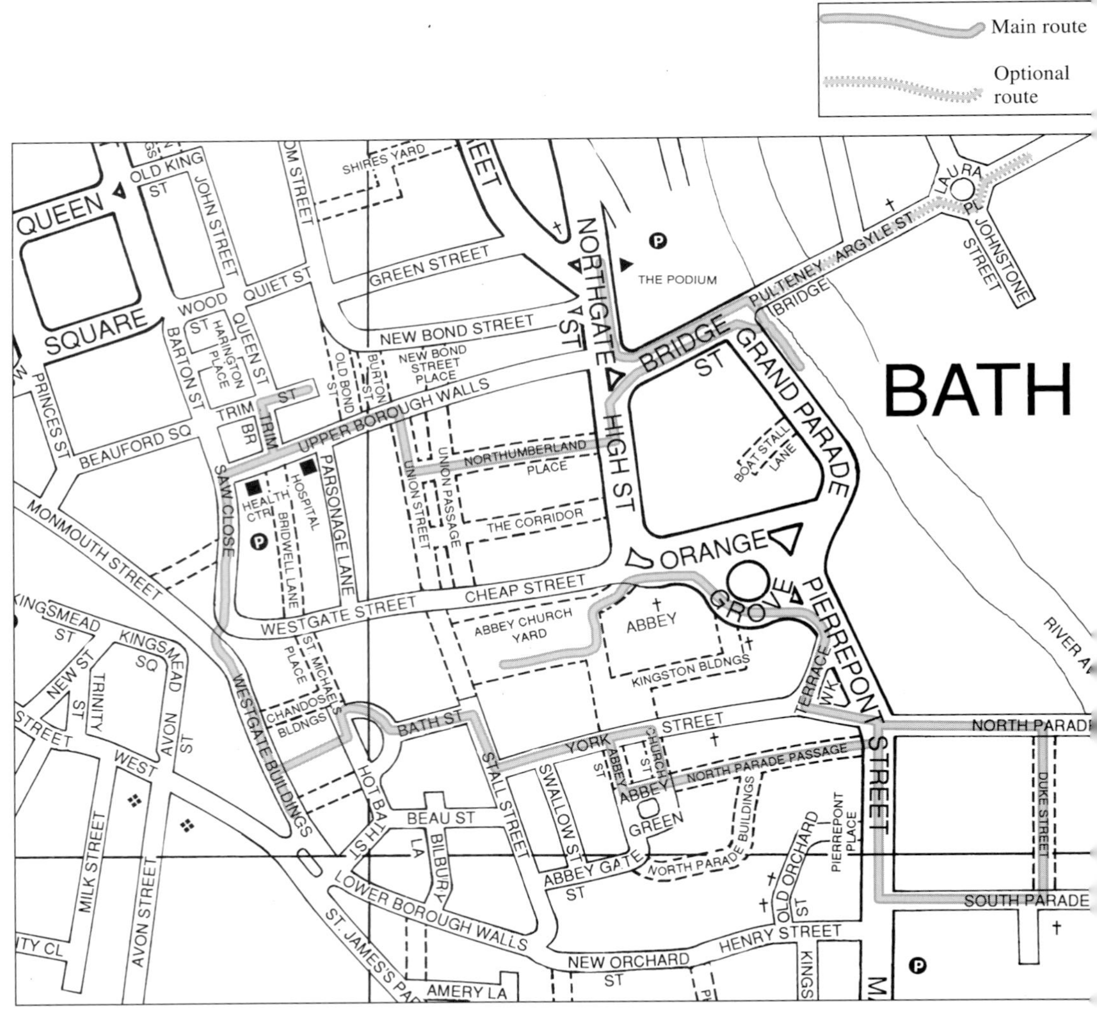

1: The City Centre

This walk explores the old core of Bath, mostly concentrating on the area once bounded by the medieval wall. It can be extended across the river into Bathwick or else linked on to Walking Tour 2. Since the route for Tour 1 is mostly flat and often pedestrianized, wheelchair users should have no difficulty (though some pavements are narrow). The text identifies buildings and features of interest reached at each stage of the walk.

Start Tour 1 in the Abbey Church Yard, facing the Pump Room with the Abbey on your left.

The hot mineral waters that made Bath into a spa rise at several points in the city, but most importantly here, where the legendary Prince Bladud was said to have discovered their curative powers. First enclosed by the Romans, the springs fed a pool sacred to the goddess Sulis Minerva whose cult was practised at a temple close to where you are standing. (Remains of the temple survive *in situ* underground and can be visited in the Roman Baths Museum.) The open-air King's Bath, which exists in reduced form immediately behind the Pump Room, was once surrounded by lodging houses for patients seeking relief by bathing. Medicinal *drinking* became fashionable only under the later Stuarts. The first Pump Room of 1706 was subsequently extended and then completely rebuilt as you now see it in 1791–5 to the design of Thomas Baldwin. Just below the pediment the Greek lettering reads 'Water is best', the equivalent of a neon sign. To the left the late-Victorian Pump Room annexe leads to the Roman Baths Museum and the great Roman bathing complex excavated in the 1880s. Left of that, the façade of the Abbey Church, notable for its carved angelic ladders, dominates the space. This Perpendicular-style building was left unfinished at the Dissolution and only completed about 1617 after national fund-raising. It succeeded a Saxon building, in which King Edgar was crowned in 973, and a much larger Norman structure which eventually became ruinous in the period up to 1500 when the diocese centred on Wells. We shall pass over the site of the former monastic close later. Meanwhile the interior is well worth visiting for its fine fan vault (partly Victorian) and rich display of monuments. The history of the Abbey can be studied further in the Visitors' Centre on the south side of the church.

Walk round the outside of the Abbey on the north, passing a temperance fountain, to the rear of the church where the Norman crossing and chancel once stood.

To reach this spot you came through what was once Wade's Passage, a Georgian short-cut lined on both sides by small shops, some of them built against the church. You now face Orange Grove, so named from the central obelisk erected to commemorate the Prince of Orange's successful water cure in 1734, and also because the area was formerly planted with trees. In the time of Beau Nash this developed into a largely enclosed square, a favourite meeting place for visitors who appreciated the convenient lodgings, gift shops, coffee house and paved walk. The nineteenth century swept most of that away. The huge Empire Hotel of 1899–1901 fills one corner and Grand Parade has opened up the whole east side. Only a re-fronted terrace of Queen Anne shops survives.

Continue past these shops, turn right into Terrace Walk and stop near the fountain on the central island.

This once-fashionable neighbourhood has also much altered. You are standing just outside the line of the city wall, running north-north-east to south-south-west at this point, on the site of Harrison's assembly rooms. First put up in 1709 and enlarged in 1720 and 1749–50, the rooms became the chief venue for the smart visiting company, scenes of heavy gambling on cards and dice and of resplendent evening balls. Secluded garden walks behind the rooms extended to the river, but were eventually superseded by Spring Pleasure Garden on the opposite bank. The profitability of Harrison's venture led to a rival establishment, Lindsey's assembly rooms, opening in 1730 at the opposite side of Terrace Walk on the site of an abandoned Stuart bowling green. Its position is marked by the junction of Terrace Walk with York Street to the right. Terrace Walk once led between the two sets of rooms and ran from Leake's well-known circulating library near Orange Grove to the Parade coffee house, opened in 1750 and now transformed into the Huntsman pub. By walking a few yards down the alley to the right of the pub you may glimpse part of the elaborate wing of Ralph Allen's town house (1727–9). The postmaster Allen grew wealthy through re-organizing the country mail system and exploiting the limestone quarries on Combe Down from which most of Georgian Bath was built. The Palladian hill-top mansion of Prior Park to which he moved in the 1730s is visible from Grand Parade near the Empire Hotel. The original 'Grand Parade', now known as North Parade, runs from near the Huntsman, at a rough right angle to Terrace Walk, and across Pierrepont Street towards the river.

In order to visit the Parades go forward on North Parade and first right along Pierrepont Street, past a modest portico that formerly led to the Orchard Street theatre (1750–1805). Cross Pierrepont Street and turn left, at the end of the block, into South Parade.

All this quarter of Bath, including the Terrace Walk neighbourhood, belonged to the Kingston (later Manvers and Pierrepont) estate, part of the spoils from the abbey holdings after the Dissolution. Bath's ambitious architect, John Wood the elder, had grandiose plans inspired by ancient Rome for this site. In the event only the Parades were achieved (1740–50), raised on extensive foundations above the damp ground and in a plainer classical style than Wood had wanted. Notice the wide pavement, as in North Parade, for promenading. At the end stairs descended to a ferry and a landing stage for pleasure boats. The rest of this area, the Ham, remained undeveloped until the next century when Brunel's GWR station arrived at the bottom of Manvers Street, and St John's Roman Catholic church was built, the fine example of Gothic Revival ahead of you. By then the Lower Assembly Rooms, where you halted earlier, had been converted, after a serious fire, into the Literary and Scientific Institution.

Return to the Huntsman by turning left along Duke Street, left again along North Parade, and over Pierrepont Street. Continue forward along North Parade Passage, noting several houses of *c*. 1622, including Sally Lunn's, on the right. Once in Abbey Green turn right by Church or Abbey Street to the junction with York Street before an open space facing the Abbey Church.

The monastic and episcopal buildings that occupied this area have all gone, though excavations have revealed foundations of some. A number of the mid-eighteenth-century premises that replaced them (including a fine house just south-west of the Abbey Church where the painter Gainsborough lived) have been demolished in their turn, leaving an open square rather larger than the original cloister. On its left the wall topped by a balustrade marks the east end of the Great Roman Bath, but other parts of the ancient thermal establishment extend below the square. These can be seen in the Roman Baths Museum, just as some of the monastic burial ground is visible in the Abbey Visitors' Centre.

Walk westwards along York Street under a high arch added during the remodelling of the spa treatment facilities in the 1880s. At the end turn right and immediately bear left into colonnaded Bath Street.

Sanctioned by the 1789 Bath Improvement Act, this street belongs to a vigorous phase of renewal in the early 1790s when Stall Street, which you have just crossed, and nearby Cheap Street were widened and partly refronted. The new Pump Room was erected around the same date and private baths built alongside with a pedimented entrance facing Bath Street. The creation of Bath Street in the old district of 'Bimbery' destroyed the medieval street pattern but produced a porticoed vista ending in the modestly sized Cross Bath, which you should now approach. This bath, still bearing traces of its former elegance, has been several times remodelled since the decades around 1700 when it was considered the most genteel place to bathe. It was popularly believed to have aided James II's hitherto childless queen to conceive in 1687, an event that precipitated the Glorious Revolution and the reign of William and Mary. The interior of the bath can be viewed from the left side. A few paces south of it and supplied by its own thermal spring stands the Hot Bath, which once had an adjoining pool for lepers. Rebuilt in 1776–8, it was further developed from *c.* 1830 into the well-equipped Old Royal Baths. The epithet 'Old' was added in 1870 on the opening of the New Royal Baths, a luxurious treatment centre on the north side of Bath Street communicating with the new Grand Pump Room Hotel round the corner in Stall Street. Both these institutions helped to stimulate a late-Victorian revival of the spa. One other former medical institution is visible from near the Cross Bath – the Royal United Hospital, seen rising behind the Hot Bath and dating from 1826. It resulted from the merger of two small infirmaries and, unlike the more famous Mineral Water Hospital, served the local community. The building now houses part of the College of Further Education.

Move behind the Cross Bath to enter Chapel Court through an arched gateway on the left. (If the gateway is locked, detour through Hetling Court, 20 yards south.) Pass through the yard, observing the buildings on either side as you go, and emerge at an iron gate into the street.

You have reached Westgate Buildings, the western boundary of the old city. The property you have just crossed belongs to the twelfth-century foundation of St John's Hospital, the oldest of several charities that supported almshouses in Bath. From 1727 the elder John Wood substantially rebuilt it during the construction of several lodging houses at the request of the Duke of Chandos to supplement the spa's accommodation for visitors. These survive in part on the east and north of the court. A short distance to the left of the gateway you have now reached, the many-gabled building beyond the small garden is an Elizabethan medical lodging, Abbey Church House, built round a medieval core.

Turn right from the gateway along the street and keep right of a new building with a dome, balcony and colonnade to stop in front of the Theatre Royal.

The old Orchard Street theatre, once a great nursery of dramatic talent, transferred here in 1805. The present low three-arched entrance partly masks a balustraded façade of the 1720s; here Beau Nash lived before moving next door to the house now occupied by Popjoy's restaurant. Sawclose, the open space in front of the theatre, took its name from a timber yard, and in the nineteenth century held weighing engines for coal and straw. The curious building with Dutch gables and a clock tower, put up in 1859–60 for the Bluecoat School, replaced the original eighteenth-century premises of this important educational charity.

Walk along the north side of this building following the line of the city wall – a section of which has been rebuilt. (Just before this, Trim Bridge leads to an arch and the carved front of 5 Trim Street, survivor of an early Georgian terrace.) Further along Upper Borough Walls you reach a largely pedestrianized street crossing.

The pedimented building on the corner bears the name of the Royal Mineral Water Hospital, opened to the elder Wood's design in 1742. Unlike other provincial hospitals of the period it catered not for local citizens but for carefully vetted patients sent from other parts of the country in the hopes of benefit from a national asset, the hot springs. Largely funded by outside contributions it nevertheless became the spa's medical centrepiece, though better-off invalids made their private arrangements when they stayed at Bath. Union Street cuts through the site of the former Bear Inn, which flanked the Hospital and long obstructed the way between lower and upper town.

Turn down Union Street and bear quickly left through Northumberland Place to come out through a passageway into High Street.

In the space from here towards the Abbey Church a traditional street market used to be held around the early Stuart Guildhall. The latter went in 1777 when Thomas Baldwin's splendid Georgian Guildhall took its place with an extensive market laid out behind. This is the columned central block of the building across the street. The wings on either side were added in the 1890s to house the technical and art schools and municipal offices, incorporating too the entrance to the much-reduced market. Unless it is in use, the chandeliered first-floor Banqueting Room, one of Bath's finest interiors, may be freely visited. It represented for the Corporation élite what the Upper Assembly Rooms were to the visiting gentry. Other rich evidence of civic life may be found in the Bath Record Office, located in the Guildhall basement.

Cross High Street, turning away from the Abbey Church, and right into Bridge Street passing along the side of the Victoria Art Gallery. Cross Grand Parade and bear right to the balustrade overlooking the River Avon.

The weir once powered fulling and corn mills on both sides of the river. It was reconstructed in 1971 with a flood control to prevent future inundations of the city downstream. Beyond the river lay Spring Garden, famous from *c.* 1740 to 1798 for summer entertainments and reached by ferry until Pulteney Bridge spanned the Avon in 1774. Designed by Robert Adam but somewhat modified since, the bridge was intended as the key to developing the Pulteneys' Bathwick estate, a speculative venture that finally got under way in the late 1780s. The large gracious suburb that was planned never fully materialized, because of the investment crisis from the mid-1790s caused by the war with France. The main achievement was the long spine of Great Pulteney Street ending in the Sydney Hotel and pleasure garden, a favourite haunt of Jane Austen who lived from 1801 to 1804 in Sydney Place opposite the garden. The hotel is much altered and now contains the Holburne Museum and Crafts Study Centre; the garden is a public park.

The Bathwick development may be visited in a detour from this walk by crossing shop-lined Pulteney Bridge. Otherwise retrace your steps up Bridge Street and turn right at the junction to stop outside the Podium, a modern shopping and café mall, which also includes the Bath Central Library with its extensive collections on local history.

You are standing just outside the former principal entrance to the city, once marked by the North Gate and its statue of the mythical Bladud. This was the location of the cloth market during Bath's heyday as a woollen textiles centre manufacturing white broadcloth. Many weavers lived in Broad Street and Walcot Street, the roads forking on either side of St Michael's church ahead of you, a satisfying tall-spired structure of 1835–7 on the site of two successive earlier churches. Several façades in Broad Street perhaps conceal earlier frontages and part of a timber-framed house exists behind one shop, a reminder that Bath was not always a wholly stone-built city. The Grammar School of 1752–4 stands halfway up the street on the left. Walcot Street recalls a yet earlier period, for it was the start of the Roman road that passed through the ancient suburb of Walcot en route for London.

Walking Tour 1 ends at the Podium. If however you wish to continue with Tour 2, now take New Bond Street westwards from the Podium to the foot of Milsom Street.

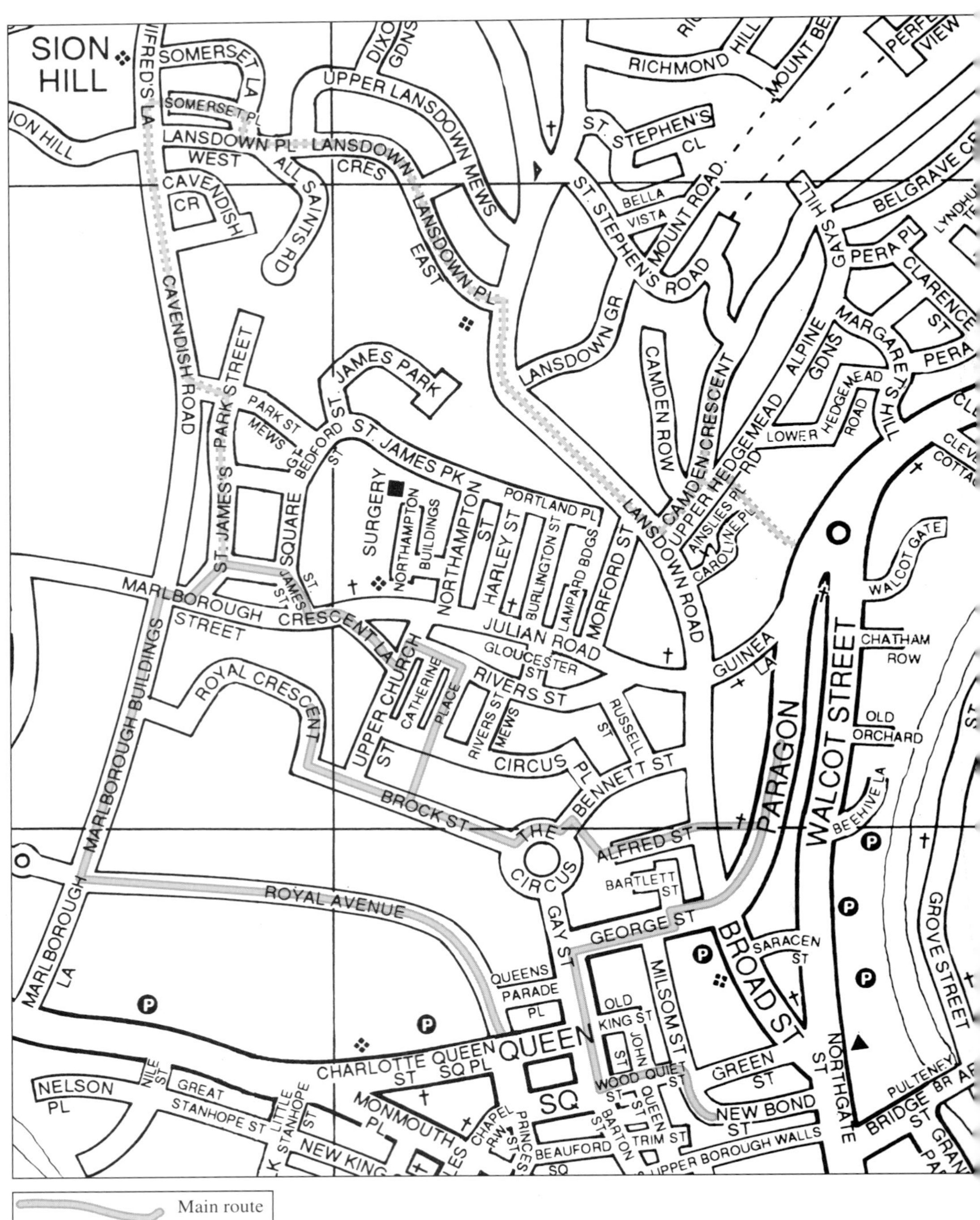

Main route

Optional route

2: The Slopes of Lansdown

This walk focuses on the expansion of Georgian Bath and visits the key sites north and north-west of the old centre. An optional detour takes in the upper crescents built from c. 1790. This route inevitably involves some uphill walking and crosses several busy roads, but apart from the detour it could be negotiated by wheelchairs.

Start Tour 2 at the bottom of Milsom Street near the corner of Quiet Street.

Since our route will not keep entirely to the chronological sequence of development, it is worth bearing in mind the four main phases: (1) 1729–39: Queen Square; (2) *c.* 1754–66: Circus, Milsom Street, George Street, Vineyards; (3) 1767–76: Royal Crescent, Upper Assembly Rooms district, Paragon; (4) 1786 onwards: Marlborough Buildings and the rapid growth of outer Walcot. These phases correspond with periods of economic optimism when the rising number of visitors and well-to-do residents encouraged speculative investment in building. Milsom Street, a spaciously conceived link between the growing upper town and the old heart of Bath, was mostly built in the mid-1760s for residence and lodging. Its immediate success, however, persuaded up-market retailers to move in and two islands of shops (only one survives) were added at the lower end in 1769–70. The Octagon proprietary chapel on the east side (now the Royal Photographic Society's central exhibition gallery) became a fashionable place of worship from 1767, and just above it a former poor-house site was filled *c.* 1782 by the bow-fronted, pedimented block of Somersetshire Buildings. New Bond Street, begun 1805, considerably improved access, and later in the century suburban omnibus services terminated near here. Before you leave do not overlook some of the fine shopfronts (for which Bath is notable) in Milsom Street and Old Bond Street.

Now follow Quiet Street and Wood Street to Queen Square.

The significance of Queen Square is not immediately apparent. To envisage it as the elder John Wood built it in 1729–39 it is necessary to wish away the traffic, to remove in imagination the lofty trees, to add a porticoed proprietary chapel at the south-west corner, and substitute a set-back house in the centre of the west side for the infill of 1830. Laid out on meadows, the square was the height of urban sophistication, one of the first unified, classical spaces of its kind in Britain. The palatial north side (best viewed from the north-east corner of the Square) introduced a new concept in domestic architecture, for it dignified and embellished a simple row of houses as never before. As the last houses were being completed on this side, the obelisk in the central garden was raised in honour of the visit of Frederick, Prince of Wales, in 1738. In terms of future development Queen Square was also influential, for it showed how the system of leasing a complete site from a landowner and then sub-letting individual plots to builders could control the overall design while sharing costs, risks and profits among many.

From the north-east corner walk up Gay Street and take the first right into George Street. Continue across the top of Milsom Street, and cross George Street at the traffic lights to the pavement opposite.

Already partly in existence by the 1730s, when the elder Wood built a short-lived royal tennis court on the south side, George Street made the T-junction with Milsom Street in the early 1760s. Edgar Buildings and Princes Buildings on the north side were built like Milsom Street on Corporation land, a sign that the city was also now concerned to realize its assets outside the walls. On the south side was the York House (later Royal York) hotel, the only additional coaching inn put up in the eighteenth century, opened in 1769 and well placed at the level end of the London road. The pavement raised over cellars on the upper side of George Street demonstrates one way in which the builders coped with sloping ground. Elsewhere they resorted to a combination of excavation and vaulting, and a system of 'stepping up' the hillside where streets ran across the contours.

Continue further along George Street, cross the foot of steep Lansdown Road at Fountain Buildings, and keep forward on another raised pavement to the Countess of Huntingdon's Chapel on the left.

The terrace you have walked past has two evocative names, first Harlequin Row from the unusual mixture of brick and stone (no longer visible) in its construction *c.* 1760–6; and then Vineyards from a productive vineyard that once covered the slope. Raised on massive foundations, the great wall of houses opposite runs from the straight row of Bladud Buildings, erected on municipal land in the mid-1750s, into the long curve of the Paragon, a private speculation begun in 1768. This plain, classically proportioned terrace contrasts with the fanciful Gothic detail of the preacher's house fronting the private Huntingdon Chapel (1765). Its light-hearted appearance nevertheless belies the seriousness of the evangelical mission attempted here to redeem fashionable Bath from its frivolity and godlessness. The chapel has recently been converted for use by the Building of Bath Museum, a revealing display on the practicalities of Georgian construction. The adjoining building exhibits the British Folk Art Collection.

Return 100 yards along Vineyards, bear right up Hay Hill, cross Lansdown Road (wheelchair users will need to cross lower down), and walk almost to the far end of Alfred Street.

One of the historical pleasures of strolling about Bath is to notice small things: incised street lettering, stone coal-hole covers let into pavements, iron brackets from the time of street lighting by oil lamps, plaques marking the residence of celebrities. No. 14 Alfred Street is a case in point. The head of King Alfred may date from the time when the controversial eighteenth-century historian, Catharine Macaulay, lived here. The ironwork includes a lamp-holder, two conical snuffers for dousing the torches that lit the way for sedan chairs at night, and a windlass for lowering weights into the basement 'area' before the house. All this neighbourhood (Alfred, Bennett and Russell Streets) went up in 1770–6 in response to the arrival of the Upper Assembly Rooms before you, which opened with a grand *ridotto* in late 1771. Though subdued on the exterior, the Rooms (restored after wartime bombing and other vicissitudes) reveal their splendour within. The three principal spaces – ballroom, octagonal card room, and tea/supper room – show how the activities of a formal evening assembly, when over a thousand people might be present, were kept functionally distinct. The Rooms still host many events, including concerts during the annual Bath Music Festival. Downstairs is the Museum of Costume, a collection of national importance. (Two other museums lie close at hand, the Museum of East Asian Art and, near the top of Russell Street, the Bath Industrial Heritage Centre, housed in the shell of a 'real tennis' court built 1776–7. Just below the Centre stands Christ Church, the first Anglican church of its type built with free seating for the respectable working-class and servant population.)

From the front of the Assembly Rooms walk round the corner westwards into the Circus.

Both the Assembly Rooms and the Circus were built by the younger John Wood, but the Circus was to his father's idiosyncratic design. The elder Wood's antiquarian interest in prehistoric stone circles appears to have promoted the plan, but it has other components and the superimposed Classical orders derive from the exterior of the Colosseum in Rome. Here they are enriched, however; the Doric, Ionic and Corinthian columns are all doubled and the carving at the first level displays many symbols of freemasonry; the acorns on the parapet may refer to the Bladud legend. This great set-piece was built in three segments over a twelve-year period, 1754–66, with Gay Street being extended up the hill to enter the Circus from the south, and Brock Street growing out to the west. The majestic plane trees were a nineteenth-century afterthought. Originally the whole space was 'pitched' with stone setts between the outer pavement and a central water reservoir, leaving an uninterrupted vista.

Brock Street at the other side of the Circus leads directly to the Royal Crescent on level ground.

The Royal Crescent (1767–74), like Queen Square and the Circus, stood initially in open fields, remnants of which are preserved (with a ha-ha to restrict grazing animals) below the sweeping arc of building. The straight row of Marlborough Buildings beyond was not begun until the late 1780s, and meanwhile Crescent Fields became a favourite promenade for the *beau monde*. Airy sites and fine vistas had become important, and whereas the Circus looked in on itself, the Crescent expansively faced the green hills across the Avon valley. Here the younger Wood developed his father's principle (of making a palace out of a line of houses) in quite dramatic style through the invention of the crescent form. Articulated by the rhythm of giant Ionic columns, the structure needed little more decoration. Originally all the doors were probably painted dark brown, there were no balcony cages, and the first-floor windows had not been lowered – a frequent procedure in the nineteenth century. The windows of No. 1 have been restored to their correct proportions and the entire house has become a museum with fully furnished period rooms. The pennant-sandstone paving, the roadway pitching, and the extensive 'areas' in front of the houses, where tradesmen would deliver to servants in the basements, are all worth noting before you move from the Crescent.

If you prefer to end the walk here, you can return pleasantly to Queen Square either along Gravel Walk (visiting a restored Georgian garden behind No. 4 Circus en route), or through Royal Victoria Park, one of the earliest amenities of its kind in the country, established in 1830. Otherwise retrace your steps a short way along Brock Street, turn left through the shopping precinct of Margaret Buildings (which formerly contained a proprietary chapel on the left), and into Catherine Place (mostly early 1780s). Exit at the north-west corner and turn left into a grassy open space.

Bath was one of several historic cities to suffer bomb damage in the so-called Baedeker raids during the Second World War. Evidence of the damage lies all around this area in demolished Georgian buildings and modern replacements, but the chief architectural victim was St Andrew's church, which formerly occupied this green triangle. Built 1870–3 to a Gothic design by Sir G.G. Scott (and with a 240-ft spire added by 1879), it was one of a score or more nineteenth-century churches and chapels that studded the Bath townscape in response to suburban growth and inter-denominational rivalry. Roman burials were found during the digging of the foundations, and a modern excavation has, not surprisingly, made other discoveries nearby, for Julian Road to your right runs approximately on the line of the Roman road heading west to the port at Sea Mills.

Proceed to the apex of the triangle and cross Julian Road. Some paces ahead a short shopping street leads into St James's Square.

This tranquil residential square, like Northampton Street just to the east, was laid out in the early 1790s, obliterating the fine gardens of Royal Crescent residents in the process. Until about 1785 little had been built north of the city 'liberties', the area of Bath magistrates' jurisdiction marked here by Julian Road. The change came with the making of Burlington Street and Portland Place further east, and the planning of large developments further up Lansdown hill soon after. The two angled streets at the top of St James's Square point indeed to these boldly sited new speculations, all part of the building fever that gripped Bath at this time, when financial credit was all too easy to obtain.

The essential part of the walk ends here. The optional extension is rewarding but is somewhat steeper and adds on nearly a mile. In any case the fine trees of St James's Square are here to be enjoyed first. If you wish to return then to the city centre, leave the square at the south-west corner, cross Julian Road to Marlborough Buildings, which you should follow down to the park. Continue to your left through the park to Queen Square and the centre.

For the extended walk you should leave St James's Square by the north-west corner and then turn left after 9 Park Street, and right at the Common into Cavendish Road. As you walk up this road notice the sophistication of Cavendish Place on your right and the use of quadrant ramping to link each house to its neighbour. Higher up the hill stop outside 1 Cavendish Crescent.

Both the Place and the Crescent are Regency buildings designed by John Pinch. Their respective starting dates of 1808 and *c.* 1814 indicate a revival of speculative building after the long slump beginning in 1793, when the outbreak of war with France unleashed a financial crisis, a collapse of credit and dozens of bankruptcies in the over-extended building trade. The war did not spell an end to Bath's popularity, however, as Jane Austen's novels testify; not until about 1830 was there much sign of decline. Cavendish Crescent is fairly austere, but a more interesting building lies across the road on the corner of Cavendish Road and Sion Hill, its name, Doric House, reflecting its Greek Revival style. It was built for Thomas Barker, a successful local artist, in 1803–5 and includes a 30-ft picture gallery. Sion Hill at the top of the High Common had recently become a fashionable address, a symptom of the new impulse for living well out of town on commanding heights.

Continue to the road crossing and climb the flight of steps slightly to the right on the opposite side.

You have reached Somerset Place, one of a handful of compositions by the unconventional John Eveleigh. The centre of the crescent is its most dramatic feature, with the two middle houses united under a massive notched and decorated pediment and further emphasized with a niche and, over the doors, mask keystones. Building started *c.* 1789 but came to an abrupt halt in the financial crash of 1793, which bankrupted Eveleigh and his associates. The crescent was completed only around 1820 and even then without all the houses planned on the west.

By following the serpentine line of Somerset Place and Lansdown Place West beyond it you will come to Lansdown Crescent. Halt opposite the archway that connects the blocks.

The spectacular setting and new taste for the picturesque that directed the winding plan are evident, though John Palmer's refined design exhibits the same kind of shallow Neoclassical detail (e.g. pilasters rather than columns) that appears also in the severer plan of Bathwick, both dating from *c.* 1788. The archway opposite was constructed about 1824 to bridge the gap between two houses just acquired by the wealthy aesthete William Beckford, who soon sold the one on the left on purchasing the second adjoining house on the right. Behind these houses Beckford landscaped his generous grounds running up Lansdown and on top planted a 154-ft tower where he installed part of his art collection. The tower, which is regularly open to the public, was the most spectacular of a number that sprouted on Italianate villas around Bath from the late 1820s onwards. Just to the right of the grassy bowl below Lansdown Crescent stood another proprietary chapel, All Saints, saving residents in the area a long Sunday trek into town.

You should now continue round the front of the crescent and follow the curve downhill to meet Lansdown Road. Turn right and keep forward past the Lansdown Grove Hotel and Lansdown Lodge to the Old Farm House pub (originally of 1690?), where you bear left into Camden Crescent. After about 100 yards cross the road to the railing at the end of a battlemented wall.

Looking back and below you have a view of Ainslie's Belvedere, a row first laid out *c.* 1760. Lansdown Road, which you have just descended, was once a perilous rocky approach to Bath (experienced by Queen Anne among others) until it was turnpiked and gradually improved in the eighteenth century. It was also the route by which visitors rode up on to the down for healthy 'airings', and also by which people reached the annual Lansdown Fair (10 August) and the racecourse (transferred to Lansdown from Claverton in 1784). The Parliamentarian defenders marched the same way in July 1643 to meet the Royalist forces at the hard-fought Battle of Lansdown during the Civil War. Camden Crescent itself was laid out off Lansdown Road around 1787 under the aegis of Earl Camden, Recorder of Bath and ex-Lord Chancellor. His coat-of-arms appears in the pediment and his elephant's head crest over the doors. As with Somerset Place the architect was John Eveleigh, and again the whole design was never completed, only this time because of unstable ground. Several landslips convinced the builders that the eastern arc of the crescent must be left unfinished with the pedimented section remaining off centre. Despite the warning of instability several streets of artisan housing later spread across the ground below the Crescent and suffered much damage in a series of landslips 1875–85, after which the area was turned into Hedgemead Park.

Return now almost to Lansdown Road and – taking great care of traffic – double back round the end of the battlemented wall. Walk a short distance along Upper Hedgemead Road to the first steps descending to the right. Follow these steps and the successive flights down to the busy London Road.

This is the heart of Walcot. In the course of the eighteenth century it was transformed from a poor village on the outskirts of Bath into a populous suburb; at the same time the once rural parish (which included Barton Farm on which Queen Square, the Circus and Royal Crescent grew up) became one of the richest investment sites in the country. The elegantly spired church was successively enlarged but could not keep pace with demand without auxiliary churches and proprietary chapels. From *c.* 1780 ribbon development began to extend along the London Road to the east and by 1791 even Grosvenor was not considered too distant for plans to build a hotel and pleasure-garden complex there to rival the intended Sydney Gardens in Bathwick. Walcot has long stood at a crucial junction of routes. Recent excavations have proved its importance under the Romans, close to a river crossing and perhaps a commercial focus well outside the religious centre associated with the hot springs.

The walk ends here. From the church the left fork down Walcot Street will eventually bring you to the Abbey Church. The right fork, bending along the Paragon, takes you to an earlier point on this walk.

Not all historic Bath can be covered in two walks and other excursions might be considered. South of the river the district of Lyncombe and Widcombe is particularly to be recommended.

The Next Steps

The prime source for the history of Bath is naturally the fabric of the city itself. The Roman past comes vividly alive at the Roman Baths Museum; parts of the medieval street plan can still be discerned in the central area; and the Abbey Church remains as a splendid memorial of the Tudor city. Otherwise most of what we see post-dates 1700. Here the great heritage of Georgian architecture and planning takes pride of place, not merely the famous set-pieces but also the extensive stock of simpler but always well-proportioned terraces reaching up and along the hillsides. Victorian and later development likewise has much to tell and deserves attention in its own right, particularly religious and industrial buildings, the evolution of routeways and the spread of suburbia. The interiors of buildings also evoke a strong sense of history: the Abbey Church, Pump Room, Guildhall, Theatre Royal and Assembly Rooms are obvious examples. Shops and restaurants occupy other listed buildings, while houses associated with famous people are often signalled by wall plaques.

Various local institutions preserve the artefacts and documentary records of the past, enabling the interpretation of Bath's history to continue and develop. Bath Central Library at the Podium houses an unrivalled collection on Bath and its region, not only books, periodicals and local newspapers but scrapbooks, cuttings, maps, and much visual and manuscript material. The Bath Record Office, located in the basement of the Guildhall, is rich in Corporation and other documents, among them a large deposit of property leases. Advice may be obtained here on access to other archives of local interest, including parish records currently held at the County Record Office in Taunton.

Although no museum traces the evolution of the city as a whole, objects, works of art and documentation concerning Bath are well represented in several museums. The Roman Baths Museum contains many excavated and other items, and the Visitors' Centre at the Abbey Church exhibits the history of the monastery and the church itself. For prints, drawings and paintings of Bath and local celebrities the chief repository is the Victoria Art Gallery. Two other museums, both sited in historic buildings, illuminate the Georgian past: the Building of Bath Museum (and study centre) in the former Huntingdon Chapel, Vineyards, shows how 'classical Bath' came into being; and the restored house at 1 Royal Crescent offers valuable insights into how the wealthier Georgians lived. Aspects of the city's often overlooked manufacturing tradition can be studied at the Bath Industrial Heritage Centre, Julian Road, which occupies what was once a 'real tennis' court. The Herschel Museum at 19 New King Street, and Beckford's Tower, Lansdown, provide worthwhile opportunities to see buildings linked with once-celebrated residents, and the grounds of Prior Park, Ralph Allen's estate at Combe Down, may also be visited in part. For information about these and other museums and sites consult the Tourist Information Centre. Details of bodies and societies concerned with the preservation and investigation of the city may be obtained at Bath Central Library.

Only a handful of the considerable number of publications on Bath can be cited here, though the booklists they often contain will suggest further reading:

Anstey, Christopher, *The New Bath Guide* (satirical verse, first pub. 1766, repr. Kingsmead Press, 1978)

Austen, Jane, *Northanger Abbey* and *Persuasion* (two famous novels partly set in 'Regency' Bath)

Cunliffe, Barry, *The City of Bath* (Alan Sutton, 1986)

—, *Roman Bath Discovered*, Rev. ed. (Routledge & Kegan Paul, 1984)

Bath History (a biennial collection of articles from 1986 onwards, now pub. by Millstream Books)

Davis, Graham, *Bath beyond the Guide Book* (vignettes on nineteenth-century Bath, Redcliffe Press, 1988)

Haddon, John, *Portrait of Bath* (Robert Hale, 1982)

Hembry, Phyllis, *The English Spa, 1560–1815* (Athlone Press, 1990)

Ison, Walter, *The Georgian Buildings of Bath*, Rev. ed. (Kingsmead Press, 1980)

Jackson, Neil, *Nineteenth Century Bath: Architects and Architecture* (Ashgrove Press, 1991)

James, P.R., *The Baths of Bath in the Sixteenth and Early Seventeenth Centuries* (Arrowsmith, 1938)

King, Austin J., and Watts, B.H., *The Municipal Records of Bath, 1189 to 1604* (Elliot Stock, 1885)

Lees-Milne, James, and Ford, David, *Images of Bath* (a comprehensive collection of Bath prints, Saint Helena Press, 1982)

McIntyre, Sylvia, 'Bath, the rise of a resort town, 1660–1800' in *Country Towns in Pre-Industrial England*, ed. P. Clark (Leicester University Press, 1981)

Mainwaring, Rowland, *Annals of Bath* (covering 1800–34, M. Meyler, 1838)

Mowl, Tim, and Earnshaw, Brian, *John Wood* (Millstream Books, 1988)

Neale, R.S., *Bath 1680–1850: a Social History* (Routledge & Kegan Paul, 1981)

Ordnance Survey, *Roman and Medieval Bath* and *Georgian Bath* (two historical maps pub. 1989)

Penrose, John, *Letters from Bath 1766–1767*, ed. B. Mitchell and H. Penrose (Alan Sutton, 1983)

Rolls, Roger, *The Hospital of the Nation* (Bird, 1988)

Smollett, Tobias, *The Expedition of Humphry Clinker* (a richly characterized novel partly set in Bath, first pub. 1771)

Warner, Richard, *The History of Bath* (R. Cruttwell, 1801)

Wood, John, *A Description of Bath* (repr. of 1765 ed., Kingsmead Reprints, 1969)

Wroughton, John, *A Community at War: the Civil War in Bath and North Somerset, 1642–1650* (Lansdown Press, 1992)

Picture Credits

The authors would like to thank the following for their permission to reproduce illustrations: Aerofilms (p. 99); Bath Abbey (pp. 18, 21); Bath Archaeological Trust (pp. 9 (top), 23); Bath Central Library (pp. 6, 12 (top), 13 (bottom), 26, 33 (bottom), 38, 39, 42, 48 (top), 54, 55, 65, 74, 75, 78, 82, 84, 85, 87, 88, 89, 91, 94, 98); Bath Industrial Heritage Centre (p. 95); Bath Museums Service (pp. 93, 96, 97); Museum of Costume (p. 52); Roman Baths Museum (pp. 2, 7, 11, 12 (bottom), 13 (top), 14, 19, 32, 90); Victoria Art Gallery (pp. 35, 41, 45, 46, 48 (bottom), 49, 50, 53, 56, 58, 59, 60, 62, 64, 66, 67, 68, 69, 70, 72, 73, 76, 79, 80, 83); Bath Record Office (pp. 24, 70); British Museum, Department of Prints & Drawings (p. 40); University of Oxford, Institute of Archaeology (pp. 4, 5, 9 (bottom), 20, 22, 27, 30, 33 (top), 37, 43). The maps on pp. 100 and 108 are reproduced from the Residents' Handbook with permission from Standbrook Guides.

Subject Index